Rearing Animal and Plant Pathogen Vectors

Rearing Animal and Plant Pathogen Vectors

Editor

Ambirsh Kumar

scitus academics

Rearing Animal and Plant Pathogen Vectors

Edited by **Ambirsh Kumar**

Printed in 2017

ISBN: 978-1-68117-026-8

Library of Congress Control Number: 2015931823

SCITUS Academics LLC,
616, Corporate Way, Suite 2, 4766,
Valley Cottage, NY 10989

www.scitusacademics.com

Notice

Contents

Preface

A pathogen or infectious agent is a biological agent that causes disease or illness to its host. The term is most often used for agents that disrupt the normal physiology of a multicellular animal or plant.

However, pathogens can infect unicellular organisms from all of the biological kingdoms. There are several substrates and pathways whereby pathogens can invade a host.

The human body contains many natural defenses against some of common pathogens in the form of the human immune system and by some "helpful" bacteria present in the human body's normal flora. Some pathogens have been found to be responsible for massive amounts of casualties and have had numerous effects on afflicted groups. Today, while many medical advances have been made to safeguard against infection by pathogens, through the use of vaccination, antibiotics and fungicide, pathogens continue to threaten human life. Social advances such as food safety, hygiene, and water treatment have reduced the threat from some pathogens.

This book provides an integrated description of methods used to rear vectors of human, higher animal, and plant pathogens in the laboratory. It deals with diverse subject areas, and contains descriptions of standard, as well as highly specialized, methods used by medical, veterinary, entomology, and plant pathology experts.

Editor

Chapter 1

Global Change and Human Vulnerability to Vector-Borne Diseases

Robert W. Sutherst

CSIRO Entomology, Indooroopilly, Queensland, Australia 4068

ABSTRACT

Global change includes climate change and climate variability, land use, water storage and irrigation, human population growth and urbanization, trade and travel, and chemical pollution. Impacts on vector-borne diseases, including malaria, dengue fever, infections by other arboviruses, schistosomiasis, trypanosomiasis, onchocerciasis, and leishmaniasis are reviewed. While climate change is global in nature and poses unknown future risks to humans and natural ecosystems, other local changes are occurring more rapidly on a global scale and are having significant effects on vector-borne diseases. History is invaluable as a pointer to future risks, but direct extrapolation is no longer possible because the climate is changing. Researchers are therefore embracing computer simulation models and global change scenarios to explore the risks. Credible ranking of the extent to which different vector-borne diseases will be affected awaits a rigorous analysis. Adaptation to the changes is threatened by the ongoing loss of drugs and pesticides due to the selection of resistant strains of pathogens and vectors. The vulnerability of communities to the changes in impacts depends on their adaptive capacity, which requires both appropriate technology and responsive public health systems. The availability of resources in turn depends on social stability, economic wealth, and priority allocation of resources to public health.

INTRODUCTION

Global change refers to the complex of environmental changes that is occurring around the world as a result of human activities. Some scientists refer to it as a huge human experiment on the Earth, for which we have little idea of the ultimate outcome, limited ways of finding out a priori, and perhaps no way of reversing. Global change is occurring across a wide range of fields, and those changes affect almost every aspect of human societies.

There have been a number of recent reviews covering aspects of global change and human health, including infectious diseases (53, 61, 117, 126, 134, 205, 206, 222, 223, 246, 249). Several reviews have specifically targeted vector-borne diseases (121, 125, 249, 270, 303, 304, 307, 318). There have not yet been thorough quantitative studies addressing the many processes at work (53,210,211,248,304,309,310). In part this is because of the complexity of the many indirect and feedback mechanisms that bear on all aspects of global change. Any consideration of one particular cause of change cannot be made in isolation because of the many interactions between the different drivers of change. As a result, appeals have been made to take a holistic approach to risk assessment and management of vector-borne diseases (117, 121, 208, 220, 268, 307,347). Unfortunately, the state of current analytical skills and data and the limited resources of the scientific community have resulted in consideration of isolated subsets of those changes in any quantitative risk assessment.

This review focuses on developing a holistic approach to the assessment of vulnerability of societies to vector-borne diseases. The aim is to assess the risks of potential changes in the status of vector-borne diseases in a changing world and to consider approaches to effective adaptation to those changes. The review presents a framework for an integrated assessment of the impacts of different global change drivers and their interactions on vector-borne diseases. The framework enables potentially important secondary interactions or mechanisms and important research gaps to be identified and provides a means of integrating targeted research from a variety of disciplines into an enhanced understanding of the whole system.

The ecology and epidemiology of vector-borne diseases can be described using the "disease triangle" of host-pathogen-environment

originally developed by plant pathologists. The disease triangle concept was extended (305-307) to emphasize the role of management in adapting to risks from invasive species and animal parasites. The risk assessment community's concept of vulnerability, as used by the Intergovernmental Panel on Climate Change (IPCC) (244), and the quarantine community's concept of pest risk analysis (146) were included. Here this combined approach is used to structure review material on vector-borne diseases of humans (Fig.1).

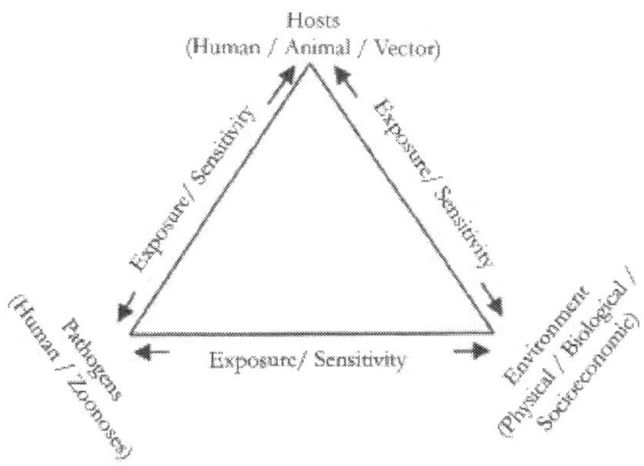

Figure1: A host-pathogen-vector-environment framework for the assessment of risks to humans from vector-borne diseases under global change.

The scheme provides a framework to guide the evaluation of risks and opportunities arising from global change effects on vector-borne diseases at a given location. It summarizes the components of the human disease complex that need to be addressed in any risk assessment. Hosts include both primary and secondary vertebrate hosts (including humans), and vectors include insects, ticks, and snails. The pathogens considered are restricted to vector-borne diseases that affect humans, including zoonoses. A broad view is taken of the environment as it affects vector-borne diseases because socioeconomic changes occurring around the world have major significance for future trends in disease patterns.

SCENARIOS OF GLOBAL CHANGE

There are a number of drivers of global change that are changing the physical and social environment on Earth to such an extent that they have the potential to influence the status of many vector-borne diseases (Fig.2). Global change drivers differ in that some, such as increases in the concentration of atmospheric carbon dioxide (CO_2) or climate change, have global origins with global impacts while others, like land use or irrigation, have local origins but are occurring on a global scale. It is important to emphasize that there is considerable uncertainty about the extent to which each of the changes will occur in the future. This is because the changes depend on human behavior and economic growth, the ability of the Earth's natural systems to act as a buffer against those changes, and the degree of skill that has been achieved in the science involved in estimating the environmental impacts of those changes.

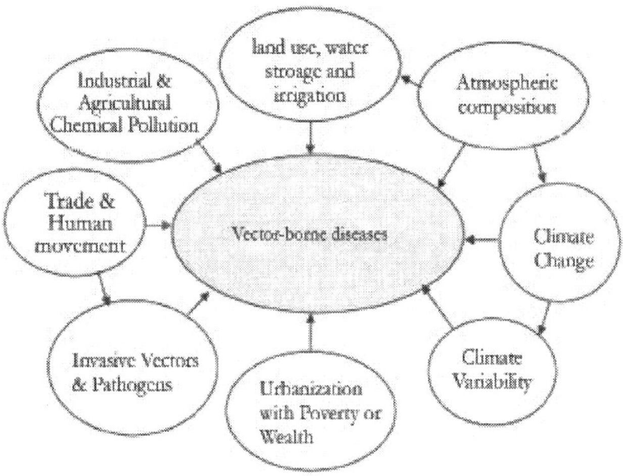

Figure 2: Drivers of global change considered in relation to potential changes in the status of vector-borne diseases.

Atmospheric Composition

The Earth's surface is kept warm by a blanket of greenhouse gases, including water vapor, CO_2 (261), methane, nitrous oxide, and some industrial gases like chlorofluorocarbons. Each gas has different warming properties depending on its structure and persistence in the atmosphere. The composition of the atmosphere has been changing over the past century, with the concentrations of these gases, except perhaps water vapor, rising as a result of the burgeoning anthropogenic activities (144). In particular, burning of fossil fuels for power and transport is transferring millions of tons of buried fossil fuels into the atmosphere each year in the form of CO_2. Livestock, rice paddies, and leakage from coal beds are also increasing the concentration of methane. There is less uncertainty about the extent of the increase in the concentrations of these gases than there is about the consequential changes in the climate. Nevertheless, changes in the concentration of $CO_2$are subject to widely different estimates that depend on assumptions about future patterns of growth in the consumption of fossil fuels. Other anthropogenic changes such as urbanization, water supply and distribution, forest clearing, agriculture, and trade issues are more predictable.

This giant undesigned and untestable human experiment with the Earth's climate and atmosphere (it is the only one that we have) has already increased the atmospheric concentration of CO_2 by almost one-third (Fig.3a) and doubled the concentration of methane in the atmosphere (Fig 3b). None of these changes in atmospheric composition is known to affect vector-borne diseases directly. However, the effects of higher concentrations of CO_2 on plants are to reduce their water loss through transpiration and to act as a fertilizer. The result is that plants produce more foliage with the same amount of water (261), provided that they do not exhaust the supply of other nutrients. Two consequences of this phenomenon that are relevant to the current consideration of the effects on vector-borne diseases are that the increased density of plant foliage will provide more favorable microclimates for insect vectors and that plant growth seasons will be extended in some situations, effectively increasing the duration of favorable microclimates each year. A further consequence in some habitats may be a larger residual amount of water being left in the soil after maturation of a crop. This could affect water tables and the speed with which soils saturate and produce surface water reservoirs suitable for breeding of mosquitoes. It follows that the increased water use efficiency of plants at high CO_2 concentrations may result in an expansion of the ranges of woodlands into lower rainfall areas with adequate soil nutrients, leading to spatial changes in the ranges of vectors in response to habitat changes (95).

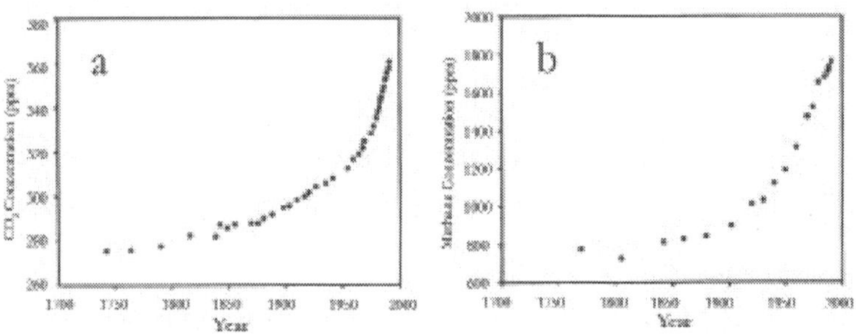

Figure 3: Changes in the concentration of the key greenhouse gases carbon dioxide (a) and methane (b) since preindustrial times. Reprinted fromhttp://www.ipcc.ch/press/sp-cop6/sld5.jpg with permission from Intergovernmental Panel on Climate Change (data archived at the Hadley Centre for Climate Prediction and Research).

Climate Change

The issue of human-induced climate change is a contentious one because it is difficult to detect a slight trend in average temperatures when it is masked by a large amount of annual variability. However, in 1996 the IPCC, an international panel of scientists commissioned to advise governments on progress in the science that underpins the understanding of climate change, stated for the first time, that "the balance of scientific evidence suggests that human activities during the last century have begun to have a discernible effect on the world's climate, causing it to warm" (140). Projected changes in the average climate depend strongly on assumptions about the relationship between the global temperature and greenhouse gases produced by human activities (144). A statistical analysis to separate solar and anthropogenic influences implied that 60% of the warming in the last 140 years was due to human activity (27). A similar analysis showed that in recent decades, the temperatures have broken out above the band of variation that has been observed over the past 1,000 years and the rate of increase is accelerating (71). This image has been referred to within the global-change community as "the image of the millennium" and provides a sobering summary of the last 200 years of human impacts on Earth. Unfortunately, one consequence of this analysis is that future rates of anthropogenic warming are expected to be greater than previously estimated because earlier analyses overestimated historical contributions from anthropogenic activity. This contributed to an update of the future scenarios for climate change (144).

These projected changes rely on extrapolation of expected trends and do not consider possible triggers that may be set off as the Earth's atmosphere warms. One phenomenon that could have overwhelming effects is a failure of the circulation of warm water from the Gulf Stream into the North Atlantic Current, which forms part of a global salt conveyer belt. The current is driven by cold, saline water sinking in giant underwater waterfalls off Labrador and Greenland, which flush the cold water back into the warm Atlantic. Global warming could cause a failure in the flushing mechanism by diluting the saline water with bursting of ice dams from melting glaciers, by increasing rainfall in the region, or by reducing the temperature gradients in the sea. In the past, this has triggered very large (up to 10°C) and very rapid (a decade or century) "flips" in climate every few thousand years, with equally rapid reversals or "flops," leading Calvin (52) to call them climate "flip-flops." The effect is to put the world into a cold-dry climate, with Europe's climate equating to present-day Siberia, with devastating consequences in terms of food supplies for the world as a whole. This would reduce risks of almost all vector-borne diseases, except perhaps flea-borne diseases, among a starving population. An equally rapid warming event would have catastrophic implications for vector-borne diseases, with rapid geographical expansion of tropical ranges affecting nonimmune populations. Since any sudden cooling will greatly reduce the risks of vector-borne diseases and a subsequent warming would be well beyond the time horizon that is relevant to the present topic, these flip-flops are noted for their wider risks but are not considered in this review.

Projected changes in rainfall are even more uncertain than those for temperature, with large differences in the climate projections from different global climate models (GCMs). The consensus is that most tropical areas, particularly over oceans, will receive more rainfall, with decreases in most of the subtropics and relatively smaller increases in high latitudes (144). The uncertainty about rainfall is increased by the potential for geographical and seasonal shifts in rainfall patterns, so that local outcomes are difficult to foresee. Readers are cautioned to interpret the following projections of changes in the status of vector-borne diseases with climate change with care. They are indicative only and are intended to alert the community to some of the steps that can be taken to insure against any deterioration in public health caused by vector-borne diseases.

There have been numerous reports of physical and biological changes in the environment that are consistent with current warming of the Earth's surface. These include an increase in the altitude of the freezing point in the tropics by 110 m (83) and the melting of tropical glaciers around the world (321). A wide range of biological effects of recent climate change has been noted (142, 219, 243, 282), including population and life history changes, shifts in geographical ranges, changes in species composition in communities, and changes in the structure and functioning of ecosystems. In contrast to the tropical effects noted above, increases in the altitudinal range of five species of trees by 120 to 375 m, together with an increase in the tree limit by 100 to 150 m, have been noted at high latitudes in the Swedish Scandes (170). Such widespread biological changes were noted by Epstein (89), who cited them in support of the notion that recent climate change could have contributed to some current changes in patterns of vector-borne diseases. The difficulty faced by researchers is how to separate such effects from the many other simultaneous influences that are usually involved.

Climate Variability and Extremes

While the primary effect of global warming will be to increase the average temperature of the Earth, the features of climate change that deserve most attention in the context of vector-borne diseases are possible changes in the frequency and severity of extreme weather events and in climatic variability. Even if the variability of the climate relative to the average remains the same, there will be disproportionate changes in the frequency of extreme events, such as fewer frosts and more floods (346) that can have large effects on disease vectors. Of further concern is the fact that the frequency of two successive extreme events is even more sensitive to small changes in the mean. The increasing temperatures will also intensify the hydrological (rainfall and evaporation) cycle (251), leading to an increased frequency and intensity of extreme weather events such as storms, floods, and droughts. Empirical evidence for such a trend is evident in a pattern of steadily increasing proportions of higher rainfall events in the United States (144).

The assumption that the variability of the climate will not change does not appear to hold (154), and it is expected that more cloud cover will increase minimum temperatures and lower the rate of increase of maximum temperatures. The result is likely to be fewer frosts and more moderate increases in the frequency of suboptimal maximum temperatures.

Analogues of Climate Change

Since the effects of climate change are difficult to study, analogues have been sought to explore the likely consequences of increases in temperature or changes in rainfall (112). They have included historical climates that show insect distributions tracking climate change (63) and different geographical locations, with the expected higher temperatures, for vectors (264). The most popular analogue is the El Niño phase of the El Niño southern oscillation (ENSO) cycle to simulate the effect of global warming. In the absence of the opportunity to observe the effect of climate change over a short period, the temporary, regional warming events associated with the ENSO cycle form an attractive analogue for climate change (37, 127). It is acknowledged that global warming is likely to lead to different combinations of changes in temperature and moisture compared with the ENSO cycle. Nevertheless, some interesting correlations have been made on the incidence of vector-borne diseases in relation to the ENSO cycle.

The ENSO has effects that are felt around the globe (112). El Niño is often associated with heat waves and drought in southern Africa and Southeast Asia including Australia, while it brings floods to the west coast of South America and to central Africa. The opposite phase, La Niña, reverses these patterns. However, enthusiasm for the use of the ENSO may have arisen during a period when the correlation of the index with summer rainfall in northeastern Australia (for example) was particularly high (Fig. 4) (51).

The reliability of the ENSO as a surrogate for climate change or as a predictive tool must be questioned in the light of the large, decade-long fluctuations in the relationship. Since the ENSO cycle plays such a dominant role in causing seasonal changes in climate, there is concern that any interaction between anthropogenic climate change and the mechanisms driving the ENSO could have unpredictable results. Unfortunately, there is already a suggestion that the severity of the ENSO cycle may be increasing, with the 1997 to 1998 event being the strongest on record (75), and it occurred simultaneously with an accelerated period of global warming since the 1970s (144).

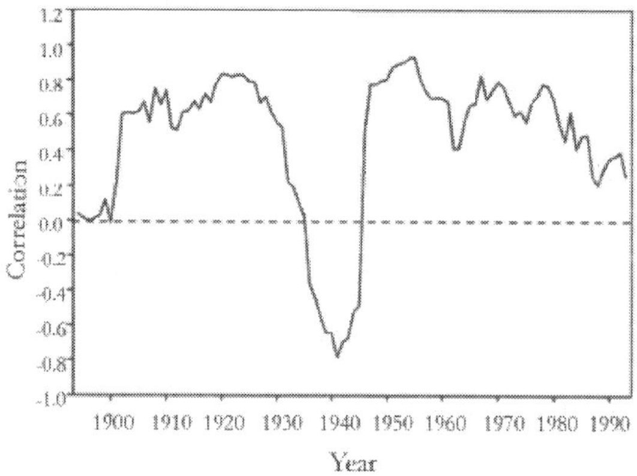

Figure 4: Long-term variation in the relationship between the ENSO index and summer rainfall in north-eastern Australia. Modified from reference 51 with permission.

Urbanization

The human population has increased from approximately 1 billion at the turn of the 20th century to 6 billion by the end of the century, and it is projected to grow to around 10 billion by 2050 (323). The world's urban populations increased from 1.7 billion (39%) in 1980 to 2.7 billion (46%) in 1997 (12) and are expected to reach 5 billion (60%) by 2030 (14). Over the next 25 years, urban populations in Africa are expected to more than double, those in Asia will almost double, and those in Latin America and the Caribbean are expected to increase by almost 50% (351). The density of humans will increase disproportionately because a higher proportion of those people will live in cities compared with today (10).

Drainage and water supplies are critical factors that determine the extent to which many diseases are either contained or propagate in urban communities. Poverty associated with rapid population growth leads to concentrations of people without the necessary infrastructure for the safe storage and distribution of water and drainage of wastewater. Used containers and tires provide breeding sites for mosquito vectors. In addition, the deteriorating public health infrastructure in many countries exacerbates the health problems (121). Each of these negative societal trends is expected to continue, and water-related issues in particular are expected to increase in importance in the developing world over the next few decades (352). On the other hand, in wealthy communities there is encroachment of residential or recreational populations into forested areas where natural hosts and vectors of vector-borne diseases exist.

Land Use, Land Cover, and Biodiversity

The burgeoning world population (326) is driving an intensification of agriculture and its spread into new areas where forests now exist. With such development comes the need for deforestation and for the storage, supply, and distribution of water for human consumption and for irrigation. World rates of deforestation in 1990 to 1995 averaged 101,724/km^2, or 0.3% per annum (12). Future projections of agricultural expansion indicate that there will be more dependence on intensive agriculture and use of irrigation where water supplies permit, with the associated habitat modification, water storage, and sanitation issues (94, 96, 118,119, 139, 173, 323). Each of these developments affects the opportunities available for breeding by vectors of diseases.

Future land cover change will occur mostly in the tropics and subtropics. It is likely to result in increases in surface temperatures of up to 2°C, with drier conditions where the land cover is reduced. In contrast to the reduced diurnal temperature range expected with greenhouse warming, future land cover change in the tropics may increase the temperature range by decreasing evaporative cooling during the day. The sensitivity of surface temperatures to future anthropogenic land cover change in the tropics is up to 1.5°C warmer than the range induced by decadal-scale interannual variability in vegetation density (80).

With changes in land use comes fragmentation of habitats, loss of biodiversity and alteration of existing vector-host-parasite relationships. The rate of species loss is now higher than at any time since the period when the dinosaurs went extinct (175). Fragmentation of habitats isolates populations with low mobility but still provides access to mobile species, thus altering the species balance in undisturbed areas. This can lead to changes in the physical environment for vectors and hence affect patterns of disease.

Industrial and Agricultural Pollution with Hormone-Disrupting Chemicals

The burgeoning industrial and agricultural chemical industries are producing thousands of new products each year. Very few are assessed for health risks, and many are being found to either mimic or disrupt the activity of hormones, especially estrogen and thyroid hormones, in humans and animals (60). Such endocrine-disrupting chemicals (EDCs) include alkyl phenols, dioxins, organochlorine pesticides, phthalates, polychlorinated biphenyls, polybrominated diphenyl ethers, and synthetic pyrethroids (167). They are found in plastics, herbicides, and pesticides that are distributed widely around the world. Apart from the potentially devastating effects on human sexual development and neurological function, there is evidence that many such chemicals also degrade immunological function (22, 69). From the perspective of risk assessments and prevention, an even greater concern is that such effects are sometimes associated only with mixtures with each other or with nitrate fertilizers in groundwater at concentrations found in groundwater across the United States (255). The side effects of these chemicals could reduce options for human adaptation to vector-borne diseases either by degrading immune responses or by withdrawal of vector control products from the market.

Trade and Travel

Increasing affluence in the developed world, combined with more economical mass transport and liberalization of international trade, is accelerating the increase in the numbers of people and the quantity of materials that are being transported around the world. Humans travel on scales from local to global. One million people are reported to travel internationally each day, and one million people travel from developed to developing countries (and vice versa) each week (106). A more recent report quoted a figure of 700 million tourist arrivals per year (115).

There were more than 14.5 million refugees worldwide at the end of 2000, 1 million more than 2 years previously (Fig. 5). From the perspective of vector-borne diseases, the most significant problems are likely to occur in Africa, with more than 3.3 million refugees, South and Central Asia, with 2.6 million, East Asia and the Pacific, with 0.8 million, and the Americas, with 0.6 million (13). In addition, a similar number of people were internally displaced within countries, usually from rural areas into cities.

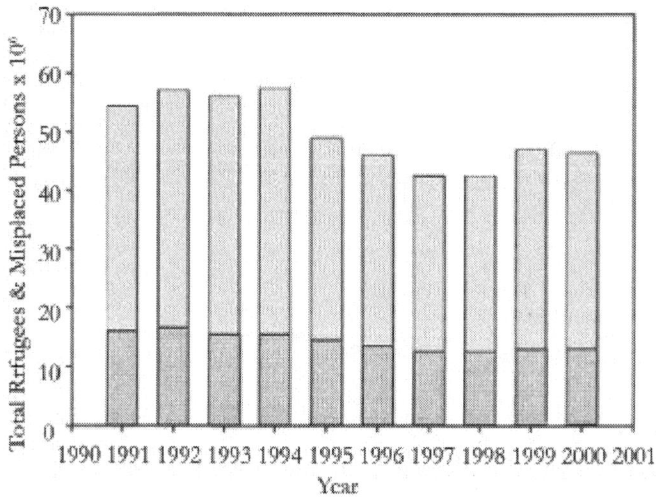

Figure 5: Numbers of refugees (light shading) and internally displaced people (darker shading) in the world in 2000. Reprinted from reference 13 with permission.

Each of these types of movements has the potential to spread disease pathogens and their vectors over long distances.

International trade in merchandise has increased three- to fourfold over the period from 1980 to 2000, with most of the increase occurring in Asia, where there was a fivefold increase in the value of exports (World Trade Organization, http://www.wto.org/english/res_e/statis_e/webpub_e.xls) (Figure 6). Inevitably, this must lead to an increase in the incidence of vectors being transported to other countries.

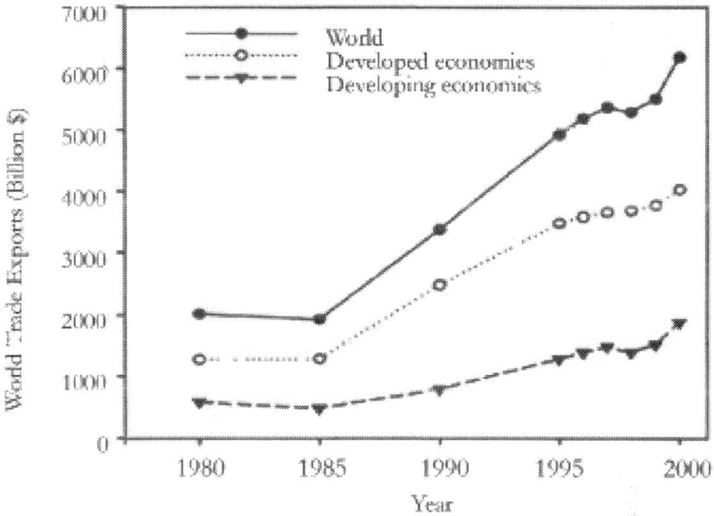

Figure 6: Volume of international trade between 1980 and 2000. Reprinted fromhttp://www.wto.org/english/res_e/statis_e/webpub_e.xls with permission from the World Trade Organization.

In this review, the risks and opportunities arising from each of these drivers of global change in relation to the vector-borne diseases are discussed, both in isolation and in combination when appropriate. The potential environmental effects of each global change driver and their additive or interactive combinations that could affect vector-borne diseases are summarized in Table 1.1. The effects are proximal causes of changes in transmission rates of vector-borne diseases. As can be seen in the second column of Table1, combinations of global change drivers tend to increase the suitability of the environment compared with the effects of each driver separately.

These include combinations of climate change, increased trade and travel, increased urbanization in poor countries, and intensification of agriculture with irrigation, deforestation, and loss of biodiversity. Few interactions reduce the risks, but any that do are likely to be related to the availability of surface water for breeding of mosquitoes under any regional drying due to changed rainfall patterns and the intensification of the hydrological cycle.

Table 1: Environmental effects of global change drivers pertinent to vector-borne diseases, and their potential biological effects Before impacts can be reviewed, it is necessary to establish a framework for assessing the risks.

Global change driver	Potential effects on vector, pathogen, and host environments	Potential effects on vectors, pathogens, and hosts
Higher CO_2 concn	Increased ambient temperature and plant biomass; range expansion of woody vegetation; longer plant growth season with humid microclimates	Increased vector longevity for the same rainfall and temperature through more humide microclimates, with possible range expansion of humid-zone vectors
Temperature increase (regional/ temporal variation)	Expansion of warm climatic zones, with longer growth seasons, less extreme low temperatures, and more frequent extreme high temperatures	Faster vector and pathogen development, with more generations per year; shorter life spans of vectors at high temperatures, reduced low-temperature mortality of vectors, and range expansion of warm-climate vectors and pathogens
Rainfall	Too uncertain and regionally variable to estimate, but increased frequency of extreme rainfall events	Altered patterns of breeding of mosquitoes, with more flushing of mosquito breeding with increased flooding
Urbanization	Increased density of human hosts, with poorer sanitation and water supply in developing countries	Higher rate of disease transmission at same vector density; more vector-breeding sites
	Increased outer urban development in or near forests in developed countries	Increased contact between humans and vectors in periurban forested areas
Deforestation	Increased human entry into forests and increased surface water from soils exposed by logging or new agriculture	More vector-breeding sites and more contact between humans and vectors
Irrigation and water storage	Increased surface water, prevention of seasonal flooding	More vector-breeding sites; reduced flushing of snails and mosquitoes
Intensification of agriculture	Increased disturbance of land and vegetation and increased surface water; reduced biodiversity	More diversity of vector breeding sites, with reduced predation of vectors
Chemical pollution	Fertilizer, pesticide, herbicide and industrial toxins and endocrine-disrupting chemicals	Impaired human immune systems
Increased trade	Increased volume of shipped goods	Increased transport of vectors, leading to "homogenization" of vectors in receptive areas
Increased travel	Increased movement of people between North and South and East and West	Increased transfer of pathogens between regions of endemicity and disease-free regions, and increased exposure of visitors to regions of endemicity

FRAMEWORK FOR ASSESSMENT OF IMPACTS TO VECTOR-BORNE DISEASES UNDER GLOBAL CHANGE

The global scientific community is faced with the huge task of assessing the likely future impacts of global change drivers on vector-borne diseases, in addition to all of the other current influences on human health, agriculture, and natural ecosystems. The numerous species and stakeholders, combined with the great variation in quality of information and data, make the task quite daunting and demand generic approaches with a hierarchy of analytical tools (315).

To develop a holistic approach to risk assessment of vector-borne diseases under global change, we need to combine the approaches developed by the different research and policy communities into a comprehensive risk assessment framework. In this review, each of these approaches is called upon to address particular issues.

The concept of vulnerability is useful for assessing risks to human societies from vector-borne diseases. It is used in the scientific and policy communities investigating the likely threats from climate change (140, 144). Vulnerability is a measure of the potential impacts of a given change, taking into account the adaptive capacity that is available to the affected system or community to respond to that change. In other words, it describes the sensitivity of the particular system of interest to vector-borne diseases, taking its adaptive capacity into account (348). The term avoids the misleading practice of considering risks in the absence of a societal response, which can give an exaggerated picture of the perceived risks. In the present context, impacts are a combination of a change in exposure of humans to pathogens with environmental change and the sensitivity of the population to that change. Adaptive capacity consists of the adaptation technologies and cultural tools and the public health infrastructure and resources that are available to implement appropriate management responses. Inclusion of a given society's capacity to implement appropriate adaptive measures discriminates between groups with disparate cultural, economic, or environmental resources that are needed to implement those measures. It helps to highlight those communities, mostly in the developing world, that are not equipped to manage the changes. The relationships of impacts, adaptation and vulnerability are shown below:

$$Vulnerability = impacts \times (1 - adaptive\ capacity)$$

$$Impacts = exposure \times sensitivity$$

$$Adaptive\ capacity = (adaptation\ products\ and\ practices) \times resources$$

Exposure

A change in the geographical distribution of a vector-borne disease has a quantal effect on the exposure of naive hosts to that disease. Such a change can come about from the movement of either a vector or pathogen to a new environment through trade, human movement, or natural means. Alternatively, it can result from climate change allowing a vector or pathogen to shift its geographical range into environments that become more suitable.

At the global level, assessment of the risks associated with different sources, pathways, and destinations of vectors and pathogens can be assessed by following the quarantine procedures that operate under international "pest risk analysis" agreements for plant health (146). Linking of global change risk assessment approaches with those used by the quarantine community has been proposed (18, 305). The procedure attempts to identify and manage risks by targeting weaknesses at the source of an infection, along the transport pathway and at the destination (Fig.7). We will see below, when considering adaptation options, that it is more difficult to manage risks when humans are the host of a vector-borne disease than when plants or animals are involved.

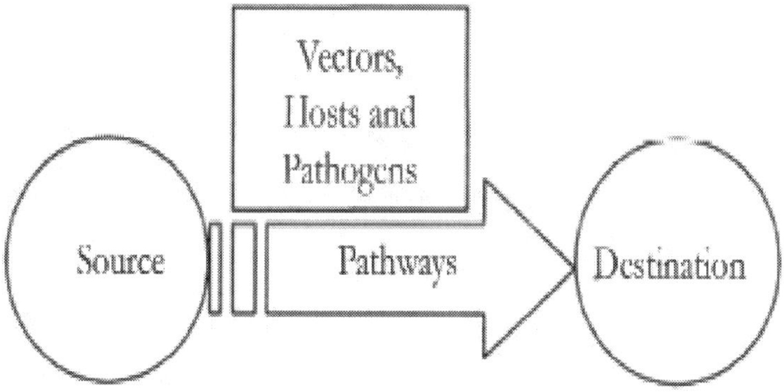

Figure 7: The plant and animal protection concept of sources, pathways, and destinations of exotic species translocations.

In the case of introduction of an exotic vector or pathogen from another continent or its spread to an area from an adjoining zone of endemicity, it is necessary to establish whether the pathogen or vector is able to persist in that new environment. The local habitat forms the template on which ecological processes operate (298). In a risk assessment, the first feature of the habitat that is usually considered is climate, partly for pragmatic reasons—meteorological data are more readily available than other types of data—but other features need to be included systematically. In the context of detection of risks of new exposure, the question is whether the species will be able to persist. This requires analytical tools with which to estimate the response of the species to the new environmental conditions. These are discussed below as part of a review of impact assessment tools. The next question relates to the sensitivity of the local population to the disease and that requires measures of the abundance of the vector and pathogen in the habitat on one hand and the immune status of the host population on the other.

Sensitivity

Sensitivity is the degree to which a system responds to an external perturbation, such as a change of temperature (144). It is essential to define clearly which attribute of a system is being used as the measure of sensitivity because different parts of any system can respond by different amounts. For example, for vector-borne diseases, the potential transmission rate may be very sensitive to a temperature change but the incidence of clinical disease may not alter if the host population is already immune. In this review, when referring to sensitivity of vector-borne diseases, we are referring to potential transmission rates. Host immunity is treated as an adaptation to infection.

Before proceeding further, it is also necessary to appreciate the nonlinear nature of many biological responses to changes in the environment. These arise from a number of features of biological systems, including thresholds such as developmental or behavioral temperature thresholds, discontinuities at the edges of the ranges of species, nonlinear responses to temperature and moisture, multiplicative effects of population growth in vectors with multiple generations each year, negative feedback associated with competition or predation as population densities increase, interactions between variables resulting in non additive effects, and the disproportionate effects of changes in the frequency of extreme events with small changes in the value of the mean. Awareness of such nonlinear effects helps to prevent surprises and so leads to more sustainable adaptation to global change. One consequence of these behaviors is the need to augment empirical and descriptive approaches, such as statistical models, with mechanistic computer simulation models (307).

The sensitivity of a human population to a given disease under global change depends on the combined responses of the pathogen, vector, and host populations. This combination has the potential to generate significant complexity. The geographical location is also a key determinant of the sensitivity of a species to environmental change. A change in the suitability of the environment within the current geographical distribution of the disease will alter the development, survival, and reproductive rates of vectors and pathogens and so affect the intensity of disease transmission and resultant exposure of the population to the disease. The extent to which the exposure changes, following a new introduction of a vector or pathogen or a change in the density of an endemic vector with climate change, depends on the position of the particular habitat relative to the potential geographical distribution of the vector or pathogen in relation to climate (Fig. 8).

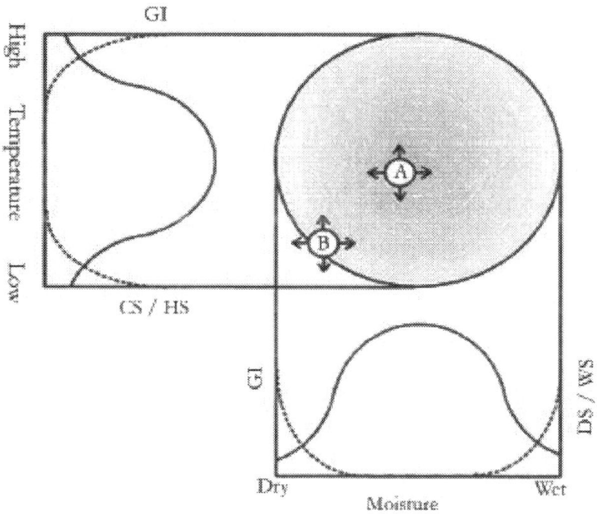

Figure 8: A conceptual model of the geographical distribution of a species related to its climatic envelope. A population (A) near the center of the climatic envelope will be subjected to variations in temperature and moisture in a more favorable range of values than will a population (B) at the edge of the envelope. GI is the CLIMEX model growth index, and CS, HS, DS, and WS are the cold, hot, dry, and wet stress indices, respectively. Reprinted from reference 305 with permission.

Computer models help to identify places where changes in the values of climatic variables are in the sensitive range of a pathogen or vector (307). This is illustrated schematically by a "climatic envelope" in Figure 8, which shows why populations at different locations within the geographical distribution of a species respond differently to a given change in the value of a climatic variable. Populations within the core of the distribution, A, in Fig. 8, defined as the zone with minimal stresses on the species (314), are relatively insensitive to a given change in temperature or moisture because the change occurs in a part of the response curve that is relatively flat. In contrast, populations in marginal parts of the distribution, B, occur where response curves are likely to be steeper and thresholds exist for some physiological processes and so are more responsive to an equal degree of change. Additionally, at or near the edges of the distribution, there is great potential for high variability in the occurrence of limiting conditions because a given change in conditions can flip a population between persistence and extinction very readily. Thus, it is evident that the underlying pressures driving the transmission dynamics of vector-borne diseases will vary more around the edges of the area of endemicity in response to climatic variability (9, 67).

Recognition of variation in the susceptibility of humans to vector-borne diseases, based either on genetic (e.g., sickle cells and malaria) or acquired immunity developed in response to exposure, is needed. The concept of herd immunity leading to endemic stability of a disease is crucial to understanding the dynamics of diseases, the likely susceptibility of populations to such diseases, and the likely consequences of interventions to reduce transmission rates (296). Since the nature of clinical symptoms differs with different transmission rates, it is essential to understand the relationships between pathogen infection, morbidity, and disease outcomes in order to plan interventions that avoid undesirable consequences. These relationships vary greatly with different pathogens, and so a case-by-case approach is necessary.

The sensitivity of a human population to a change in exposure depends on the immune status of the population. Diseases affect human health most severely when there is initial contact resulting from humans entering new habitats, from a spread of disease organisms and their vectors, or from temporary surges in transmission rates during abnormal seasonal conditions, for example. In such cases, naive, nonimmune populations are especially susceptible to epidemics of acute disease.

The rate of disease transmission leads to different disease patterns, such as that for pathogens to which humans can acquire immunity, like malaria (Fig.9). On a spatial scale, the graph represents a cross-section of Fig.8. At high transmission rates, a condition known as endemic stability is created, whereby most hosts are immune, creating herd immunity (C). Around the edges of the area of endemicity there are areas with intermittent epidemics of disease (B), which are referred to as endemically unstable areas. These frequently cause the greatest concern because they involve nonimmune hosts that are particularly susceptible to infection in a high-risk environment. The disease is absent from areas (A) that do not provide suitable environmental or socioeconomic conditions for transmission. These areas may be too cold or too dry for the pathogen or vector to develop and survive during the unfavorable season, or they may have human living conditions, such as insect screens or air conditioning, that prevent contact with the vectors. In areas with very high transmission rates, the hosts may succumb to acute forms of the disease if their health is in any way impeded, creating an "overload" condition (D). In the case of dengue, subsequent infection with a different serotype greatly increases this latter risk by causing additional clinical effects with hemorrhagic symptoms (153).

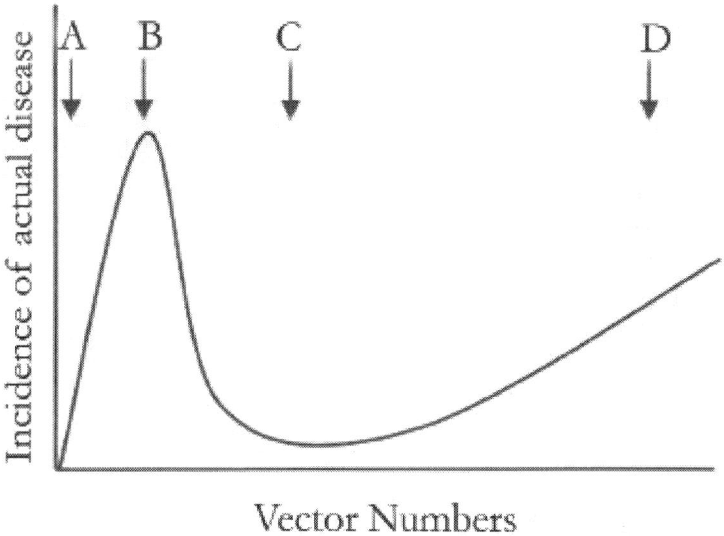

Figure 9: Conceptual model of the relationship between the incidence of human disease and disease transmission rates as determined by vector densities. A, establishment/extinction/eradication zone; B, epidemic/acute-disease zone; C, endemic stability/chronic-disease zone; D, overload/acute-disease zone.

Once we have defined the extent to which a population is likely to be exposed to a vector-borne disease under global change and have also assessed its sensitivity, we are able to derive a measure of the likely impact on the population, in the absence of any intervention to manage that risk as part of an adaptation strategy. This provides us with a baseline measure of risk against which we can estimate the benefits of different options to adapt to the risks.

Impacts

Two approaches have been recommended for analyses of likely impacts of climate change used by the IPCC (244). These are referred to as the top-down and bottom-up approaches. Many authors have used climate change scenarios generated by GCMs as a means of investigating likely impacts of vector-borne diseases (147, 208, 209, 212, 280). The alternative approach relies on sensitivity analyses of a range of climatic variables, and was preferred by Sutherst (304, 307) on the grounds that the climate change scenarios are too immature and changeable to be of lasting value. The use of sensitivity analyses covering the broadest range identified by the global climate modelers avoids the problem of rapid dating that occurs with scenarios. On the other hand, when calculating the net present value of future costs, it is necessary to attach a date to the sensitivity analyses so that discounting can be applied. The two approaches have been combined into a risk management approach (151).

Climate change and trade and transport in particular have the potential to affect the geographical distribution of vectors. While climate change alters the immediate environment of a vector, translocation to a new region presents similar and probably greater changes for vectors. Such changes need to be studied by using geographical-scale approaches. Sutherst (305) presented a conceptual framework for studying the effects of climate on the distribution and abundance of species and how they are affected by climate. As shown in Fig. 8, populations respond differently to a given change in a climatic variable depending on where they are situated in relation to their climatic envelope.

Integrated assessment frameworks to bring some of these elements together are under development (53, 205,248) but do not yet incorporate local environmental circumstances (220). A framework for analyzing impacts on parasites has been described (307) based on theoretical ecology and the framework outlined above. The adoption of political ecology as a framework for analysis of emerging infectious diseases has also been advocated (217). The discipline incorporates social, economic, environmental, and biological components to present a holistic approach. Each of these approaches needs a set of analytical tools.

Tools for risk assessment under global change have been reviewed elsewhere (220, 312). A wide range of approaches have been applied to the assessment of risks for humans to vector-borne diseases under global change. They have ranged from the use of historical analogues (121, 267, 269, 270), and geographical analogues (264) to a variety of statistical (193, 194, 280) and modeling (189, 205, 210, 212, 248, 304, 307,312, 315) tool and models combined with fuzzy logic or rules (68). Historical events are helpful in providing pointers to potential causes of changes in status of diseases (269) but usually suffer from a lack of firm data, sometimes leading to uncertainty in interpretation.

Each technique has limitations, but the most important considerations are the need to apply basic scientific principles (55, 304, 311). Using independent data to test the resultant models, complying with the limitations of chosen analytical or descriptive tools and data sets, and avoiding parameterization of models based on data sets with very narrow ranges of variation can achieve compliance. Often, apparently accurate statistical models fail to demonstrate predictive ability when tested against independent data rather than data derived by dividing a set of data and using one set for fitting and the other for testing the models (262, 278, 279). In addition, popular statistical models, like logistic regression and discriminant functions, rely on pattern matching with meteorological data and so cannot cope with novel climates or with extrapolation to other locations with different patterns of temperature and rainfall, even though they may describe the current range of a species quite accurately. Hence, such descriptive techniques are suited only to answering questions that involve small incremental changes in conditions within the existing ranges.

The ranges and relative abundance of two important African malaria vectors, *Anopheles gambiae* sensu stricto and *A. arabiensis,* have been related to temperature and a ratio of potential evaporation to rainfall as a measure of moisture availability (193). The population at risk from lymphatic filariasis in Africa was also related to these climatic variables (194). Using a combined model and rule-based approach, thresholds for temperature and rainfall have been inferred by using observations from areas of Africa with different malaria transmission patterns (68). The CLIMEX model (304, 311, 313) incorporates a hydrological model to describe the availability of moisture and so accounts for the effects of changes in temperature, rainfall, and evaporation when assessing risks from climate change. It automatically takes any temperature-moisture interactions into account when provided with appropriate meteorological data that include relative humidity or equivalent readings. CLIMEX has been used widely for risk assessments under climate change (303, 304,307). The malaria transmission factors, biting and entomological inoculation rates, were predicted in Kenya using a soil moisture model (250). The model substantially improved the prediction of biting rates compared to rainfall, explaining up to 45% of *A. gambiae* biting variability and 32% of the variability of *A. funestus*when given different time lags.

Each species of vector has characteristic climatic requirements (194, 304) and vector competence for a given biotype of parasite (344) (29). This flags the need to keep each element of the disease triangle (Fig. 1) in mind because the climatic requirements of each vector-pathogen combination needs be taken into account in order to develop a realistic measure of risk (48, 304). Incorporation of species-specific vectorial capacity into global risk assessments has started (208). Integrated assessment frameworks are being developed to bring some of these elements together, with applications to malaria, dengue, and schistosomiasis (53, 205, 220,248, 315). The use of spatial tools, such as geographical information systems and landscape ecology, in studies of vector management and global change effects on vector-borne diseases has been advocated (43,97, 159).

Benchmarks for Measuring Impacts

To detect impacts of global change, we need monitoring data for a number of environmental and disease related variables covering long time series. While historical records of disease incidence provide a valuable basis for detecting a change in transmission patterns, we also need to monitor concurrent environmental and social conditions. This provides benchmarks against which to measure the likely impacts of changes in any given variable.

Temperature is one such variable that varies systematically with latitude and altitude. The effect of altitude on temperatures is approximately equivalent to 5.7°C/km of elevation. The expected altitudinal range shift with increasing temperatures can be calculated using the formula (183)

$$T = Tc - 0.006h$$

Where T is the screen temperature at height h (meters) and T_c is the equivalent at sea level. Thus, ignoring regional variations in sensitivity to global warming, for each 1°C increase in the global temperature there will be a potential increase of ~170 m in the elevation of a given transmission rate of vector-borne diseases. Warming over the past century has been ~0.6°C (144). Thus, reported changes must be within the range of 100 m to have credibility. For example, one credible report is of an increase in height of the freezing point in the tropics of ~110 m (83).

Similarly, expected latitudinal shifts in species ranges with global warming can be expected to be broadly consistent with effects of latitude on temperatures. The approximate formula (183)

$$Tc = \left[27 - 0.008A^2\right]$$

Where T_c is the long-term sea level temperature at latitude A, describes the difference in temperature between that latitude and the equatorial temperature. Thus, on average, there is an approximate difference in temperature of 0.6°C per degree of latitude. Hence, range shifts of about 1.7° of latitude or 200 km can be expected for each 1°C increase in global temperatures. Again, a rise of 0.6°C in the last century can be expected to have been accompanied by range shifts of ~118 km. These figures provide a benchmark against which to relate reported changes in the distribution of vector-borne diseases with respect to global warming, but they need to be related to local modifying factors that create different microclimates and so change the actual area at risk.

Similar benchmarks need to be provided for all other environmental and social variables, with rigorous interpretation of historical events that have often been poorly documented or misinterpreted.

Climate change has the potential to change the intensity of transmission of vector-borne diseases in addition to altering the exposure to the diseases by shifting the geographical distributions, as shown above. The extent to which the disease is sensitive to changes in transmission rates depends on a number of variables, including the responses of vector and pathogen to changes in the particular range of temperature or moisture concerned, and the immune status of the host population. Ideally, it would be useful to have a readily measurable benchmark against which to assess reported claims of involvement by climate in observed changes in the status of established vector-borne diseases. Unfortunately, the species-specific nature of the transmission dynamics of each pathogen renders that more difficult than the task of benchmarking changes in geographical distributions. However, it is still possible to match geographical locations with similar intensity of transmission by using models such as CLIMEX. Alternatively, mathematical models of the biological processes in the transmission cycle (also called mechanistic models) can be used to infer the sensitivity of the transmission rates of vector-borne diseases to changes in climate (189, 210, 212, 307). The major advantage of dynamic models over nonmathematical approaches or statistical models is that they are able to detect surprises or so-called emergent properties of systems that arise from discontinuities, such as thresholds or nonlinearities in biological processes.

IMPACTS

The effects of individual global change drivers on the biology of vectors and disease pathogens are summarized in Table 1. The combined effects of simultaneous changes in some of the drivers are examined below. Information comes from IPCC (144) and the general literature on the biology of vectors. In general, the projected changes are negative for human societies, since they tend to favour increases in transmission of vector-borne diseases. Such generalizations need to be treated cautiously because the outcomes are very location specific. The main reason for the trend with climate is that most of the endemic vector-borne diseases are tropical and so global warming and intensification of water storage and irrigation will naturally create a tendency to expand the range into temperate zones and increase the rate of reproduction of vectors in cooler parts of the range. Some complementary reductions in ranges and reproductive rates can be expected in the hottest parts of the current ranges. These tendencies will be exacerbated in some cases by increased rates of dispersal of the pathogens and vectors in human-mediated transport, and opportunities for intensification of transmission will increase as human population densities increase. On the other hand, many adaptive responses are possible, and if there is an improvement in public health facilities, they are likely to counter most of the changes favoring vectors and pathogens.

Climatic and nonclimatic global change drivers, such as human movements, land use and irrigation, and drug or pesticide resistance, can have large effects on disease transmission. Since some environmental changes are global but vary on a regional scale, the degree of exposure of each human-vector-pathogen system will vary with both the driver involved and the geographical location. The risks associated with each type of change need to be addressed on a disease-by-disease and location-by-location basis. An assessment of relative risks associated with each disease and global change driver is needed to prioritize the allocation of resources to adaptive measures. Such a rating system does not exist at present, and its production will require inputs from panels of experts. While most projected environmental changes appear to favor water-breeding vectors, temperature effects on other types of vectors are likely to be local and less severe.

While humans have different exposures to vector-borne diseases under each global change driver, the disease systems also vary in their sensitivity. The extent to which the incidence of a disease is sensitive to a nominated change at a particular geographical location depends on the interaction of the disease organism, its vector, its host population, and the environment (Fig. 1). The global change drivers are likely to have their greatest effect by influencing the numbers and seasonal patterns of activity of the vectors or by moving or accelerating the development of the pathogens. The degree of contact between hosts, vectors, and pathogens and the immune status of the host population will also be sensitive to change.

In most historical instances, the resurgence of diseases can be related to local ecological changes that favored increased vector densities or host-vector contacts, reintroductions of pathogens, or breakdown of vector control measures (121, 270). Development projects such as irrigation and water storage, urbanization, and deforestation have resulted in changes in communities of vectors, with increased population densities of certain species that led to the outbreaks of vector-borne diseases. Increased travel and transport have introduced infectious agents and vectors into new areas. The advent of global-scale environmental changes in recent decades has been an additional risk. The next sections review the evidence for the effect of environmental change on the key vector-borne diseases with likely future global change scenarios.

Atmospheric Composition

An indirect effect of increasing concentrations of CO_2 in the atmosphere is that the water use efficiency of plants is increased. Under good climatic and nutritional conditions, this will result in larger plants that provide more humid shelter for insect vectors and for plant pathogens. However, since plant growth under field conditions is often limited by factors other than water, such as nutrients, there is likely to be a generally higher water table and soil moisture content than occurs at present, unless global warming results in reduced rainfall or substantially increased evaporation (261). Such conditions are conducive to an increase in the frequency of pools of open water that provide suitable habitat for mosquito breeding. This would have consequences for both freshwater- and fouled-water-breeding mosquitoes and the diseases that they transmit.

Climate Change

Climate change has the potential to alter the average exposure of human populations to vector-borne diseases by changing the geographical distribution of conditions that are suitable for the vectors and disease pathogens. An increase in global temperatures will result in an expansion of warm temperature regimens into higher altitudes and latitudes. Any associated changes in rainfall in tropical and subtropical zones will also render habitats more or less suitable for vectors. In addition, the implications of the asymmetrical increases of temperature with global warming (154) for the epidemiology of vector-borne diseases need to be clarified. Greater effects can be expected from the extended relaxation of limiting effects of low temperatures on vector survival, behavior, and disease transmission in cold-limited climates than from smaller and less frequent increases in extreme maximum temperatures. These changes would make temperate environments more receptive to many tropical vector-borne diseases while having less negative effects on tropical environments.

Extreme climatic events have major effects on the transmission rates of vector-borne diseases. In the light of expectations that climate change will increase the frequency of such events disproportionably, such extreme events may emerge as a more important feature of climate change than are changes in average climatic conditions. They are therefore considered in more detail below.

There have been a large number of studies and reviews of the sensitivity of vector-borne diseases to climate change (37,40,49,50,61,62,82,84,88-90,110,121,123,125,126,134,164-166,169,186-189,191,192,206,209,215,220-223,225,228,230,245,246,249,264,266,267,269,27-0,295,303,307,309,310,335,350). The results have led to quite different perceptions of the role of climatic change and other factors in historical patterns of disease incidence.

The coherent pattern of the retreat of tropical glaciers, an upward shift in the freezing isotherm in the tropics, increases or decreases in the geographical ranges of temperate or Arctic species, respectively, at higher latitudes, earlier spring migration and breeding by birds, and earlier seasonal activity of insects have been cited as examples of impacts of gradual global warming (90, 125, 126, 243, 282). The observations were claimed to be consistent with increasing global temperatures and with model predictions. Taken together, these phenomena provide strong evidence that climatic changes in recent decades are already affecting up to 50% of the species examined in a survey of the literature (243, 282). There is no reason to believe that vector-borne diseases are exceptions to this experience of small and gradual changes in seasonal activity and expansion of ranges to higher altitudes and latitudes. The issue for workers in the field is to establish adequate baseline data on seasonal transmission patterns, prevalence of disease and geographical distributions, benchmarks to monitor and assess the consistency of changes with known physiological processes, and sufficiently accurate monitoring data in strategic locations to be able to detect the changes as they occur around species range boundaries initially. Only then will the medical community be able to separate the subtle effects of climate change on vector-borne diseases from the more obvious effects of other factors.

A number of authors have raised the possibility that global warming may have played some part in the recent range expansions and outbreaks of vector-borne diseases (37, 40, 89, 90, 125, 163, 186, 188, 197). Two types of climatic effects could theoretically have been involved. First, changes like the ones observed for other species of plants and animals referred to above will gradually increase the transmission rates in cooler climates and so extend transmission into previously disease-free areas while slowing transmission in areas that become too hot. In some cases, realization of this expectation with vector-borne diseases will be different for other species because often the vectors are already there but the pathogens have been eliminated. Second, changes in the intensity of extreme climatic events will alter the patterns of epidemics. Any change in the intensity and frequency of extreme climatic events may take decades to detect against a background of insufficiently long historical records and high climatic variability with ENSO-like events, and it is probably too early to invoke this effect in any historical events.

Other authors (34, 121, 136, 266, 270, 294), citing historical outbreaks and identifying the largest current signals in a set of data, concluded that other factors were more important than climate and questioned the veracity of claims (90, 197, 206, 223) that anthropogenic climate change could have contributed to the epidemics. For example, it has been suggested (34) that replacement of forest by agriculture provided new habitats for breeding of mosquitoes at Usambara in Tanzania, rather than local temperatures rising as a result of land clearing, as was previously suggested (214). The role of climate change in an outbreak of malaria in Rwanda (197) was questioned because it coincided with a change in detection methods that was more likely to explain the jump in reported incidence of infections (270). Opposing interpretations of historical temperature data in East Africa, based on interpolated meteorological data (235), led to different interpretations of the role of global warming in the observed increase in incidence of malaria in recent decades (136, 247; J. A. Patz, M. Hulme, C. Rosenzweig, T. D. Mitchell, R. A. Goldberg, A. K. Githeko, S. Lele, A. J. McMichael, and D. Le Sueur, Letter, Nature 420:627-628, 2002). A negligible role was seen for global warming in the resurgence of vector-borne disease in Latin America, Africa, and Asia in the past two decades (121, 266, 270, 294). It was claimed to be inappropriate to use climate-based models to predict future prevalence because climate plays a small role in disease outbreaks (270). That view does not take sufficient account of the role of climate in determining the underlying seasonal phenology or geographical distributions of vectors and pathogens. Neither does it recognize the contribution of climate-based modeling in allowing researchers to extrapolate results from one geographical location to another. What has been missing from the global change studies is adequate inclusion of non-climatic variables in the analyses, which reflects the difficulty in building and maintaining global databases of local environmental changes.

In a more pragmatic view, global warming was considered to be unlikely to cause major epidemics of tropical mosquito-borne disease in the United States (121) and Australia (48) as long as the public health infrastructure and living conditions remain the same. It is not surprising that the role of climate change in historical events has been contentious because the extent of the changes is only just beginning to be large enough to be distinguished from natural variability and the events were not sufficiently well documented to ensure that all variables could be accounted for. Despite the differences in emphasis and focus on historical or future events, all authors agree that there are multifactorial causes of change in the incidence of vector-borne diseases. Land use events will be more important in the short term, but climate change has the potential to be important in the longer term.

Climate change will affect both the invertebrate vectors and the development of pathogens in those vectors. Basic biological considerations indicate that with global warming, the duration of the growth season will increase, allowing more generations of vectors each year in cooler areas. Development is prevented at low temperatures, but as temperatures rise, a race develops between parasite development and accelerated mortality of the vector. The winters will be shorter and less severe and so will reduce the mortality rates of species of vectors that are currently limited by low temperatures. Other temperate species of vectors are insensitive to winter conditions in some environments (270). In some environments, temperatures will rise to levels where the mortality rates of the vectors are so high that they die before being able to transmit a pathogen. Changes in future moisture regimens are much more uncertain.

Malaria

(i) Exposure and sensitivity

Most of the analyses of the impacts of climate change on vector-borne diseases have been aimed at malaria, consistent with the dominant global impact of that disease. The initial emphasis has been focused on the direct effects of changes in temperature on development of the parasites and longevity of the adult mosquitoes. This reflects the ease of investigating temperature effects rather than their relative importance compared with other drivers of change. Small increases at low temperatures were shown to increase the risk of transmission disproportionately, and it was concluded that vulnerable communities in malaria-free areas or those with unstable malaria are likely to be at increased risk of future outbreaks (189). An increase of 12 to 27% in the epidemic potential of malaria transmission compared with current areas of endemicity has been projected as an indication of the sensitivity of malaria to climate change (209).

Modeling studies indicate that higher temperatures will lead to an increase in the population that is exposed to malaria as a result of an expansion of the geographical distributions of vector-borne diseases into higher altitudes and latitudes (49, 50, 189, 192, 211-213, 248). A mathematical model, designed to identify malaria epidemic-prone regions, was used to explore possible changes in epidemiology with projected global climate change in the African highlands (192). It was assumed that free water for breeding sites would be available when higher temperatures occur because water is not currently limiting. Most malaria epidemics in the endemically unstable highlands are due to *Plasmodium falciparum,* the cause of the most severe form of clinical malaria. A plea was made to accord these areas special status and recognize them as having a high risk under climate change.

Europe has experienced significant warming in recent decades, and there is evidence of climatic effects in the northern spread of tick vectors in Sweden (165). Nevertheless, the current geographical range of malaria in Europe is much smaller than its potential range as shown from historical records (148, 149, 191, 269, 303). In many regions the vectors are present but malaria transmission does not occur because the pathogens have been eliminated. An increase in average temperature has the largest effect on epidemic potential where parasite development is limited by low temperatures in temperate areas, consistent with the conceptual models in Fig. 8 and 9. Infected mosquitoes introduced through airports are also likely to survive longer in the future if there is increased rainfall and will therefore enhance the problem known as airport malaria (295).

A claim that Australia was highly vulnerable to malaria under climate change (233) has been refuted (48,332). The suitable area is determined mostly by the climatic requirements of the only highly competent vector, *A. farauti,* rather than the temperatures required for the development of malaria parasites (48, 304). The CLIMEX model was used to determine the area at risk of malaria after an increase in temperature, so any reduction in soil moisture due to increased evaporation at the higher temperatures was factored into the calculation. An increase of 1.5°C was expected to allow *A. farauti* to colonize Gladstone, a town on the east coast of Australia 800 km further south of its current range limit, with islands even further south being potential habitats. The results exceed the benchmark for the effects of such a temperature rise and illustrate the need to consider localized effects of topography on likely range expansions. Whether this potential is realized will depend on many other variables, particularly the state of the public health system. More recently, the mosquito has been detected at Mackay, 2° south of the previous southernmost record near Townsville (328). The finding confirmed earlier unpublished records and is not thought to relate to any change in temperatures.

Both the direct and indirect effects of increased temperature on anopheline mosquitoes, malaria parasites, and their hosts have been examined (295). It was concluded that the most likely effects of climate change would be on the availability of surface water for larval habitats. It may also be assumed that any increase in the density of foliage of plants growing in an enriched CO_2 atmosphere will provide more favorable shelter for adults of some species of mosquitoes, extending their longevity. If the residual soil moisture also increases as the water use efficiency of plants increases, there may also be an increase in the amount of surface water during the season and the expanded range of sheltered habitats referred to above. These scenarios are still highly speculative.

A descriptive, statistical model was used to challenge claims that the global distribution of *P. falciparum*malaria is likely to increase significantly under climate change (280). Several comments about this analysis are necessary. First, it was claimed that little change is likely in the area at risk because those areas, which become more receptive with higher temperatures, will suffer increased moisture deficits. This point had been noted previously (148), but as we saw above, moisture-related climate change scenarios are still too uncertain to be useful. The complicated relationship between the incidence of malaria and floods and droughts makes the task even more difficult. Second, the current distribution of "malaria," used to define the current global area at risk, was not very specific and the analysis did not take into account the different climatic needs and vector competence of the 50 or more species of mosquitoes, of which about half are considered to be primary vectors (344). This is critical, as is evident in Australia, where the area at risk has been shown previously to differ vastly when estimated using the responses of the only highly competent vector, *A. farauti,* or of the *P. falciparum* pathogen (Fig. 10) (48).

The global area currently at risk of malaria transmission greatly exceeds the area of endemicity because the pathogens have been eliminated from large parts of the world but the vectors remain and pose a threat if reinfected (148). Third, the assumption that adaptation measures in developed countries would prevent the spread of malaria is vulnerable to social unrest and economic decline, such as have occurred in Eastern Europe and central Asia.

Finally, statistical models are inappropriate tools for extrapolating geographical distributions because they rely on pattern matching of meteorological data and so cannot cope with novel climates that arise with climate change (168, 304). A credible global risk assessment of malaria must consist of an aggregation of regional assessments, taking into account their local differences in vectors, pathogens, and current disease status, and must be developed using dynamic simulation models rather than statistical models.

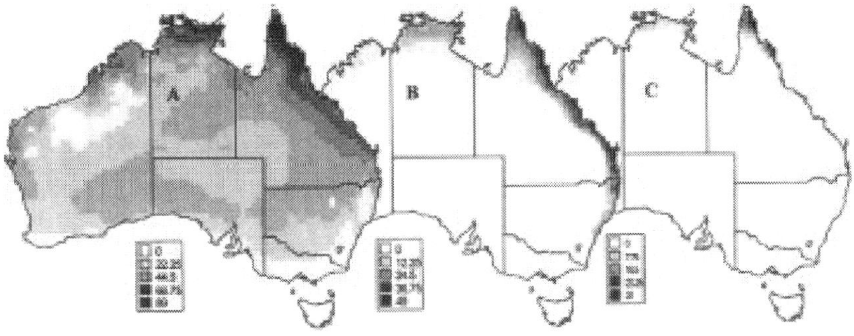

Figure 10: (A) Comparison of the estimates of areas at risk from *P. falciparum* malaria in Australia, based on the pathogen only, related to temperature for development. (B) As for panel A but including moisture limitation for mosquito breeding. (C) As for panel A but including the restriction imposed by the distribution of the only highly competent malaria vector, *Anopheles farauti,* as limited by climate. Modified from reference 304 with permission.

The complexity of assessments of risks from vector-borne diseases, in different geographical ranges and different habitats, is further illustrated by some elegant work on nonvector mosquitoes. The temperature regimen interacts with the annual cycle of day length at 50°N latitude in North America, affecting not only the seasonal phenology of the mosquito species (*Wyeomyia smithii*) but also its genetic composition. The critical photoperiod that triggers diapause decreased by over 30 min between 1972 and 1998 with increasing temperature (42). This resulted in the mosquitoes remaining active for an extra 9 days in the warmer climate. Hence, some species are able to adapt very rapidly to changes in their environment and the outcome in any particular ecosystem will depend on the relative ability of each species to track the multiplicity of changes in any environment. The example emphasizes a dimension of species adaptation to change that has been given insufficient attention in global change research, namely, polygenic inheritance of adaptive characters. There is often a large amount of genetic variation present in populations that allows them to adapt rapidly to year-to-year variation in seasonal conditions (317) and hence to climate change.

(ii) Extreme climatic events and malaria transmission.

Since most climate-related vector-borne disease events occur when there is a marked deviation from average climatic conditions, it is important to determine the impact of the predicted increase in extreme climatic conditions on the incidence of these diseases. If the climate change scenarios are correct and there is a trend toward more extreme climatic events, there is a need to apply a different form of analysis in order to define the changes in the frequency and intensity of such events. Ecologists have identified appropriate statistical tools (101), but these tools have not yet been applied to vector-borne diseases. In the meantime, it is possible only to access qualitative analyses of such events.

Referring again to Fig 8, it is evident from theory that changes in temperature or moisture will trigger the greatest responses from vector-borne diseases in geographical regions where transmission is most sensitive to change around the edges of geographical distributions. Here we examine some examples of epidemics or lulls in transmission arising from extreme climatic events, which are summarized in Table 2. They range from droughts that dry out rivers into ponds, which provide favorable breeding sites for mosquitoes (38, 41, 200,256), to floods that either cause malaria epidemics in arid areas (195) or, conversely, wash away vector populations in humid environments, temporarily suppressing breeding in some habitats while increasing it in others (25, 190). Temporary periods of high temperature can overcome the cold limitation of parasite development in vectors at high altitudes in the tropics (105).

Table 2: Examples of the effects of extreme climatic events on the incidence of malaria[a]

Avg rainfall	Event
Low	Epidemic — El Niño high temperatures and rainfall in cool-dry, high-altitude areas of Pakistan (37)
	Epidemic — high rainfall: arid or semiarid areas of Kenya (6), Gujarat (3), Punjab (41)

	Epidemic — high temperatures and rainfall: tropical highlands with little moisture deficit (Kenya [234], and Uganda highlands [184])
	Epidemic — high rainfall with La Niña 1988: extended area of endemicity on northeastern coast of Venezuela (23)
	Lapse in transmission — flooding: hot-wet areas with flooding that washes away breeding sites (Usambara [190], South Africa and Mozambique 2000 [25])
High	Epidemic — drought: humid areas with ponding of rivers (Sri Lanka [41], Colombia [39, 256], drought in Venezuela [36])

[a]Note that in each case other factors may be involved.

It is instructive to compare these observations with the major outbreak of the tick (*Boophilus microplus*) vector of a malaria-like parasite, *Babesia,* of cattle, at Mt. Tamborine in Australia during a warm El Niño year (Fig. 11) (302). Animal examples are often useful to illustrate some features of human vector-borne diseases epidemiology because the data are more detailed and may be less severely affected by interventions to curtail transmission. With an average warm season maximum temperature that was 1.6°C above the long-term average at this temperature-limited location, four times as many ticks were produced and the highest daily infestation increased from ~200 to over 1,400 per animal. The increase was caused by the compound growth of three generations, magnified by the accelerated development rate of eggs that enabled many more to hatch before the onset of winter. Such changes are likely to be experienced in areas where vectors have several generations each year and there is weak density-related mortality. This illustrates the important point that there is the potential for disproportionately large increases in the rates of disease transmission with small increases in temperature in cool-limited habitats (189). It gives some credence to claims that higher temperatures may have contributed to some recent epidemics of malaria (37, 38, 41, 128), but that does not imply that these effects are related to climate change. The above results illustrate how extremes of high temperatures and both high and low rainfall have the potential to have profound effects on the incidence of malaria (163). Whether or not higher temperatures per se have been responsible for some of the historical outbreaks referred to earlier is uncertain, given the concurrency of other events and unquantified data for all significant variables involved.

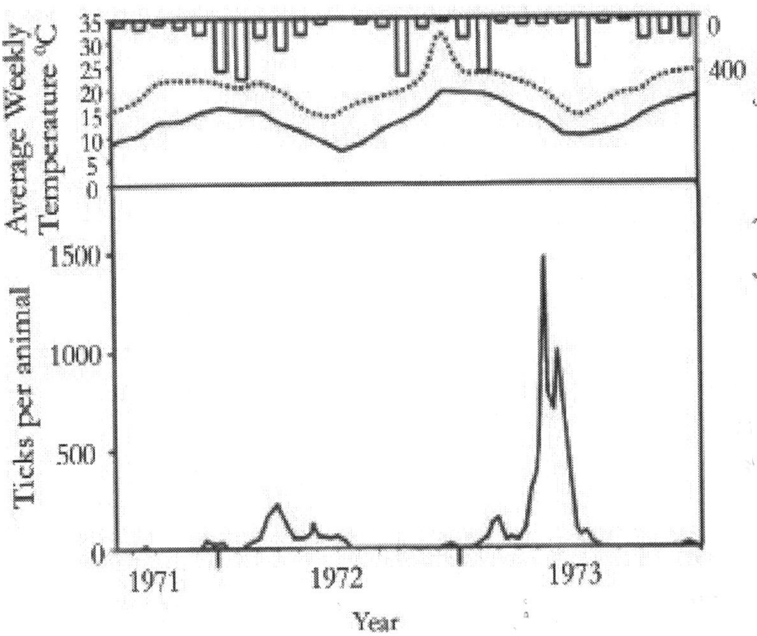

Figure 11: Numbers of the tick vector (*Boophilus microplus*) of the bovine malaria-like parasites *Babesia* spp., at Mt Tamborine, Australia, over 2 years with different temperatures in 1971 to 1973. Modified from reference 302 with permission.

The challenge for scientists is to translate climate change scenarios, with their higher average temperatures and intensification of the hydrological cycle, into meaningful measures of malaria transmission. It is not yet clear what effect the projected increase in intensity of rainfall and evaporation, combined with fewer but heavier rainfall events, will have on mosquito breeding sites, but the above incidents suggest that there will be more variability in transmission rates. Hydrological studies are needed to determine the probabilities of changes in the habitats of mosquitoes that will affect their breeding opportunities. Working with soil moisture instead of rainfall and evaporation is essential to achieve more accurate results.

Vector-Borne Diseases other than Malaria

(i) Exposure and sensitivity.

Few climate change risk assessments have been reported for diseases other than malaria. A summary of those studies is given below.

The complex, mediating effect of climate on the transmission of vector-borne diseases is well illustrated by the work on *Culex tarsalis* Coquillett, the primary vector of St. Louis encephalitis (SLE) and Western equine encephalomyelitis (WEE) in the western United States (264). The survival of mosquito larvae in aquatic environments is severely reduced at higher temperatures, and the survival rate of the adults also declines. Hence, the viruses are involved in a race to complete their development in the adult mosquito before it dies. At 32°C the mosquito is able to restrict the development of WEE virus but not that of SLE virus. High summer temperatures in southern California are therefore likely to break the transmission of WEE. In cooler areas, the higher summer temperatures would curtail the survival of adults of *C. tarsalis* and overwintering survival could alter because they go into diapause. Thus, increases in temperature, of the order projected under climate change, have the potential to extend the northern range of both viruses and to reduce the southern range of WEE virus. On the other hand, some temperate species of mosquitoes, such as *C. pipiens,*are insensitive to variation in the winter conditions that occur in the southern United States (265).

Schistosomiasis is a snail-borne disease that is increasing in incidence as a result of the provision of water storage facilities. The transmission potential of *Schistosoma* spp. is sensitive to climate change around the edges of current areas of endemicity (209). These authors expected the epidemic potential of schistosomiasis to decrease by 11 to 17% with global warming due to higher mortality rates of miracidia, cercariae, and the snail vectors. Health impacts of climate change were expected to be most pronounced in populations living in less economically developed, temperate areas in which endemicity is currently low or absent.

Dengue fever epidemics occur around the tropics, but, perhaps because they are usually urban events driven largely by the availability of the virus and man-made waste acting as water containers for breeding by the vector *Aedes aegypti,* there appears to be a smaller climatic influence on the disease than occurs with other arboviruses. Higher temperatures can accelerate the transmission of diseases such as dengue even during low rainfall periods because artificial water storage containers are favored breeding sites for *A. aegypti* in particular. The results of modeling indicate that global warming can be expected to increase the latitudinal and altitudinal range of dengue and extend the duration of the transmission season in temperate locations as well (81, 98, 147, 209). An increase in temperature-related transmission intensity can also be expected to increase the number of secondary infections of young people who are the most susceptible to dengue hemorrhagic fever and shock syndrome (147). Further insight into the likely effects of global warming on dengue transmission is provided by experience with periods of extreme temperatures associated with the ENSO cycle, as discussed below.

Visceral and cutaneous forms of leishmaniasis are transmitted by a group of biting flies known as sand flies, the main genus of which is *Phlebotomus.* The reservoir hosts are rodents and dogs, and the disease is usually associated with rural environments, where the sand flies breed and shelter in rodent burrows. The disease occurs widely in the tropics, in semi-arid regions in particular. Two studies have indicated potential changes in the geographical distribution of the vectors. Modeling studies in southwest Asia have indicated potential range expansion of *Phlebotomus papatasi* with global warming (70). In Italy, visceral leishmaniasis caused by *Leishmania infantum* is prevalent in the milder parts, where it is transmitted by *P. perniciosus.* Low temperature appears to be one of the main factors preventing its spread into northern Europe (169). *P. perfiliewi,* suspected of transmitting cutaneous leishmanisais, is found in regions with more extreme high and low temperatures. Increases in temperature are likely to accelerate the development of the leishmania organisms but inhibit *P. perniciosus;* therefore, the outcomes are not clear. Little change is expected with the cutaneous form.

There have been studies of the effect of climate change on tsetse flies, including *Glossina morsitans,* a vector of human trypanosomiasis, in Africa (278). Unfortunately, the analyses involved descriptive, statistical models, fitted to very geographically limited data sets, and so they do not have predictive value (304). Given the extent of interactions between species of *Glossina* and the replacement of displaced species by others, a meaningful assessment of the likely changes in the distribution and abundance of tsetse flies and the incidence of trypanosomiasis needs to take them into account (116), in addition to the likely direct effects of such climatic changes on the *Glossina* flies and their habitats.

Chagas› disease, caused by *Trypanosoma cruzi,* is transmitted by the triatomid bug, *Triatoma infestans,* in rural areas with poor housing in South America. Analogue and simulation models were used to indicate that the population growth of the vector in Argentina would be slowed with global warming and so the risks from that disease would be reduced (49).

A marked northward spread of *Ixodes ricinus* has been observed over the past two decades in Sweden (186,188). The increased range of about 100 km and higher incidence of tick-borne encephalitis transmitted by *I. ricinus* between the early 1980s and mid-1990s were closely related to warmer summers and winters in the 1990s compared with the previous three decades (188). There were consistent direct and indirect relationships between climate and disease incidence, and a model was developed to predict changes in disease incidence based on bioclimatic thresholds. The extent of the biological changes is also consistent with our benchmark (see above) for responses to increases in temperature in the past century.

In Australia there are a number of mosquito-borne viruses that currently cause diseases of various severity in the human population (286). An attempt to evaluate the risks of these diseases under climate change was made difficult by the great uncertainties about the future direction of the change in rainfall. Some GCMs were indicating increases, while others gave opposite results, and the directions also changed in summer and winter. There is also insufficient understanding of the biology of the many vectors involved and the roles of their habitats and alternate hosts (286).

(ii) Extreme climatic events and vector-borne diseases other than malaria.

Much less work has been done on relating the incidence of vector-borne diseases other than malaria to extreme climatic events. Some such events are summarized in Table 3. They show that extremes of both high and low rainfall are correlated with the incidence of mosquito-borne diseases in different environments. Causation has not been proven.

Table 3: Examples of effects of extreme climatic events on the incidence of vector-borne diseases other than malaria

Avg rainfall	Event
Low	Epidemic: Rift Valley fever affecting humans in arid northeastern Kenya after heavy rain (195)
	Epidemic: dengue fever with heavy rainfall in Malaysia (99) and the South Pacific, but introduction of virus is more important (129)
	Epidemic: Ross River virus outbreaks after summer floods if nonimmune native hosts are available (200)
	Epidemic: Murray Valley encephalitis in heavy-rainfall year in northern Australia (237)
	Epidemic: ponding of rivers during drought causing SLE and Japanese encephalitis in Papua New Guinea (200)
High	Epidemic: dengue in the Western Pacific in early 1998 during the latter part of an El Niño cycle (11), with higher than average sea surface temperatures in the central Pacific
	(http://iri.columbia.edu/climate/ENSO/background/monitoring.html) virus introductions also important.

[a]Note that in each case other factors such as fluctuating host immunity may be involved.

The relative insensitivity of dengue fever transmission to climate suggests that the incidence will vary little with climatic variability. In practice, there is sparse information in the field, although the dengue outbreaks in the Western Pacific in 1998 (11) occurred when the negative, El Niño phase of the ENSO was in place, with high temperatures in the area (http://iridl.ldeo.columbia.edu). A study in the South Pacific found a variable correlation between dengue and the

ENSO. However, the population density and amount of travel between islands, transferring the virus from place to place, appeared to have a large effect (128), consistent with other observations on the dominant roles of socioeconomic and political factors in dengue transmission (81).

Murray Valley encephalitis is an arbovirus disease that is endemic in the tropics in Australia, with reservoirs of infection in water birds. Infrequent, severe epidemics of Murray Valley encephalitis occur in temperate southeastern Australia after heavy rainfall and flooding, and the ENSO has been proposed as a predictive tool (237).

Ross River virus, which causes epidemic polyarthritis, is transmitted by a large number of species of mosquito, and its life cycle can involve different species of intermediate hosts, including kangaroos. The disease is distributed throughout Australia and Papua New Guinea. Heavy rain or flooding, which leads to increased breeding of mosquitoes, can cause outbreaks of the disease (200) provided that other conditions are suitable. These include the availability of a reservoir of uninfected, vertebrate hosts and suitable seasonal temperatures.

Urbanization

The higher human population densities and lack of the necessary urban infrastructure in tropical regions in particular have profound effects on the transmission potential of diseases (123, 221). Dense urban development with poor infrastructure is widespread in the developing world and leads to increases in the incidence of human diseases that need large human populations to persist and wastewater for the vectors to breed (123). The deteriorating public health infrastructure in many countries exacerbates the problem. Vectors of dengue fever and yellow fever are able to exploit artificial sources of water such as water storage pots, tires, or old containers in garbage. Polluted wastewater also provides a suitable breeding environment for *Culex* mosquitoes that transmit lymphatic filariasis (199) and arboviruses such as SLE virus in the United States and Rift Valley fever virus in Africa (292). Meanwhile, rural-urban migration is credited with leading to a new pattern of infection referred to as urban schistosomiasis (329). On the other hand, the reduction in the incidence of Chagas› disease with urbanization has been alluded to above in relation to climate change.

Land Use, Land Cover, and Biodiversity

The effects of environmental change on emerging parasitic diseases have been reviewed recently (249). Examples were cited of upsurges in malaria with deforestation in Africa, Asia, and Latin America, where the diversity of vector species ensures that there is continuing transmission, because habitat changes favor different species of mosquitoes. The types of vegetation and ground cover determine the vector species that occurs following deforestation, with natural and human-built water storage facilities playing a major role. Agriculture has pervasive local effects on vector-borne diseases by affecting the availability of breeding sites for different species of vectors (229). A number of land use issues that affect the incidence of vector-borne diseases have been identified, including deforestation, land cultivation, and various water storage, distribution, and irrigation structures and practices (64, 105, 229, 231, 303). They can be expected to continue to affect the future patterns of those diseases as the land use changes accelerate. For example, clearing of cattail marshes in Africa for cultivation removes breeding sites for *Anopheles funestrus,* but cultivation of papyrus swamps and deforestation provide open, sunlit water that is suitable for breeding by *A. gambiensis* (231). Cultivation of irrigated rice can either increase the incidence of malaria greatly or have no effect when the vector is *A. funestrus* in mainland Africa (66, 174). Similar differences in the responses of different species of mosquito to irrigation were observed with malaria vectors in Sri Lanka (7). Forecasting the consequences of changes in environmental management requires the involvement of multidisciplinary teams in the planning and implementation of the projects (230).

Deforestation combined with industrial, residential, and agricultural development in the Amazon has had widespread effects on the species of anopheline mosquitoes present and on the rates of transmission of malaria (316). The most significant effects were altered breeding grounds and shelter for the mosquitoes, which changed the intensity of contact with humans. Notable was the great diversity of effects in different regions; however, changes that favoured *Anopheles darlingi,* the most efficient malaria vector, were the most important.

The implications of a number of environmental changes associated with rural development have been investigated. Forest penetration has involved humans in viral and leishmanial zoonoses and has introduced*Onchocerca volvulus* into Central and South American forests. Clearing of forests for agricultural developments such as rubber plantations in Malaysia has resulted in increases in malaria, and there has been a spread of the snail vectors of schistosomiasis into forests. In Indonesia the incidence of lymphatic filariasis was reduced by forest clearing and development, which exposed the mosquito breeding sites to sunlight (182). Similarly, clearing is used to control malaria in Asia by reducing the breeding of *Anopheles balabacensis* (229). However, deforestation can increase the breeding of sun-loving *Anopheles* vectors of malaria in Africa, as mentioned above (229).

An "edge effect" changed the patterns of transmission of trypanosomiasis and loiasis in West Africa. Occupation of land, with the resultant change in vegetation cover, affected the transmission dynamics of triatomine vectors of *T. cruzi,* phlebotomine transmission of leishmaniasis, and tsetse fly transmission of *T. rhodesiense* (64). Each of these effects are destined to continue as deforestation continues apace around the tropics.

Water storage reservoirs, from jars to dams, and irrigation practices provide breeding sites for mosquito vectors of several viral and protozoan diseases including malaria, while large, still water bodies are particularly well suited to the breeding of snail vectors of schistosomiasis. There has been a changing incidence and geographical distribution of schistosomiasis, partly due to human migration, new irrigation and water impoundments, particularly in Africa, and successful eradication in some countries (30, 56). Ecological changes resulting from the building of the Aswan Dam in Egypt have resulted in a shift from predominantly*S. haematobium* to *S. mansoni*. There was a massive outbreak of *S. mansoni* in northern Senegal, due to intense transmission, after the construction of the Diama dam on the Senegal river and the Manantali dam on the Bafing river, Mali (297). The Three Gorges Dam in southern China is expected to increase the transmission of *S. mansoni* over a vast area by preventing annual flushing of the snail vectors (180).

Some of the effects of various water-related activities on vector-borne diseases have been summarized (229). They include reduction in the incidence of dracunculiasis by controlling the *Cyclops* intermediate hosts in drinking water; artificial lakes that drown the breeding habitats of *Simulium* spp. (vectors of onchocerciasis) while creating new habitat for *Anopheles* vectors of malaria and filariasis and snail hosts (*Biomphalaria* and*Bulinus* spp.) of schistosomiasis; dam spillways providing larval habitats for *Simulium* spp., resulting in artificial foci of onchocerciasis in West Africa; heavily vegetated irrigation canals that provide habitats for*Anopheles* spp. and snails; and irrigated rice fields that provide habitats for *Anopheles* and *Culex* spp., including *C. tritaeniorhynchus,* an important vector of Japanese encephalitis virus.

A complex relationship exists between irrigation and malaria incidence in Africa (143). In environments with small populations of mosquitoes, increased numbers of vectors following the introduction of irrigation can increase the incidence of malaria in areas of unstable transmission, such as the African highlands and on the fringes of deserts. However, irrigation has little impact on malaria transmission for most of sub-Saharan Africa, where it is stable. The lower incidence of malaria in some communities with irrigation than in surrounding areas was explained by a combination of changes in the species composition of the mosquitoes and better protective measures made possible by increased wealth of the community.

Irrigation in two large-scale agricultural areas of western Kenya facilitated the transmission of malaria throughout the year by providing habitats for the two main vectors (111). At Ahero, *Anopheles arabiensis*was most abundant when the rice crop was immature, followed by *A. funestus* when the crop was mature. At Miwani, populations of *A. gambiae* peaked during the long rains whereas the proportion of *A. arabiensis*was greatest during the dry season.

Malaria incidence increased in the Usambara Mountains in Tanzania, following forest clearing to make way for tea plantations and later for agriculture (34, 214). Immigration of malaria-infected laborers from the surrounding lowlands spread the disease in the highlands. Interpretation of these historical changes in the incidence of malaria around Amani has been the subject of continuing debate, and the data have been extensively quoted as an example of the effects of higher local temperatures, resulting from land clearing, on the transmission of malaria. Reiter (270) favored an explanation based on the social changes associated with immigration of infected workers. Reports of the history of malaria in the area have recently been reinterpreted (34). The earlier increases in incidence were explained by intensive agriculture providing more breeding sites for the mosquito vectors that were previously uncommon in this highland habitat. A recent resurgence of malaria in the area was attributed to widespread development of resistance of the parasites to chloroquine. The same explanation was provided by Shanks et al. (294) for the dramatic increases in malaria cases since 1965 at tea plantations in the western highlands of Kenya.

The effect of land use change on malaria transmission was investigated at Kabale in the southwestern highlands of Uganda from December 1997 to July 1998 (185). Mosquito density, biting rates, sporozoite rates, and entomological inoculation rates were compared between eight villages near natural papyrus swamps and eight villages near swamps that had been drained and cultivated. Associated microclimatic conditions were also compared. There was a nonsignificant tendency for all malaria indices to be higher near the cultivated swamps. The numbers of *A. gambiae* sensu lato were associated with higher temperatures near the cultivated swamps, which resulted from the change in land cover.

The increasing incidence of malaria in Africa has been attributed to the growing reliance on corn as a staple food crop (356). In the absence of corn pollen, the silt-laden puddles of water, in which the *A. arabiensis*mosquitoes breed, are very low in nutrients. Corn pollen provides a rich and widespread source of nutrients for mosquito larvae. This could contribute significantly to increasing vector population growth during the flowering season of the crop, which corresponds to the increase in the numbers of mosquitoes in Ethiopia. It was suggested that the force of transmission of malaria in sub-Saharan Africa might be reduced if maize plantings were removed from the immediate vicinity of homes, as apparently was required in Rhodesia some decades ago.

Lyme disease in the northeastern United States and tick-borne encephalitis in Europe are increasing problems as human settlements encroach on forested areas (123). Emergence of Lyme disease, caused by the spirochete *Borrelia burgdorferi*, has been attributed partly to reforestation of outer suburban and agricultural areas in the northeastern United States (21). There were concurrent moves to conserve native fauna, particularly the white-tailed deer, *Odocoileus virginianus*, which are suitable hosts for adults of the tick vector, *Ixodes dammini* (21).

White-footed mice, *Peromyscus leucopus,* provide suitable hosts for burgeoning populations of the tick larvae (100), which are efficient vectors of *B. burgdorferi* (172). However, habitat fragmentation also reduces biodiversity and so leads to a preponderance of these mice. The disease "dilution effect," from the tick larvae feeding on less competent hosts, is lost, with the result that a large proportion of the larval population become infected (240). Infected nymphs then pose the major threat to humans. The ticks have recently been found to transmit other bacteria that may cause similar symptoms, such as *Babesia microti* and unnamed *Borrelia, Ehrlichia,* and *Bartonella* species (91, 337).

As just observed, natural biodiversity of hosts can reduce the transmission of vector-borne diseases, and there is also substantial information indicating the importance of natural enemies in controlling vectors of disease (57). This topic has been studied widely, and biological agents have been exploited for biological control (176, 285). Most of the effort has been directed against aquatic Diptera. The natural-enemy component was shown to be responsible for significant population reduction and to be indispensable to integrated control approaches. Outbreaks of malaria in Venezuela 1 year after ENSO-related droughts may have been caused by the death of the natural enemies of the mosquito vectors during the droughts (36).

This sampling of the large literature on the effects of land use on vector-borne diseases gives an indication of the diversity of changes and of the wide range of effects that they have on a number of vector-borne diseases. It also illustrates the difficulty facing researchers in trying to extract generalizations from such disparate observations and to create global databases in order to predict future global trends and impacts.

Endocrine Hormone Disruptors

It would be remise not to at least mention the risk that is posed to human health in general, and threats from vector-borne diseases in particular, by the global contamination of even the most remote habitats with EDCs. Of particular concern in the present context is the listing of synthetic pyrethroids as active EDCs (113) because they are being used so widely in agriculture and in impregnated bednets to prevent malaria. At present there have been no records of reduced immunity involving vector-borne diseases (22, 76), but observations of the impairment of the immune system by currently recorded groundwater concentrations of mixtures of agricultural chemicals across the United States is a warning sign (255). Health and safety issues receive less attention in developing countries, and such pollution with industrial and agricultural chemicals is widespread. The traditional reliance on natural immunity to diseases such as malaria and schistosomiasis in the developing world may be under threat. The paramount importance of herd immunity to malaria, in particular, in protecting populations from acute disease makes any such decline of immunity dangerous.

Trade and Travel

There are a number of different dimensions to the movement of people and materials around the world that affect the distribution and incidence of vector-borne diseases. People can either act as carriers of pathogens into new environments or accidentally translocate vectors in transport vehicles. People can also become victims of vector-borne diseases when they travel to new countries where they are exposed to diseases for the first time. Such people are usually naive to the disease, and thus morbidity and mortality rates are relatively high. Some examples of past incidents are listed as an indication of the potential for future spread of vector-borne diseases as trade and travel increase with globalization of trade and increasing wealth.

Movements of people, materials, or vehicles have been responsible for short- and long-distance transfer of several disease vectors (109) (Table 4). *Aedes albopictus,* a vector of dengue, was transported from Japan into the Americas and Europe (135, 161, 287), *Ochlerotatus japonicus,* a vector of arbovirus, was carried from Japan into the United States (253), and *Ochlerotatus camptorhynchus,* a known vector of Ross River virus, was moved from Australia into New Zealand (156). The worldwide migration of insecticide resistance genotypes of mosquitoes is an excellent example of the extent to which vectors have been spread around the world (263).

Table 4: Examples of vectors and vector-borne diseases that have been spread around the world naturally or aided by human activity

Invader species	Destination	Source	Pathway
Vectors			
Aedes albopictus	Americas, Pacific	Japan	Second-hand tires
Ochlerotatus japonicus	North America	Japan	Shipping likely
C. pipiens (pesticide resistant)	Global	Asia	Multiple
Ochlerotatus camptorhynchus	New Zealand	Australia	Unknown
Pathogens			
West Nile virus	United States	Middle East	Unknown
Dengue virus (122, 124)	Americas, Pacific and most tropical countries, Australia	Asian source increased greatly with population increase, urbanization, and decline of vector control and public health infrastructure.	Human air travel
Japanese encephalitis virus	Southeast Asia, Australia	Far East and Southeast Asia	Migratory birds and dispersal of vectors
Plasmodium spp. (including drug resistant strains) (44, 47, 203, 207, 214, 259)	Widespread	Southeast Asia and western Pacific	Humans
Rift valley fever virus	Egypt	Sudan	Trade in livestock (87)
Ross River virus	Fiji and Pacific Islands (114), New Zealand (121, 202)	Australia	Humans

The global spread of vector-borne diseases is being driven not only by human activities but also by natural forces. Vector-borne diseases have been spreading for centuries, and the shifts in their geographical distributions are an integral part of the epidemiology of the diseases. Human sleeping sickness, caused by *Trypanosoma brucei gambiense* and *T. brucei rhodesiense,* entered Kenya in about

1901 and the 1950s, respectively. The former disease was eradicated by attacking *Glossina fuscipes* with DDT, but the latter disease still persists in the Lambwe Valley in Western Kenya (338). Japanese encephalitis virus and related mosquito-borne viruses have caused outbreaks in Malaysia and India, but the source of the virus is unknown (86, 320, 333). The virus also spread into north Queensland, Australia, in 1995, apparently either by natural wind-borne transfer of infected mosquitoes, perhaps *Culex annulirostris,* from Papua New Guinea (273) or in migrating birds (132).

Increasing travel opportunities, population pressures in rural areas, and natural disasters and civil unrest are increasing the numbers of people traveling and being exposed to vector-borne diseases (65, 293). Each year, 20 million people visit malarious areas, and there are 10,000 cases of imported malaria in the European Community alone, most of which are caused by the more virulent *P. falciparum* (115). The types of human movements that influenced the incidence of malaria in different regions are summarized in Table 5. They show the variety and geographical range of such movements. Travelers have carried pathogens into other countries (258), including malaria into several countries (44, 47, 203, 207, 214, 259) and dengue viruses of all four serotypes into many countries but particularly the western Pacific, South Asia, and South America (124), and Ross River virus into Fiji and other islands in the Pacific (114, 284) and into New Zealand (121,202).

Table 5: Types of movements associated with malaria problems in different regions of the world[a]

Type of movement	Region		
	Americas	Africa	Asia
New settlements for agriculture or mining	Central America, Amazon		Southeast Asia and western Pacific
Populations displaced by war, civil unrest; refugee migrations		Central Africa	Middle East, Central Asia
Resettlements		Ethiopia, East African highlands, Madagascar	

Population movements in response to exceptional rain		Dry savanna, desert fringes, southern Africa	Indian subcontinent

[a]Data from reference 259.

Genetic variation in both disease competence in vectors and virulence of pathogens adds another dimension to the observed spread of vector-borne diseases around the world. In particular, dengue virus and its vector, *Aedes aegypti,* exhibit major variation in virulence and competence, respectively, in different geographical strains (301). Two molecular groups of the mosquito, with different geographical origins, varied in susceptibility to the dengue virus. A domestic form, *A. aedes aegypti,* from Southeast Asia, the South Pacific islands, and South America, had high dengue virus infection rates compared with a sylvan form, *A. aedes formosus,* from West Africa and some Indian Ocean islands. This is resulting in an expansion of the geographical range and changes in the epidemiology of the disease (93).

The potential impact of the spread of vectors and pathogens around the world greatly exceeds that of potential range expansions under climate change. While the latter are incremental increases, the former can change the risk level of a whole continent (304) by introducing a competent vector for the first time. Similarly, the above example of dengue fever illustrates how the introduction of a pathogen into new areas where competent vectors already exist has caused massive disease epidemics.

Interactive Effects of Global Change Drivers

While each of the drivers of global change will have effects on the transmission of vector-borne diseases, the combined effects have the potential in some cases to multiply the risks. The portion of the world that is becoming climatically suitable for tropical vectors with global warming is increasing. Possible higher tropical rainfall combined with higher CO_2 concentrations may offset greater evaporation at higher temperatures, so that both factors will tend to increase the amount of surface water available for breeding by mosquitoes in the expanded area that is made suitable for breeding by the increase in temperatures. Higher temperatures will not only increase evaporation but also accelerate development of pathogens and reduce the longevity of vectors. These counteracting climatic changes will have a significant effect on the demand for irrigation, which itself will be driven by the need to intensify agriculture to feed the burgeoning human population in the developing world. While increased urbanization will raise the density of human populations, global population growth will also increase the total numbers of people at risk. Globalization of trade and movement of goods and people are accelerating, and the intensity of contacts between humans is increasing in the emerging megacities with inadequate water supply, sanitation, and public health infrastructures.

These combined forces suggest a tendency toward increased risks of spread and transmission of vector-borne diseases. The greatest risks from global change appear to be associated with mosquito-borne diseases, particularly malaria and dengue fever. The greatest potential impacts probably lie in the interactions between invasions of vectors or pathogens from tropical and subtropical regions into an expanded receptive zone and increasing urbanization and poverty in developing countries. This latter effect is illustrated by the spread of dengue into the Americas since 1980 (121). On the other hand, as discussed below, social changes and adaptive management have the potential to counter many of these negative influences, provided that resources are redirected into public health.

Summary of Potential Impacts on Key Vector-Borne Diseases

Perceptions of the risks of the different global change drivers affecting vector-borne diseases vary according to the method used for assessment of those risks. Biologists often adopt a reductionist approach and try to isolate each variable and define its influence on the system concerned, even if the effect is small. Economists assess the relative importance of each of the variables and are not concerned with small or future effects (243). Biologists are concerned with small effects that may become larger in the future. They are also concerned with nonlinear and often disproportionate responses to small changes in (say) temperature around threshold developmental temperatures, for example (307). This dichotomy of views is also evident in the community investigating global change and risks of vector-borne diseases. Theoreticians and modelers have tended to emphasize the effects of climate change because it is part of a large global activity, it is tractable, and it can be supported by sound physiological data from the laboratory. Systems scientists and ecologists are anxious to take holistic approaches to global change issues, as evidenced by the The Amsterdam Declaration on Global Change (http://www.sciconf.igbp.kva.se/Amsterdam_Declaration.html), but are frustrated by a lack of tools to integrate physical and social systems, data on local effects, and social structures that facilitate that type of research. Public health practitioners, on the other hand, have been more concerned with weighing the risks from each source under current conditions. While all agree that there are many factors affecting the status of each disease, it is difficult to generalize across regions, as we saw in Fig. 8, and the more subtle effects of small changes in climate, for example, are difficult to isolate and quantify. However, that does not mean that climate change will not be a major concern in the future, since numerous modeling studies forecast significant changes in phenology and vector numbers with increasing temperatures in cooler environments. Practitioners also argue that the vectors are usually already present in areas adjacent to current zones of endemicity but the pathogens are not, suggesting that more emphasis needs to be placed on analysis of the pathogen part of the triangle in Fig.1. Practitioners may also be dismissive of modeling because they do not appreciate the significance of nonlinearity of responses such as that shown in the field observations in Fig. 11. We need to remember that the ecology of vector-borne diseases is highly complex and defies simplistic analyses (270).

It is evident that changes in human population growth, modification of the environment for agriculture, and trade and travel are important current influences on vector-borne diseases. The development of resistance in both vectors and pathogens and the deterioration of public health infrastructure and sanitation are major contributing factors to a deteriorating global problem of dengue and malaria in particular. In future, accumulating residues of EDCs may also emerge as a major issue in the maintenance of human immunity to vector-borne diseases. These latter factors represent failures of management rather than direct increases in risks from environmental changes. They portend problems with future efforts at adaptation. It is sobering to find that more people are dying from malaria today than 30 years ago (254). Future risks may arise from much more subtle effects from uncertain directions such as anthropogenic climate change and variability, and EDCs, but only time and more research will clarify those risks.

FRAMEWORK FOR DESIGNING ADAPTATION OPTIONS UNDER GLOBAL CHANGE

Adaptation is the process by which the potential impacts are reduced by applying a range of management options (Fig. .12). To ameliorate the impacts of vector-borne diseases on human health under global change, societies will need to implement adaptive strategies. General guidelines for the design of adaptation to climate change have been developed within the IPCC (244) and are equally applicable to other global change drivers. Responses to climate change can be either autonomous (automatic as part of daily business) or planned (when the adaptation strategies require deliberate policy decisions) (144). Adaptive responses have also been classified as being behavioral, engineering, or administrative/legislative (245). Here a specific approach is presented for adaptation to changes in vector-borne diseases under global change. Sustainable management of vector-borne diseases depends on a holistic approach, incorporating measures that address vectors, pathogens, hosts, and their interactions with each other and the environment. This means putting management at the center of the host-vector-disease triangle (Fig. 13).

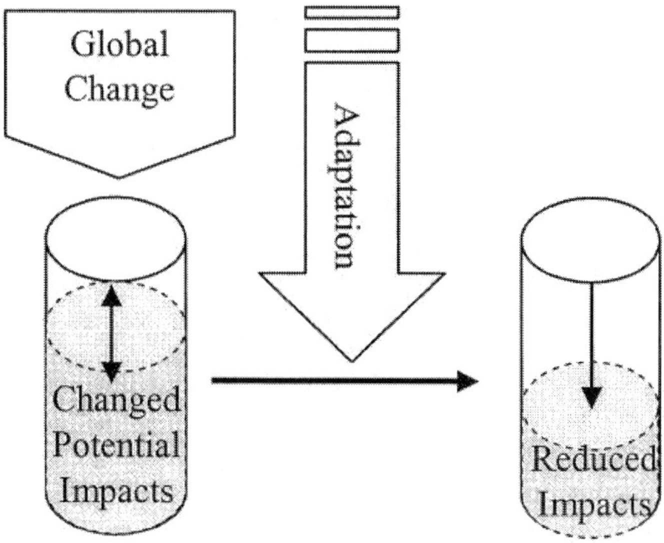

Figure 12: "Adaptation" reduces potential impacts by applying technology.

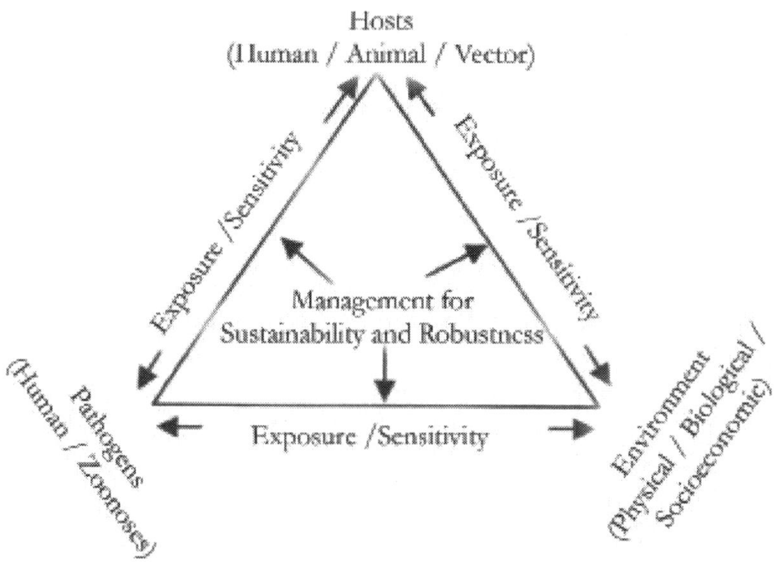

Figure 13: The host-pathogen-vector-environment triangle including management interventions to minimize the vulnerability of humans to vector-borne diseases under global change.

Without foresight in relation to new technologies, an assessment of the options that are currently available for future adaptation to global change will need first to identify the current and past practices that have been found to be effective in managing the risks from vector-borne diseases. We can then explore their potential for use as tools with which to facilitate the adaptation of human societies to the changing risks from vector-borne diseases under global change. Specific future technologies are impossible to anticipate due to the aggregate creativity of the many human minds available to generate new ideas.

Successful control of vector-borne diseases depends on three capacities: effective surveillance to provide feedback on progress (assuming that benchmarks have been established), community ownership of the new measures, and a viable public health infrastructure to deliver the services (181). Recognition of the problem requires some measures of change to be fed back to the community to raise awareness of the issue. These are provided by indicators, suitably chosen to maximize the visibility of the changes taking place (17). Suitable indicators also provide feedback to the community on the progress associated with adoption of the new approaches to manage the necessary changes. Without this feedback, recognition of the problem and adoption of new approaches are likely to be too slow to avoid some disasters. Thus, while monitoring or surveillance activities are considered by many scientists to lack challenge, they provide the key to motivation for change (17).

Implementation of adaptive measures is likely to be successful only if effective service delivery systems (123) are integrated with existing management practices (144). Early intersectorial involvement is essential in planning for rural development based on epidemiological guidelines (64).

Adaptation depends on adoption of innovative approaches or products to prevent or control vector-borne diseases in a changing environment. This, in turn, needs promotion of new approaches, critiques of current practices, and facilitation of change, which always has a cost that needs to be outweighed by the benefits provided by the new technology (17). The attributes of management tools that make them more likely to be available for adaptation to global change in the decades ahead are important in identifying future options. Each adaptation option needs to be evaluated against specific objectives by using criteria such as effectiveness and constraints (244) or sustainability and robustness (309). A multidisciplinary group of scientists involved with global change developed a set of criteria with which to evaluate adaptation options (309, 310). The criteria addressed the issue of sustainability and robustness of current management options. The robustness of each option needs to be determined in order to ensure that the technique or product is able to perform under variable conditions. Each approach is also evaluated in terms of its sensitivity to changes in the timing, intensity, and spatial movement of the target species under global change. Their sustainability is based on their likely susceptibility to a number of risks such as the development of resistance, economic viability, and changes in both societal values and environmental awareness. In summary, their performance needs to meet standards set by using the accounting concept of the "triple bottom line" (http://www.sustainability.com/philosophy/triple-bottom/tbl-intro.asp). Some of the key principles of sustainability are to think long-term, to understand the system, to recognize natural limits to human population growth, to protect nature and the services that it provides such as natural enemies of disease vectors, to transform the way we do business by guiding development without growth in the use of resources, to be fair to each other, to nature, and to future generations and, in so doing, reduce risks to all, and, finally, to embrace creativity in order to develop novel ways of adapting to change (17).

Social values change over time and vary in different communities and so may determine the acceptability of a given adaptation option. For example, attitudes to safety and effects on the environment have changed greatly over the past few decades. The key to successful adaptation is considered to be the provision of information to managers in order to allow them to fine-tune control practices to track environmental changes. This would be based on a menu of available procedures and products, together with analytical tools to assess their potential impacts and likely benefits. Such a hypothetical decision support system (DSS) (Fig. 14) could then be coupled directly to the Internet to ensure efficient delivery of relevant and timely information to stakeholders. The DSS consists of computer simulation models of each of the target and non-target components of the environment that are affected in either a beneficial or adverse way by a proposed product or practice. Sustainable strategies must minimize adverse effects of chemical residues on human health and the environment. Thus, an environmental lifecycle assessment, in which the effects of a product or practice are defined from cradle to grave, forms one pillar of any information system that is used to guide the sustainable management of vector-borne diseases. Such an analysis of the product would cover the period from invention to disposal, including effects on all target and nontarget species (157). As discussed above, particular concern currently exists about the many industrial and agricultural EDCs. Sustainable management of both vectors and pathogens also demands additional measures to delay the selection of resistance genes that shorten the useful life of so many pesticides and drugs.

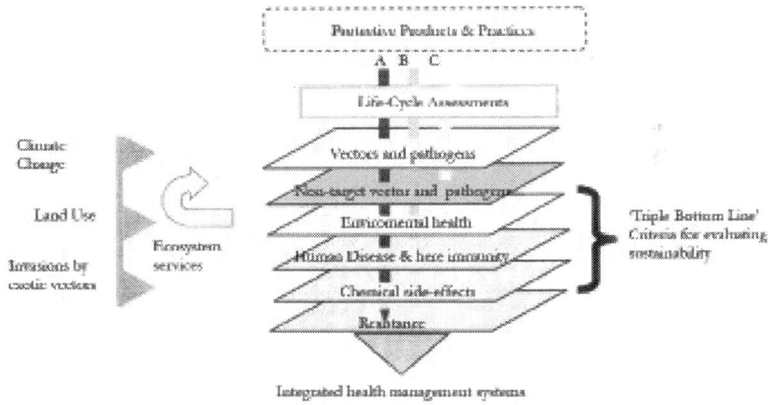

Figure 14: Decision support system to guide the design or sustainable and robust management strategies for adaptation to changes in the status of vector-borne diseases with global change.

Historical patterns of vector ecology and disease transmission have traditionally been used as a basis for the design of management strategies in public health and in agriculture. That has been possible only because environmental conditions, such as the climate, were relatively constant from year to year. With climate change, this no longer applies because there is a trend of change over time. In future, adaptation is going to have to rely on interpretative and predictive tools that can track and anticipate the future conditions and allow the user to tune the adaptation strategy accordingly. These tools will be mechanistic computer simulation models that can both predict and explain the biological responses of vectors, pathogens, and humans to the specific environmental change (305, 315).

Designers of management strategies for vector-borne diseases must also consider the broader implications for communities of any intervention in terms of herd immunity (296). In the case of malaria, there is the potential to alter clinical patterns in areas of endemic infection by creating populations that are non-immune to a disease when decreased transmission reduces immunity of both the existing population and future children (227). In the event that there is a lapse in the effectiveness of the disease control program, these non-immune hosts are likely to be at high risk of severe infections associated with resurgent disease transmission in areas where infection is normally endemic (Fig 9). This raises some very difficult ethical questions. Who should receive treatment? What is the balance of benefits and risk from immunity and debilitating effects of chronic infection? Who should be responsible for any ensuing increases in the risks of more severe clinical disease in the community? What constitutes a safe approach when some members of a community may benefit at the expense of others?

The risk of severe clinical symptoms with successive infections with viruses like dengue fever virus are important. Prior infection with one serotype predisposes the patient to the dangerous dengue hemorrhagic fever when subsequently infected with another virulent serotype (153). This creates the opposite effect to immunity and emphasizes the need to take a preventative approach. The need to consider whole systems when planning interventions is illustrated further by the increased production of adults of *Aedes aegypti* after removal of a proportion of larvae from rearing containers with limited food supplies (2). Crowding of larvae reduced the overall production of these mosquitoes.

It is necessary to identify causes of any changes in effectiveness of a given strategy over time because they could be incorrectly attributed to one of several possible causes such as selection of resistance genes, operator error, changes in observational procedures, or changing seasonal phenology due to climate variability or long-term climate change (121, 270, 307). The proposed DSS would have to include computer models of the biological, physical, and sociological processes involved in determining the transmission rates of pathogens for each disease. There have not yet been many studies to design options for adaptation to changes in the risks from vector-borne diseases (224, 307). Some models have been designed to guide the interpretation and on-site management of vector-borne diseases affecting humans (81, 97, 98).

The skill of climatic forecasting is increasing and promising some opportunities to provide advance warning of some high-risk situations associated with the ENSO cycle, for example (127, 201, 237, 238). However, the ENSO is thought to be a chaotic system that is difficult to predict, and its effects on rainfall can be very variable over short distances (306). In addition, as discussed above, the correlation between the ENSO and climatic variables has varied greatly over time (Fig.4) (5, 51), making it less reliable than some recent experiences would suggest. Therefore, the ENSO is likely to provide information of limited reliability to add to that available from existing tools, such as systematic monitoring and modeling based on direct relationships between biological and climatic variables, that are available to entomologists at present (306). The most useful ENSO-type information would be that which is relevant to forward planning in order to ensure adequate supplies of drugs or pesticides to meet any increase in vector populations (306).

Additional or alternative means of forewarning of impending increases in disease transmission are provided by surveillance systems as an integral part of a public health infrastructure (286). For example, monitoring of *Anopheles gambiae* mosquitoes in houses was suggested as a means of warning of impending malaria epidemic conditions (185). Such monitoring will automatically take into account any changes in the phenology of the vector and so will be a highly efficient component of an adaptation strategy for climate change. The use of geographical information systems to enhance the spatial and temporal resolution of surveillance data provides further opportunities for efficiencies (35, 97). Of course, explanations for changing patterns will still be needed to interpret the causes of these changes and avoid inappropriate responses (307).

Vector-borne diseases will continue to be a problem because of the adaptability of pathogens and vectors to drugs and pesticides, respectively, and the difficulties of managing vector control programs through decentralized health systems when external activities can increase vector numbers and hence the rate of disease transmission (228). It is essential to understand the factors that increase the transmission of disease in order to prevent outbreaks of diseases, as well as to provide a basis for their effective control (117). However, a more pessimistic view is that the current world circumstances juxtapose people, parasites, plants, animals, and chemicals in a way that precludes timely adaptation (347). The combination of increasing human movements and major changes in the physical environment is responsible for the unexpected spread of diseases via many different pathways. Vector-borne diseases are emerging or resurging as a result of changes in a number of different fields, but particularly as a result of the failure of preventive strategies and their replacement by emergency responses to disease outbreaks (123). Diseases have resurged as a consequence of insecticide and drug resistance, demographic and societal changes, and genetic changes in pathogens. Such forces of change are integral components of the pattern of global change taking place around the world.

The likely sustainability of the currently available approaches can be evaluated using a range of scenarios for the future. Formal means of generating and evaluating future scenarios are also needed (290). Sensitivity analysis is a more practical planning and design approach for the design of adaptation strategies than is the use of climate change scenarios because solutions require the design of strategies that are insensitive to climatic perturbations rather than being optimal for a particular amount of change that is specified in a given scenario (304).

A comprehensive review of experiences with the available methods of control of vector-borne disease is beyond the scope of this paper, but some indication of the current status of the field is necessary to provide a platform on which to develop a sound approach to adaptation to environmental change.

ADAPTATION OPTIONS

Legislative

Many deliberate policy changes could be implemented to enable us to adapt to the impacts of vector-borne diseases under global change. They involve legislation or administrative actions to respond to changes in distributions of vectors, diseases, and human hosts. The measures include changes of monitoring, case detection, diagnosis and reporting, public information and education, knowledge capture and management using information technologies such as remote sensing and mapping with geographical information systems (138, 239), climate forecasting, computer modeling, quarantine surveillance, early-warning systems, and mass vaccination programs. Most of these activities are integral components of any effective preventative health system and so ought to be implemented to meet current needs. While eradication is an idealistic goal, it is usually either unattainable or unsustainable, judging from past efforts with malaria in particular (349).

The failure of some vector or disease eradication programs has been attributed to a lack of funds (242). Efforts to eradicate malaria with insecticides failed in many regions due to the withdrawal of DDT, the development of resistance to the pesticides, or the reintroduction of the mosquitoes from other areas (349). Partial success was achieved with eradication of the main vector of dengue fever virus, *Aedes aegypti,* with successes in southern, temperate zones of Australia but failure in the Americas after initial success in Central America and Brazil (121).

There have, however, been some impressive results from concerted and coordinated efforts to minimize the transmission of vector-borne diseases over large areas. These have relied on suppression of the vector populations or saturation treatment of the pathogens. Eradication of malaria was successful in most of Europe by using DDT, removing breeding sites by draining swamps, and encouraging the keeping of cattle in proximity to homesteads in order to provide an alternative host for the mosquitoes of the malaria pathogens (191, 269, 358). However, in Ethiopia there was an increased incidence of malaria in children sharing the same house with cattle, therefore, there needs to be some distance between the livestock and human housing (108). In South America, eradication of the *Anopheles gambiae* mosquito from northeast Brazil in the 1930s was a significant watershed in the history of malaria control (241). More recently the global Roll Back Malaria campaign, being conducted by agencies of the United Nations during the decade from 2001 to 2010, has launched a concerted effort to halve the incidence of malaria around the world by using a combination of vector control and early treatment of infections in vulnerable populations (271).

Pesticide-based vector control programmes greatly reduced the incidence of onchocerciasis (or river blindness) in West Africa and Chagas› disease in South America (228) by reducing populations of the*Simulium* and *Triatoma* vectors, respectively. In West Africa, eradication of onchocerciasis by aerial spraying of the breeding sites of *Simulium* in fast-flowing rivers was successful in several countries. Further attempts, involving mass treatments of several million people with ivermectin, were initially hindered by a lack of coordination until the advent of the African Programme for Onchocerciasis Control in 1995 (92). Widespread treatment of the human population with ivermectin also reversed anterior-chamber lesions, but there were some adverse reactions to ivermectin treatment when people were heavily coinfected with *Loa loa*(102). There is optimism that similar approaches can be applied to eradicate lymphatic filariasis in India by using diethylcarbamazine and ivermectin (10).

Long-term success in eradication of the reduvid bug, *Triatoma infestans,* has been achieved in the State of Sao Paulo, Brazil (275). Control of Chagas› disease, caused by *Trypanosoma cruzi,* was achieved by suppressing the vectors with insecticides and providing improved housing. In contrast, eradication of domestic *T. infestans* failed in an area of Santiago del Estero in Argentina (289). It is hoped that Chagas› disease can be controlled by using a combination of insecticides and control of blood banks in South America (10).

In Africa, eradication of the tsetse fly (*Glossina* spp.) vectors of human and animal trypanosomiasis has met with mixed success because the fly tends to reinvade areas that have been cleared unless development follows and permanent vegetation-free buffer zones are maintained (133, 338). Stronger links between tsetse control policy and rural development, with intersectorial participation, are essential (64). This means that eradication of vectors such as the tsetse fly must be a slow and cautious process (24). Failures to eradicate*Glossina pallidipes* from parts of Africa, including the Lambwe Valley in Kenya, has led to persistent outbreaks of human trypanosomiasis. In Uganda, a resurgence of human sleeping sickness was associated with encroachment of the dense, exotic shrub *Lantana camara*. The epidemic was stopped by the use of insecticide-impregnated tsetse traps. Social resistance to the clearing of bush in valleys and later civil war has led to a catastrophic increase in the incidence of epidemics of sleeping sickness caused by *Trypanosoma rhodesiense* in Zaire and

Central Africa, as public health programmes have failed (228, 260). Environmental concerns related to land degradation and loss of wildlife following successful eradication of the tsetse fly in regions of Africa reduce the attractiveness of eradication of the fly from unfarmed land (133). Where human trypanosomiasis is concerned, the case is much more compelling. Recent attempts have been made to promote area-wide eradication of tsetse flies in Africa following success on a small island in Zanzibar (158). These initiatives have been questioned on historical, ecological, logistical, and financial grounds (281).

Engineering and Behavioral

The usual engineering or behavioral response by affected individuals to vector-borne disease is to change their behavior at crucial times or to use one or more of a wide range of options to control either the vector or the pathogen or both. Some personal behavioral responses include avoidance of exposure to vectors by staying indoors at dawn and dusk and wearing protective clothing. Routine responses by communities, as part of everyday operations in response to a perceived increase in climatic variability, could include tuning tactics in a surveillance program to detect earlier infections that may initiate outbreaks. Engineering options for vector control include habitat modification, insect screens, bednets, biological control, pesticides, repellents, and more effective integration of these approaches. Targeting of pathogens with drugs or vaccines also provides options to reduce transmission and to reduce symptoms. To identify the tools that have the greatest potential for use to address global change, it is necessary to evaluate their future sustainability and robustness under a wide range of conditions (309). Some of the options that are currently available are rated for these attributes in Table 6. Preventative measures based on environmental management rate highly in terms of their robustness, but their potential sustainability is limited by their demands on management. To date, no approach has been successful without social stability and maintenance of an effective public health system.

TABLE 6: Sustainability (socially, economically and environmentally) and robustness under global change (resilience to changed environment, timing, spatial movements, habitat change) of some available methods of vector and disease prevention and control[a]

Product or practice	Disadvantages	Advantages	Sustainability	Robustness
Engineering				
Biological vector control with parasites, predators, pathogens	High exploration and testing costs, risk of nontarget impacts, effectiveness varies from nil to total suppression, usually needs regular "inundative" releases	'Free' vector suppression once established, minimal side effects if highly specific, minimal maintenance	++++	+++
Drugs	Adverse side effects, drug resistance, high recurrent costs	Prophylactic or therapeutic; rapid response	++	++++
Pesticides	Pesticide resistance, nontarget impacts, high recurrent costs	Rapid response, high effectiveness	++	++
Vaccines	Ineffective against key protozoa and viruses, short protection from molecular vaccines, time lag in responses	Simple implementation, safe technology, lifetime protection in some cases	++++	++++
Management of environment or housing	Reduction of vector breeding or exposure to vectors, competing interests, Manipulation is temporary, high cost and demands on management	Modification has long-term effectiveness, low maintenance costs	+++	++++
Integration of vector and disease management	Complex to implement, adoption is low	Many of the above	+++	+++
Administrative				
Quarantine, surveillance, education	Large infrastructure needed, high maintenance costs, low reliability	Benefits large areas and populations	++	++
Behavioral				
Avoidance of exposure use of repellents	Adoption is low, complex to manage, variable effectiveness	Long-term effect, moderately high efficacy	+++	+++

[a]Ratings scaled from a base of 0 to a maximum of ++++.

Management of Vector-Borne Diseases by Vector Control

A range of chemical, biological, trapping, and environmental management techniques are available for the control of disease vectors (64, 329, 334). The incidence of Japanese encephalitis in East Asia has been greatly reduced by a combination of mass vaccination of children, improved living conditions, reduced use of water with new rice cultivars, and rehousing and relocation of piggeries to prevent mosquito feeding and reduce contact with human populations (141, 152, 355). Improvement of housing, water supplies, and sanitation and the return of livestock to provide alternative hosts for anopheline mosquitoes are also valuable. Entomopathogens have proved to be effective against mosquito larvae when used as biopesticides (171), but they have not shown adequate recycling capacity or ability to provide toxin-bearing spores on the water surface, and so they have limited capability as biocontrol agents (79). The use of biological pesticides (biopesticides) in the form of*Bacillus thuringiensis* and *B. sphaericus* reduced the incidence of malaria in Managua, Nicaragua, by 90% from 1996 to 2000 (15) and by similar amounts in Hubei Province in China (357) and Maroua in Cameroon (20). Several of the above authors emphasized the need for a good knowledge of the location and dynamics of breeding sites, the biology of the mosquitoes, and improved formulations of *Bacillus* spp.

Biological control has the potential in some cases to provide long-term, low-cost control of vector populations that are sustainable under a range of circumstances. Natural solutions for vector-borne diseases are preferable to the use of artificial chemicals, which are prone to failure due to the development of resistance, are costly and demanding on management, and often have deleterious side effects on humans and on the environment (196, 330). Biological control of mosquito populations by using natural enemies is a well-established practice and is based mostly on predatory fish (254, 334). Success has been achieved against *Aedes aegypti,* a vector of dengue fever, in specific situations like Australian wells and gold mines by using inundative releases of the copepod *Mesocyclops aspericornis* (285). However, biological control does have risks to the local fauna if it is not carefully evaluated before being implemented. The mosquito fish, *Gambusia affinis,* selectively removed the early instars of predacious insects (including *Notonecta unifasciata, Buenoa* sp., *Belostoma flumineum,* Odonata, dytiscids, and *Tropisternus lateralis*) in rice fields in California (28). This increased mosquito survival, but simultaneous removal of zooplankton by *Gambusia*reduced mosquito survival. In addition, introduced *Gambusia* strains have caused irreversible impacts, reducing the native fish fauna (16, 232). Thus, there is scope for considerable improvement in the practice of biological control of disease vectors and in the range of situations in which it can be applied.

Preventative measures are preferable and include the design of water reservoirs to avoid areas of shallow water that are suitable for breeding of mosquitoes (150). Sound design and maintenance of dam spillways and irrigation canals can reduce the incidence of vector-borne diseases (229). Alternating wet-dry irrigation of rice is credited with reducing the incidence of both malaria and Japanese encephalitis in areas where the vector mosquitoes breed in rice fields (329).

Since no treatment of or vaccination for dengue is available, mosquito control is the only way to reduce the incidence of dengue around the world (276). Environmental management to remove breeding sites is very efficient and is a core strategy when dealing with container-breeding mosquitoes like *A. aegypti.* Other mechanical methods can also be very effective in controlling mosquito breeding in specific situations (216). A reduction of 99.7% was achieved in the number of infective bites by *Culex quinquefasciatus* carrying larvae of *Wuchereria bancrofti,* by covering the surface of wet pit latrines in the town of Makunduchi, Zanzibar, with expanded polystyrene beads and mass treatment of the population with diethylcarbamazine to reduce the incidence of microfilariae.

There are good historical examples of successful use of environmental management to control malaria for prolonged periods in selected areas (327). A package of control measures was used, consisting of vegetation clearance, modification of river boundaries, drainage of swamps, application of oil to open water bodies, and house screening. This was combined with the use of quinine and mosquito nets on part of the population to reduce malaria incidence in Zambian copper mines by 70 to 95% for a period of 20 years. The use of insecticide-impregnated bednets for control of malaria is recognized as a potential means of reducing morbidity and mortality in children (228, 254) and is a cornerstone of the global Roll Back Malaria campaign. The bednets have produced dramatic reductions in the number of cases of malaria in regions such as southern China (354) and in child mortality in trials in sub-Saharan Africa (160), and their use is being extended widely. However, there is evidence that the nets are much less effective during general use by communities compared with during trials. Suboptimal community use of bednets and resistance to insecticides may reduce the sustainability of bednets, although they have been shown to continue to reduce malaria even when resistance has developed in populations of *A. gambiae* senau stricto (78). An emerging concern referred to above is that some synthetic pyrethroids, such as permethrin and cypermethrin, may act as EDCs (164) and threaten the sustainability of this approach. Recommended future directions in vector control include environmentally safe insecticides, new approaches to vector control, and training programs for health care workers (123).

Management of Vector-Borne Diseases by Targeting the Pathogens

The second approach to the control of vector-borne diseases is to prevent or treat infections of the pathogens by using drugs or vaccines.

(i) Chemotherapy

Together with vector control, chemotherapy has provided the foundation for the control of vector-borne diseases for decades. Chemotherapy is a vast topic, and it is appropriate here only to note that there have been some major contributions from the use of drugs, as described above, as part of combined drug and vector control programmes but that there are limits to the sustainability of such drugs. The two main constraints are that most people in the developing world cannot afford the cost of modern drugs and that pathogens have a propensity to develop resistance to most drugs that have been used on a wide scale. Malaria, in particular, has become resistant to every drug that is currently available in Asia (254). Therefore, there are questions about the future role of chemotherapy in the control of vector-borne diseases. In the case of malaria, concerns about the maintenance of the efficacy of old and new antimarlarial drugs dominate current thinking (254).

(ii) Vaccines

Vaccines are the preventative panacea that medical practitioners dream about. There has been apparent success with a Japanese encephalitis vaccine in east Asia (329), as described above in relation to vector control. Mass vaccination of children provided the basis for the integrated program.

Unfortunately, to date vaccines have not shown promise against protozoan pathogens like *Plasmodium* or*Trypanosoma,* metazoan parasites like *Schistosoma,* or viruses like dengue fever virus, for a variety of reasons. Protozoa have proved particularly difficult to control with vaccines because of their capacity to vary their antigens and so avoid recognition by the immune system of the host. Despite this, there was optimism about the prospects for an effective vaccine against malaria, mixed with recognition of the significant constraints that remain due to the antigenic polymorphism exhibited by wild parasite strains and the genetic restriction of immune responses (300). Priorities for research include the need to understand the mechanism of immunity to malaria, the search for antimalarial vaccines, and the potential completion and delivery of benefits from the malaria genome project (254). While naturally acquired immunity can protect against acute malaria infections, practical vaccines are many years away and so is the necessary infrastructure to deliver the vaccines in Africa (272). Loss of natural immunity following radical drug cures highlights the conundrum faced by health care workers in that prevention or drug-based cures of natural infections can leave populations without the natural immunity that currently protects them from acute infection (299).

No vaccine is available for leishmaniasis, and a major vaccine development program, aimed initially at cutaneous leishmaniasis and employing a range of molecular tools, is under way (131). International efforts to create a schistosomiasis vaccine have offered little hope of early success (31). The feasibility of producing an effective vaccine against a parasite that is so well adapted to its host that it can survive in host tissue for decades has been challenged, and the need for a vaccine has been questioned when chemotherapy is very effective and the primary needs are to provide safe water, sanitation, education, and access to good public health facilities (120). Vaccination against the bacterium *Borrelia burgdorferi*, a causative agent of Lyme disease, is controversial, with claims of adverse reactions and reactivation of past infections (336). Dengue virus has several different serotypes that do not respond to the same vaccine. Indeed, prior infection with one strain predisposes the patient to dengue hemorrhagic fever and a vaccine developed against any single strain has the risk of enhancing virus replication (153). The burgeoning molecular biology industry may yet create a raft of novel tools and techniques to protect against such parasites (254), but the short protective periods of tested recombinant vaccines is an obstacle to their effectiveness in creating stable epidemiological situations.

As the examples above have shown, success depends on integration of different approaches aimed at both the pathogen and the vector. This lesson needs to be learned by every new generation of researchers and policy makers to avoid the temptation to seek simple solutions based on magic bullets.

Adaptation of Control Measures for Vector-Borne Diseases in Response to Global Change

Responses to changes in the timing and intensity of disease transmission under global change need to be designed a priori to enable them to be proactive rather than reactive, as illustrated by the preventative vaccination against rabies in North America (274, 283). This calls for a thorough understanding of the biogeography and epidemiology of each disease in the local area at risk. High-risk areas and communities need to be identified in order to focus efforts toward adaptation of the existing disease management programs. Some indication of the needs for modification of current management tools, in order to accommodate global change, are summarized in Table 7. All techniques and approaches need to be tuned to make them more flexible and adaptable to a changing environment, as shown by the low success rate with their current application around the world. This demands a more knowledge-based, rather than product-based, approach.

Table 7: Indicative changes needed to some vector and pathogen control methods in order to address changed risks from environmental change and international trade and travel

Global change	Changes in vector and pathogen control methods[a]							
	Pesticides	Biological control	Environmental management	Traps/ Bednets	Quarantine	Public health infrastructure	Drugs	Vaccines
Environmental change	++ (different seasonal vector populations, resistance)	++ (variation in effectiveness around edges of distribution)	+ (integrated management of breeding sites)	+ (change pesticides if involved)	+ (low efficiency)	++ (preventative measures, delivery systems)	++ (resistance)	++ (efficacy, antigenic variation)
Trade and transport	+ (exotic-vector ecology and resistance)	++ (import new agents for exotic species)	+ (different exotic-vector ecology)	+ (exotic species with new behaviour)	++ (capacity to monitor the volume of migration and traded goods)	++ (incursion prevention and response capability)	++ (new resistance profile)	++ (strain variation)

[a]0, business as usual; +, minor tuning; ++, significant alteration. Issues related to changing needs are in parentheses.

Adaptation to climate change requires a combination of monitoring, interpretation of field observations based on an understanding of the system involved, and adjustment of existing management actions to accommodate the changes in geographical distribution, seasonal numbers, and timing of vectors (307). As discussed above, it is critical that the cause of changed transmission rates is determined to avoid inappropriate responses based on assumptions about the cause of failure (307). Provision of protection for the most sensitive human populations, without acquired immunity to the pathogen concerned, will be a priority. These people will be found in the vicinity of the altitudinal and horizontal boundaries of the geographical distribution of the species when the variation in climate leads to exceptional divergence from average conditions. They are likely to be found among the most underprivileged communities.

In the case of local environmental changes brought about by local disturbances such as introduction of dams and irrigation or deforestation, there are less likely to be qualitatively different risks, and so implementation of current management practices will be appropriate.

Adaptation to Invasions by Exotic Vectors and Pathogens

A holistic approach will address the risks from exotic invasions by managing the sources, pathways, and destinations of exotic vectors and vector-borne diseases (Fig.15). As in the case of transported plant and animal material, there are potential opportunities to apply rigorous risk management procedures to minimize the risk of entry of exotic species into new environments. Risks at each step can be managed by taking appropriate steps to reduce the chances of a vector passing through barriers to new locations. This requires steps to be taken to reduce the chances of an infection at the source from entering international transport, to reduce its chances of survival in transit, and then to prevent its entry into and establishment at the destination. Failing these measures, there are sometimes options to contain or eradicate the infection if it is detected very quickly. Otherwise, it is usually only possible to alleviate the effects if the vector or pathogen becomes established widely before blocking measures can be put in place. Such measures must be compatible with the current laws of the World Trade Organization. This means that they must be based on justifiable cost-benefit analyses, with the application of the concept of "acceptable" rather than "minimal" risk to the decision about whether to allow the entry of a product (146).

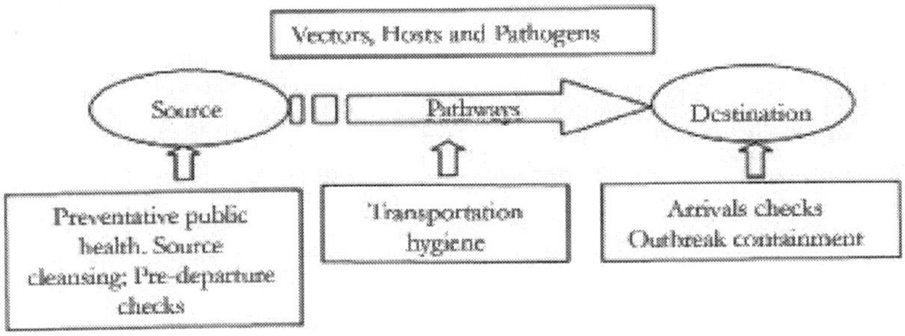

Figure 15: The plant and animal protection concept of sources, pathways, and destinations with adaptation measures to manage the changes arising from global change drivers.

There are no technical reasons why such criteria cannot be applied to vectors of human vector-borne diseases. On the other hand, there are large social deterrents to applying them to humans themselves to avoid transporting the pathogens as they travel. This distinguishes human vector-borne diseases from diseases of plants and other animals and means that the risks of expansion of the geographical distributions of human vector-borne diseases exceed those of the diseases of plants and animals. Therefore, it is more difficult to manage the risks when humans are the host of a vector-borne disease. If the health of humans, agricultural systems, and natural ecosystems are going to be maintained, it will be incumbent on the World Trade Organization to reconsider the weighting given to economic, public health, and environmental considerations to minimize the risks whenever possible.

Management of vector-borne diseases at the source of infection requires measures to be taken to remove the pathogen and/or vector from the environment, as discussed above. This has been achieved successfully in many countries in relation to malaria and human yellow fever, but there has been less success with dengue virus (123). Measures included vaccination of humans for yellow fever and control of pathogens with drugs, combined with vector management, for malaria or vector management alone for dengue fever.

Identification and management of pathways of infection have been less successful, judging by the continuing arrival of exotic vectors into new countries. This is illustrated by the numerous reports cited above of historical spread of vector-borne diseases around the world. Regulatory responses have included the treatment of waste tires with chemicals or biological control agents and increased surveillance at ports of entry.

Surveillance has been increased to reduce the risk of establishment of exotic species, but results with vectors of human diseases and the disease organisms themselves continue to show how difficult it is to achieve total exclusion (8, 121, 135). Quarantine services in recipient countries (destinations) focus their effort on inspections on arrival and on surveillance and responses to infections when the barrier fails. The examples cited in relation to the management of pathways illustrate the failure of the management of both sources and destinations to prevent the dispersal of exotic diseases and their vectors. The hope must be that dispersal rates are reduced enough to delay the spread of these diseases by useful amounts.

Threats to Sustainability of Adaptation Options

Resistance

Drugs and pesticides are used widely to reduce the transmission of diseases, and there has been a long history of the development of resistant strains. Changes in the genetic susceptibility of vector-borne diseases and of their vectors have the potential for profound effects on the ability of public health systems to adapt to the impacts of some diseases under global change.

Drug resistance has been an ongoing problem for decades and has formed the subject of many reviews (10,33, 59, 73, 162, 198, 226, 236, 322, 339-343, 345). Resistance genes continue to be selected in malaria organisms (34, 203), causing resurgences in disease incidence. The international spread of multiple drug-resistant malaria organisms in Southeast Asia has been attributed largely to movements of civilians during civil disturbances (293).

Similarly, insecticide resistance in mosquitoes continues to threaten efforts to prevent transmission (19, 46,72, 171, 349). Insecticide-impregnated bednets, traps, and lethal targets are effective, but the early detection of resistance to pyrethroids in bednets emphasizes the low sustainability of any approaches that depend solely on pesticides (64). Resistance in mosquitoes appears to have arisen from both agricultural (4, 74, 242) and urban (4, 331) exposure. Resistance has been reported to permethrin and deltramethrin in *Anophales gambiae* in West Africa (54). As in the case of drug resistance, such pesticide resistance genes are being dispersed widely around the world (177, 263).

Unexpected side effects can arise from the selection of resistance genes. It has been reported (218) that insecticide resistance inhibited the vectorial capacity of mosquitoes that transmit *Wuchereria bancrofti*. Prasittisuk and Curtis (257), on the other hand, found in an experimental system that selection for resistance to DDT in *A. gambiae* had no effect on the susceptibility of the mosquito to a *Plasmodium* sp. in rodents.

Strategies for managing the selection of pesticide resistance in disease vectors have been derived mainly from those designed by entomologists working on agricultural or veterinary problems. Sutherst and Comins (308) first coined the terms "saturation" and "moderation" to describe two opposite strategies. The former attempts to minimize the size of the vector or pathogen population and hence the probability of generating resistance genes. The latter attempts to minimize the selection pressure applied by any single produce or practice by adopting an integrated approach, referred to as integrated pest management. These approaches built on the pioneering work of Georghiou and Taylor in the 1970s, which was summarized by Georghiou (107), who also expanded the saturation/moderation options to include management by multiple attack. This applies to the use of chemical rotations or mixtures, which can be applied to give either moderation or saturation depending on the concentration and intensity of use.

The balance of opinion is that resistance needs to be managed by avoiding a magic-bullet (saturation) approach that intensifies selection and adopting multipronged measures (moderation) that reduce the need for the use of any one chemical (32, 198, 226, 252, 288, 319, 341).

Human Safety and Non target Effects of Vector Control

The widespread use of pesticides in vector control has inevitably had its effects on both the local human population and local fauna. The early effects of DDT on bird life are well known, but the replacement chemicals were also not without their risks (204). For example, efforts to control dengue fever by controlling the vector, *Aedes aegypti*, with organophosphorus insecticide led to three poisonings and reduced cholinesterase levels in 53 out of 2,391 people sampled from the local population in southern Brazil (291).

Pesticides applied on soil at recommended levels rarely had a detrimental effect on microbial populations in temperate wetland rice fields. They did affect invertebrate populations, inducing the blooming of individual species of floodwater zooplankton and reducing populations of aquatic oligochaetes in soil. The observations raise concerns about the long-term effects of pesticides on microorganisms, invertebrates that are important to soil fertility, natural enemies of rice pests and mosquitoes, and biodegradation of pesticides (277).

The nontarget effects of biological control agents for mosquitoes have been noted above. Chemical control of*Simulium, Glossina,* and *Anopheles,* the vectors of onchocerciasis, trypanosomiasis, and malaria, respectively, and of the snail intermediate hosts (*Bulinus* and *Biomphalaria*) of *Schistosoma* can have effects on the fauna of aquatic environments. For example, chemicals used in the control of *Simulium* had several environmental impacts on nontarget invertebrates and fish when used in the Onchocerciasis Control Programme of West Africa (178). The nontarget effects of area-wide spraying with chemical pesticides for the control of tsetse flies in Africa have been reduced in recent times, with more selective use of insecticide-treated cloth targets and selective spraying of resting sites with low-drift sprays (85).

Community Health and Public Health Infrastructure

The capability of a society to adapt to global change depends not only on the technical options that are available but also on the human resources that the society can bring to bear to address the issue. Prevention of outbreaks of many vector-borne diseases requires an operational public health system. These resources depend on the economic and public health of the society, so that developing countries have far fewer options available to them than do developed countries. On top of this handicap, several developing countries, particularly in Africa and Asia, are experiencing an erosion of their economic capacity due to the epidemic of AIDS (26), with serious implications for their capacity to manage both human health and agriculture as a result of the loss of able-bodied workers (130, 325). Human trypanosomiasis, caused by *T. brucei gambiense* or *T. brucei rhodesiense,* is increasing in East Africa, where containment measures for tsetse fly vectors (*Glossina fuscipes*) have declined in effectiveness with political unrest and demands placed on the health budgets by AIDS (1). Such a human immunodeficiency virus-induced shortage of labor and capital poses risks for efforts to maintain public health under global change and particularly the containment of trypanosomiasis, for which vegetation must be cleared regularly to remove shelter for tsetse flies (303, 307).

Social disturbances such as wars and civil unrest cause public health services to fail, with resultant outbreaks and spread of infectious and vector-borne diseases, particularly malaria (45, 58, 293, 324). During the war in Nicaragua from 1983 to 1987, population movements and resettlement into rural areas, where preventive care was not available, caused epidemics of malaria and other diseases. The incidence of malaria increased in the war zone in Nicaragua, while there was a large decrease in incidence in the non-war zone (103, 104).

By now it should be evident that risk assessments without consideration of adaptation options give an incomplete picture of the risks from global change. Adaptation is an ongoing process in human societies, and continuing effort needs to be focused on updating management practices to respond to the changing environment. The next section discusses how a measure of risk from impacts can be combined with fine-tuning of adaptive management measures to develop measures of societal vulnerability to each driver of global change.

Adaptive Capacity of Different Social Groups

This review of the adaptation options available to manage vector-borne diseases under global change highlights the many technologies available. In order to exploit them, societies need to have the cultural, economic, and environmental resources to implement the necessary programs. The combination of technologies and resources defines a community's adaptive capacity to respond to vector-borne diseases under global change. We have seen how successful control of vector-borne diseases depends on effective surveillance, community ownership, and a viable public infrastructure (181). Adaptive capacity is clearly related to economic and social development and stability. As such, we can readily determine the capacities of different nations and community groups to adapt to the changes in vector-borne diseases under global change. Documentation of those communities is beyond the scope of this review.

FRAMEWORK FOR ASSESSMENT OF VULNERABILITY

Now that we have identified the key potential impacts of vector-borne diseases under global change and are able to evaluate adaptation options, the next step is to obtain measures of vulnerability of targeted communities. This is done by combining impacts and adaptation options with the adaptive capacity of the affected communities into measures of social vulnerability (Fig.16).

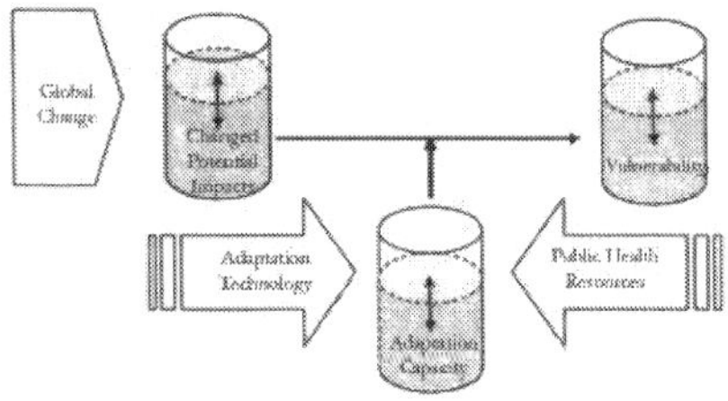

Figure 16: "Vulnerability" is determined by the extent of change in potential impacts and the adaptive capacity of the affected community.

Examples of some likely increases in vulnerability of different communities to vector-borne diseases under different global changes are given in Table 8. There is very large potential for the vulnerability of urban populations in developing countries to dengue fever and dengue hemorrhagic fever to increase as increasing population densities in megacities outstrip the capacity of the authorities to build appropriate public health infrastructure. In the case of malaria, drug and insecticide resistance, increased irrigation in agriculture, and global warming each have the potential to increase the vulnerability of communities in developing countries. Accelerating travel between developed and developing countries will increase the incidence of airport malaria, but existing public health services should be able to contain its spread and prevent local transmission. Lyme disease also has the potential to increase in affluent developed countries as populations seek more leisure in forested areas where animal conservation is increasing. Adaptive behaviors and use of repellents provide simple solutions to that problem if transmission rates are reduced by maintaining biodiversity.

Table 8: Potential for change in the vulnerability of human societies in some representative situations of key vector-borne diseases[a]

Vector-borne disease	Potential for:			
	Change in exposure	Change in sensitivity	Adaptation	Change in vulnerability
Malaria				
Tropical lowlands	++ (resistance, movement)	++ (resistance, irrigation)	+	+++
Tropical highlands	++ (resistance, movement, climate change)	+++ (resistance, climate change, agriculture)	+	++++
Temperate developed	+ (climate change, movement)	+ (climate change)	+++	+
	+ (climate change)		+	++
Temperate developing		++ (climate change)		
Dengue fever				

Urban developed	+ (movement)	+ (waste)	+++	+
Urban developing	+++ (water services)	+++ (water services, waste)	+	+++++
Rural	+	+ (waste)	+	+
Lyme disease				
Urban wealthy	++ (reforestation, behavior)	++ (behavior)	+	+++

[a]Plus signs indicate potential changes; the extent of potential change is indicated by the numbers of plus signs.

The key measures that are needed to reduce the vulnerability of different communities around the world, by managing the impacts of each global change driver are as follows. (i) Raise standards of living in developing countries to protect their inhabitants and to indirectly reduce the risks to inhabitants of developed countries. (ii) Reinstate a preventative approach to public health as the foundation of control of vector-borne diseases. This will include ongoing monitoring as well as management of vector breeding sites, avoidance of contact with vectors in housing, and changes in human behavior patterns. (iii) Build the adaptive capacity of communities to be more flexible and responsive to changing conditions. (iv) Adopt holistic approaches to account for unforeseen as well as intended consequences of human actions in cultural, economic, and environmental dimensions. (v) Adopt a knowledge-based approach to the management of vector-borne diseases, based on comprehensive decision support systems (Fig. 14). Place emphasis on clarifying the causes of problems rather than on treating the symptoms (179). (vi) Manage surface water in cities and in agriculture to reduce breeding sites for insect, molluscan, and crustacean vectors of disease. (vii) Strengthen international sanitary procedures for movement of human pathogens and vectors around the world. (viii) Avoid intrusions into old-growth forests. (ix) Protect natural biodiversity to ensure that natural enemies of vectors are encouraged. (x) Support research (134) to clarify likely trends by collecting baseline data, define the biological and genetic processes involved, and their relationships with environmental variables by using mechanistic computer simulation models, build a knowledge base and predictive tools for adaptation, and create new protective products and services for resource-poor communities.

The key to reducing societal vulnerability to the health impacts of climate change is to enhance existing public health infrastructure and intervention programs (121, 224). Sustainable management strategies for vector-borne diseases must either create or preserve herd immunity or implement sustainable preventative measures. When programs fail after extended periods, the scene is set for epidemics of disease among populations that have lost their immunity. Even with sustainable technologies, human societies will remain vulnerable to vector-borne diseases as long as there is a risk of an interruption in the protective program. This only emphasizes the cruel reality for many people in the developing countries that are either socially or economically unstable. In the longer term, only improved living conditions will deliver a sustained reduction in vulnerability to environmental health hazards.

CONCLUSIONS

Global change is a vast field that covers most human endeavors, and so it is impossible to cover the topic comprehensively in a single review such as this. The rates of change of all aspects of human and environment-related actions are accelerating. This gives rise to numerous opportunities for unexpected or enhanced risks from vector-borne diseases, arising from the interaction between different types of change such as climate, patterns of travel, unplanned expansion of megacities, and intensification of agriculture. There are increasing risks of the spread of vector-borne diseases from developing to developed countries as globalization further accelerates the pace of movement of goods and people around the world. Already there is a trend of increasing global incidence of severe diseases such as malaria and dengue fever. This has arisen largely from declining public health infrastructures, development of resistance to drugs and insecticides, and reliance on reactive treatment rather than prevention.

On the other hand, there are examples where large-scale interventions have been successful in greatly reducing the incidence of vector-borne diseases, such as onchocerciasis in West Africa and Japanese encephalitis in East Asia.

Acknowledging the gross simplifications, a summary of the current status of knowledge and beliefs about future trends in relation to vector-borne diseases under global change is given in Table 9. There are significant uncertainties surrounding some of the risks, but for others the trends are clear and the outcomes are predictable. This should be enough to galvanize the global community to restore public health systems, reinstate preventative measures, and take up the opportunities to reduce the risks of spread of these diseases.

Table 9: What we know, what we can expect, what we do from here, and how successful our efforts might be

Global change	What we know	What we can expect	What we do from here	How successful our efforts might be
Climate and atmospheric greenhouse gases	The rates of increase of concentrations of greenhouse gases are accelerating.	Double to treble the concentration of CO_2 by the end of the century.	Stop transferring coal, oil, and gas from the ground into the air by burning fossil fuels.	The global consumption juggernaut is almost unstoppable, but moves toward sustainability are being made.
Climate change	Global average temperatures have increased by over 0.5°C over the past half-century, but warming is not evenly spread.	Further increases in temperature of 1-6°C (144) during the next century, with changed geographical ranges, seasonal patterns, and intensity of transmission of vector-borne diseases.	As above. Develop and implement adaptation measures, including better monitoring, predictive systems, and preventative measures, to anticipate changes. Most emphasis in developing countries.	As above. Adaptations are feasible given awareness, resources, political will, social stability, and development.
	The frequency of extreme hot days has increased, and that of cold nights has decreased	Trend to continue, with altered vector breeding and disease transmission rates.	Develop and implement adaptation measures as above.	Adaptation is feasible as above.
	Vector and pathogen development rates increase with temperature; vector longevity decreases.	Altered disease transmission rates.	Develop and implement adaptation measures as above.	Adaptation is feasible as above.

	The frequency of extreme high rainfall events has increased.	Future rainfall patterns are likely to vary regionally, affecting vector phenology.	Develop and implement adaptation measures that are resilient to variation in rainfall.	Adaptation is feasible as above.
Travel and trade	Air travel has increased greatly over the past decade, with more north-south travel. The volume of trade has increased by 3- to 4-fold from 1980 to 2000.	International travel and globalization of trade should accelerate, with resultant increases in the spread of vectors and pathogens.	Reduce the incidence of disease in developing countries, strengthen sanitary measures on shipping and aircraft, and increase the integrity of border security in importing countries.	Adaptation is feasible as above, but emphasis needs to be on reducing sources of infection in developing countries.
Urbanization	Human population has increased from ≈1.5 to 6 billion in the last century, and there has been a strong move into cities.	Human population growth and urbanization will continue in the developing world, intensifying disease transmission rates.	Improve sanitation and public health facilities, and increase the standard of living in developing countries to enable adaptation measures to be implemented.	Adaptation is feasible as above.
Land use	Water storage, irrigation, and deforestation have increased hugely in recent decades.	Accelerating water storage and use of irrigation; major problems arising with supply, disposal, and quality of water, providing vector-breeding sites. Deforestation continues to provide new breeding sites.	Design water storage facilities to avoid shallow water, use drip irrigation, build water disposal infrastructure in cities.	A huge, expensive challenge, but with multiple benefits.

Adaptation must be based on a sound understanding of the causes of changed transmission patterns in each situation, in other words on an understanding of the whole vector-pathogen-host-environment system. This calls for a systems approach with comprehensive and testable predictive models to remove the subjectivity from qualitative judgements. Adaptation measures must be culturally, economically, and environmentally sustainable, and they must be able to retain their effectiveness in the face of strong environmental variation or social disturbance; i.e., they must be robust. Biological approaches based on either host resistance or natural enemies tend to be more robust because they have in-built flexibility and avoid the need for extra contributions by human management, which is so often the weakest link.

The vulnerability of communities depends as much on their capacity to prevent or respond to increases in disease transmission as it does on the risks themselves. Therefore, the key to reducing the incidence of vector-borne diseases is to increase the standards of living in developing countries and the allocation of resources to preventative measures in both developing and developed countries. A distinction needs to be made between growth and development (17). Growth in the density of human populations and their associated demands for resources and production of wastes has natural limits. It is ultimately limited by land for food production, water, renewable and nonrenewable resources, and social stability. Development, on the other hand, refers to improvements in human health and personal development. The success of globalization in advancing living standards by providing services that enhance health and well-being, rather than material goods, will play a large part in reducing the vulnerability of disadvantaged communities. A global focus on provision of public health facilities and preventative measures rather than material consumption will be a faster route to reducing the incidence of vector-borne diseases and one step toward saving the human race and the world's biological life from future catastrophe.

ACKNOWLEDGMENTS

My thanks to Rod Mahon and Richard Russell and two anonymous referees for helpful comments on the draft manuscript. Rick Bottomley assisted with the bibliography and illustrations, and Gunter Maywald provided support for the CLIMEX model.

REFERENCES

1. Abaru, D. E. 1985. Sleeping sickness in Busoga, Uganda, 1976-1983. Trop. Med. Parasitol. 36:72-76.
2. Agudelo-Silva, F., and A. Spielman. 1984. Paradoxical effects of simulated larviciding on production of adult mosquitoes. Am. J. Trop. Med. Hyg. 33:1267-1269.
3. Akhtar, R., and A. J. McMichael. 1996. Rainfall and malaria outbreaks in western Rajasthan. Lancet348:1457-1458.
4. Akogbeto, M., and S. Yakoubou. 1999. Resistance of malaria vectors to pyrethroids used for impregnated bednets, Benin, West Africa. Bull. Soc. Pathol. Exot. 92:123-130.
5. Allan, R., J. Lindesay, and D. Parker. 1996. El Niño southern oscillation and climatic variability. CSIRO Publishing, Collingwood, Australia.
6. Allan, R., S. Nam, and L. Doull. 1998. MERLIN and malaria epidemic in north-east Kenya. Lancet351:1966-1967.
7. Amerasinghe, F. P., P. H. Amerasinghe, J. S. M. Peiris, and R. A. Wirtz. 1991. Anopheline ecology and malaria infection during the irrigation development of an area of the Mahaweli project, Sri Lanka. Am. J. Trop. Med. Hyg. 45:226-235.
8. Anderson, J. F., T. G. Andreadis, C. R. Vossbrinck, S. Tirrell, E. M. Wakem, R. A. French, A. E. Garmendia, and H. J. Van Kruiningen. 1999. Isolation of West Nile virus from mosquitoes, crows, and a Cooper's hawk in Connecticut. Science 286:2331-2333.
9. Andrewartha, H. G., and L. C. Birch. 1954. The distribution and abundance of animals. University of Chicago Press, Chicago, Ill.
10. Anonymous. 1996. Four TDR diseases can be eliminated: TDR News 49:1-5.
11. Anonymous. 1998. Dengue in the WHO western Pacific region. Wkly. Epidemiol. Rec. 73:273-280.
12. Anonymous. 2000. World development report 1999/2000. World Bank, Washington, D.C.
13. Anonymous. 2001. *In* T. Damstra, 50 years later, refugee flight

on the rise, international support waning. Refugee reports. U.S. Committee for Refugees 22:1-9.

14. Anonymous. 2001. World urbanization prospects. The 2001 revision. ESA/P/WP.173. United Nations, Geneva, Switzerland.

15. Anonymous. 2001. Zapping mosquitoes with biopesticides. Pestic. News 54:9.

16. Arthington, A. H., and L. N. Lloyd. 1989. Introduced poeciliids in Australia and New Zealand, p. 333-348. *In* G. K. Meffe and F. F. Snelson, Jr. (ed.), Ecology and evolution of livebearing fishes (Poeciliidae). Prentice-Hall, Inc., Englewood Cliffs, N.J.

17. AtKisson, A. 1999. Believing Cassandra. Chelsea Green Publishing Co., White River Junction, Vt.

18. Baker, R. H. A., C. E. Sansford, C. H. Jarvis, R. J. C. Cannon, A. MacLeod, and K. F. A. Walters. 2000. The role of climatic mapping in predicting the potential geographical distribution of non-indigenous pests under current and future climates. Agric. Ecosyst. Environ. 82:57-71.

19. Bang, Y. H. 1985. Implications in the control of malaria vectors with insecticides in tropical countries of south east Asia. J. Commun. Dis. 17:199-218.

20. Barbazan, P., T. Baldet, F. Darriet, H. Escaffre, D. H. Djoda, and J. M. Hougard. 1998. Impact of treatments with *Bacillus sphaericus* on *Anopheles* populations and the transmission of malaria in Maroua, a large city in a savannah region of Cameroon. J. Am. Mosq. Control Assoc. 14:33-39.

21. Barbour, A. G., and D. Fish. 1993. The biological and social phenomenon of Lyme disease. Science260:1610-1616.

22. Barnett, J. B., T. Colborn, and M. Fournier. 1996. Consensus statement from the work session on 'chemically induced alteration in the developing immune system'. The wildlife/human connection. Environ. Health Perspect. 104(Suppl. 4):807-808.

23. Barrera, R., M. E. Grillet, Y. Rangel, J. Berti, and A. Ache. 1999. Temporal and spatial patterns of malaria reinfection in northeastern Venezuela. Am. J. Trop. Med. Hyg. 61:784-790.

24. Barrett, J. C. 1989. Tsetse control, land use and livestock in the

development of the Zambezi Valley, Zimbabwe: some policy considerations. Network paper 19—African Livestock Policy Analysis Network: International Livestock Centre for Africa, Addis Ababa, Ethiopia.

25. Bateman, C. 2000. Flood disease control—moving smartly to save lives. South Afr. Med. J. 90:330-331.
26. Becker, C. M. 1990. The demo-economic impact of the AIDS pandemic in sub-Saharan Africa. World Dev. 18:1599-1619.
27. Beer, J., W. Mende, and R. Stellmacher. 2000. The role of the sun in climate forcing Q. Sci. Rev.19:403-415.
28. Bence, J. R. 1982. Some interactions of predaceous insects and mosquitofish *Gambusia affinis:* a review of some recent results. Bull. Soc. Vector Ecol. 7:41-44.
29. Bennett, K. E., K. E. Olson, M. D. Munoz, I. F. Fernandez-Salas, J. A. Farfan-Ale, S. Higgs, W. C. Black, and B. J. Beaty. 2002. Variation in vector competence for dengue 2 virus among 24 collections of*Aedes aegypti* from Mexico and the United States. Am. J. Trop. Med. Hyg. 67:85-92.
30. Bergquist, N. R. 2002. Schistosomiasis: from risk assessment to control. Trends Parasitol. 18:309-314.
31. Bergquist, N. R., and D. G. Colley. 1998. Schistosomiasis vaccines: research to development. Parasitol. Today 14:99-104.
32. Bia, F. J. 1992. Malaria prophylaxis: taking aim at constantly moving targets. Yale J. Biol. Med. 65:329-336.
33. Bjorkman, A., and P. A. Phillips-Howard. 1990. The epidemiology of drug-resistant malaria. Trans. R. Soc. Trop. Med. Hyg. 84:177-180.
34. Bodker, R., W. Kisinza, R. Malima, H. Msangeni, and S. Lindsay. 2000. Resurgence of malaria in the Usambara mountains, Tanzania, an epidemic of drug-resistant parasites. Global Change Hum. Health1:134-153.
35. Booman, M., D. N. Durrheim, K. LaGrange, C. Martin, A. M. Mabuza, A. Zitha, F. M. Mbokazi, C. Fraser, and B. L. Sharp. 2000. Using a geographical information system to plan a malaria control programme in South Africa. Bull. W. H. O. 78:1438-1444.
36. Bouma, M. J., and C. Dye. 1997. Cycles of malaria associated with El Niño in Venezuela. JAMA278:1772-1774.

37. Bouma, M. J., C. Dye, and H. J. Van der Kaay. 1996. Falciparum malaria and climate change in the Northwest Frontier Province of Pakistan. Am. J. Trop. Med. Hyg. 55:131-137.

38. Bouma, M. J., R. S. Kovats, S. A. Goubet, J. St. H. Cox, and A. Haines. 1997. Global assessment of El Niño's disaster burden. Lancet 350:1435-1438.

39. Bouma, M. J., G. Poveda, W. Rojas, D. Chavasse, M. Quinones, J. Cox, and J. Patz. 1997. Predicting high-risk years for malaria in Colombia using parameters of El Niño Southern Oscillation. Trop. Med. Int. Health 2:1122-1127.

40. Bouma, M. J., H. E. Sondorp, and H. J. Van der Kaay. 1994. Health and climate change. Lancet343:302.

41. Bouma, M. J., and H. J. van der Kaay. 1996. The El Niño Southern Oscillation and the historic malaria epidemics on the Indian subcontinent and Sri Lanka: an early warning system for future epidemics?Trop. Med. Int. Health 1:86-96.

42. Bradshaw, W. E., and C. M. Holzapfel. 2001. Genetic shift in photoperiodic response correlated with global warming. Proc. Natl. Acad. Sci. USA 98:14509-14511.

43. Brenner, R. J., D. A. Focks, R. T. Arbogast, D. K. Weaver, and D. Shuman. 1998. Practical use of spatial analysis in precision targeting for integrated pest management. Am. Entomol. 44:79-101.

44. Bruce-Chwatt, L. J. 1968. Movements of populations in relation to communicable diseases in Africa.East Afr. Med. J. 45:266-275.

45. Bruce-Chwatt, L. J. 1985. Mosquitoes, malaria and war, then and now. J. R. Army Med. Corps131:85-99.

46. Bruce-Chwatt, L. J. 1987. Malaria and its control: present situation and future prospects. Annu. Rev. Public Health 8:75-110.

47. Bruce-Chwatt, L. J. 1988. History of malaria from prehistory to eradiation, p. 1-59. *In* W. H. Wernsdorfer and I. McGregor (ed.), Malaria: principles and practice of malariology, vol. 2. Churchill Livingstone, Edinburgh, United Kingdom.

48. Bryan, J. H., D. H. Foley, and R. W. Sutherst. 1996. Malaria transmission and climate change in Australia. Med. J. Aust. 164:345-347.

49. Burgos, J. J., S. I. Curto de Casas, R. U. Carcavallo, and I. G. Giron. 1994. Global climate change influence in the distribution of some pathogenic complexes malaria and Chagas' disease in Argentina.Entomol. Vectores 1:69-78.

50. Burgos, J. J., S. I. Curto de Casas, R. U. Carcavallo, and A. Martinez. 1994. Malaria and global climate change in Argentina. Entomol. Vectores 1:123-135.

51. Cai, W., P. H. Whetton, and B. Pittock. 2001. Fluctuations of the relationship between ENSO and northeast Austalian rainfall. Climate Dyn. 17:421-432.

52. Calvin, W. H. 1998. The great climate flip-flop. Atlantic Monthly 281:47-64.

53. Chan, N. Y., K. L. Ebi, F. Smith, T. F. Wilson, and A. E. Smith. 1999. An integrated assessment framework for climate change and infectious diseases. Environ. Health Perspect. 107:329-337

54. Chandre, F., F. Darrier, L. Manga, M. Akogbeto, O. Faye, J. Mouchet, and P. Guillet. 1999. Status of pyrethroid resistance in *Anopheles gambiae sensu lato.* Bull. W. H. O. 77:230-234.

55. Chatfield, C. 1995. Model uncertainty, data mining and statistical inference. J. R. Stat. Soc. Ser. A158:419-466.

56. Chitsulo, L., D. Engels, A. Montresor, and L. Savioli. 2000. The global status of schistosomiasis and its control. Acta Trop. 77:41-51

57. Christie, M. 1954. A method for the study of larval populations of *Anopheles gambiae* and other pool-breeding mosquitoes. Annu. Trop. Med. Parasitol. 48:271-276.

58. Cleaver, H. 1997. Malaria and the political economy of public health. Int. J. Health Serv. 7:557-579.

59. Coetzee, M., D. W. K. Horne, B. D. Brooke, and R. H. Hunt. 1999. DDT, dieldrin and pyrethroid insecticide resistance in African malaria vector mosquitoes: an historical review and implications for future malaria control in southern Africa. S. Afr. J. Sci. 95:215-218.

60. Colborn, T., D. Dumanoski, and J. P. Myers. 1996. Our stolen future: are we threatening our fertility, intelligence and survival? A scientific detective story. Dutton, New York, N.Y.

61. Colwell, R., P. Epstein, D. Gubler, M. Hall, P. Reiter, J. Shukla, W. Sprigg, E. Takafuji, and J. Trtanj. 1998. Global climate change and infectious diseases. Emerg. Infect. Dis. 4:451-452.

62. Cook, G. C. 1992. Effect of global warming on the distribution of parasitic and other infectious diseases: a review. J. R. Soc. Med. 85:688-690.

63. Coope, G. R. 1995. The effects of quarternary climate changes on insect populations: lessons from the past, p. 29-48. *In* R. Harrington and N. E. Stork (ed.), Insects in a changing environment. Academic Press, Ltd., London, United Kingdom.

64. Coosemans, M., and J. Mouchet. 1990. Consequences of rural development on vectors and their control. Ann. Soc. Belge Med. Trop. 70:5-23.

65. Coosemans, M., and A. Van Gompel. 1998. Arthropods vectors of diseases. What is the risk for travellers of being bitten? Of being contaminated? Bull. Soc. Pathol. Exot. 91:467-473.

66. Coosemans, M., M. Wery, B. Storme, L. Hendrix, and P. Mfisi. 1984. Epidémiologie du paludisme dans la plaine de la Ruzizi, Burundi. Ann. Soc. Belge Med. Trop. 64:135-158.

67. Cox, C. B., and P. D. Moore. 2000. Biogeography: an ecological and evolutionary approach. Blackwell Science, Malden, Mass.

68. Craig, M. H., R. W. Snow, and D. le Sueur. 1999. A climate-based distribution model of malaria transmission in sub-Saharan Africa. Parasitol. Today 15:105-111.

69. Crisp, T. M., E. D. Clegg, R. L. Cooper, W. P. Wood, D. G. Anderson, K. P. Baetcke, J. L. Hoffmann, M. S. Morrow, D. J. Rodier, J. E. Schaeffer, L. W. Touart, M. G. Zeeman, and Y. L. Patel. 1998. Environmental endocrine disruption: an effects assessment and analysis. Environ. Health Perspect. 106(Suppl. 1):11-56.

70. Cross, E. R., and K. C. Hyams. 1996. The potential effect of global warming on the geographical and seasonal distribution of *Phlebotomus papatasi* in Southwest Asia. Environ. Health Perspect. 104:724-727.

71. Crowley, T. J. 2000. Causes of climate change over the past 1000 years. Science 289:270-277.

72. Curtis, C. F. 1996. Options for the control of malaria vectors. Pestic. Outlook 7:20-24.

73. Curtis, C. F., N. Hill, and S. H. Kasim. 1993. Are there effective resistance management strategies for vectors of human disease? Biol. J. Linn. Soc. 48:3-18.

74. Curtis, C. F., J. E. Miller, M. H. Hodjati, J. H. Kolaczinski, I. Kasumba, and I. Denholm. 1998. Can anything be done to maintain the effectiveness of pyrethroid-impregnated bednets against malaria vectors? Philos. Trans. R. Soc. Lond. Ser. B 353:1769-1775.

75. Dai, A., K. E. Trenberth, and T. R. Karl. 1998. Global variations in droughts and wet spells—1900-1995. Geophys. Res. Lett. 25:3367-3370.

76. Damstra, T., S. Barlow, A. Bergman, R. Kavlock, and G. Van Der Kraak. 2002. Global assessment of the state-of-the-science of endocrine disruptors. World Health Organization, Geneva, Switzerland.

77. Dansgaard, W., S. J. Johnsen, H. B. Clausen, D. Dahljensen, N. S. Gundestrup, C. U. Hammer, C. S. Hvidberg, J. P. Steffensen, A. E. Sveinbjornsdottir, J. Jouzel, and G. Bond. 1993. Evidence for general instability of past climate from a 250-kyr ice-core record. Nature 364:218-220.

78. Darriet, F., P. Guillet, R. N›Guessan, J. M. C. Doannio, A. Koffi, L. Y. Konan, and P. Carnevale.1998. Impact of resistance of *Anopheles gambiae s.s.* to permethrin and deltamethrin on the efficacy of insecticide-treated bednets. Med. Trop. 58:349-354.

79. Das, P. K., and D. D. Amalraj. 1997. Biological control of malaria vectors. Indian J. Med. Res.106:174-197.

80. Defries, R. S., L. Bounoua, and G. J. Collatz. 2002. Human modification of the landscape and surface climate in the next fifty years. Global Change Biol. 8:438-458.

81. Deubel, V., and F. Rodhain. 1999. Climate variations and dengue fever: direct and indirect impacts.Med. Maladies Infect. 29:289-295.

82. Dhanapala, A. H. 1998. Sensitivity of malaria potential transmission to climate change in Sri Lanka.Asian Profile 26:283-292.

83. Diaz, H. F., and N. E. Graham. 1996. Recent changes in tropical freezing heights and the role of sea surface temperatures. Nature 383:152-155.

84. Dobson, A. 1992. Global warming and potential changes in host-parasite and disease-vector relationships, p. 201-217. *In* R. Carper, R. L. Peters, and T. E. Lovejoy (ed.), Global warming and biological diversity. Yale University Press, New Haven, Conn.

85. Douthwaite, R. J. 1992. Non-target effects of insecticides used in tsetse control operations. World Anim. Rev. 70-71:8-14.

86. Easton, A. 1999. Outbreak of Japanese encephalitis hits Malaysia. Br. Med. J. 318:893.

87. El-Rahim, I. H. A. A., U. A. El-Hakim, and M. Hussein. 1999. An epizootic of Rift Valley fever in Egypt in 1997. Rev. Sci. Tech. Off. Int. Epizoot. 18:741-748.

88. Epstein, P. R. 1998. Global warming and vector-borne disease. Lancet 351:137.

89. Epstein, P. R. 2000. Is global warming harmful to health? Sci. Am. 283:50-57.

90. Epstein, P. R., H. F. Diaz, S. Elias, G. Grabherr, N. E. Graham, W. J. M. Martens, E. Mosley-Thompson, and J. Susskind. 1998. Biological and physical signs of climate change: focus on mosquito-borne diseases. Bull. Am. Meteorol. Soc. 79:409-417.

91. Eskow, E., R. Vemkitesh, S. Rao, and E. Mordechai. 2001. Concurrent infection of the central nervous system by *Borrelia burgdorferi* and *Bartonella henselae*. Evidence for a novel tick-borne disease complex. Arch. Neurol. 58:1357-1363.

92. Etya›Ale, D. E. 1998. Mectizan as a stimulus for development of novel partnerships: the international organization's perspective. Ann. Trop. Med. Parasitol. 92(Suppl. 1):S73-S77.

93. Failloux, A. B., M. Vazeille, and F. Rodhain. 2002. Geographic genetic variation in populations of the dengue virus vector *Aedes aegypti*. J. Mol. Evol. 55:653-663.

94. Falkenmark, M. 1997. Meeting water requirements of an expanding world population. Philos. Trans. R. Soc. Lond. Ser. B 352:929-36.

95. Farquhar, G. D. 1997. Carbon dioxide and vegetation. Science 278:1411.

96. Fischer, G., and G. K. Heilig. 1997. Population momentum and the demand on land and water resources. Philos. Trans. R. Soc. Lond. Ser. B. 352:869-889.

97. Focks, D. A., R. J. Brenner, D. D. Chadee, and J. H. Trosper. 1999. The use of spatial analysis in the control and risk assessment of vector-borne diseases. Am. Entomol. 45:173-183.

98. Focks, D. A., E. Daniels, D. G. Haile, and J. E. Keesling. 1995. A simulation model of the epidemiology of urban dengue fever: literature analysis, model development, preliminary validation, and samples of simulation results. Am. J. Trop. Med. Hyg. 53:489-506.

99. Foo, L. C., T. W. Lim, and R. Fang. 1985. Rainfall, abundance of *Aedes aegypti* and dengue infection in Selangor, Malaysia. Southeast Asian J. Trop. Med. Public Health 16:560-568.

100. French, J. B., W. L. Schell, J. J. Kazmierczak, and J. P. Davis. 1992. Changes in population density and distribution of *Ixodes dammini* Acari: Ixodidae. J. Med. Entomol. 295:723-728.

101. Gaines, S. D., and M. W. Denny. 1993. The largest, smallest, highest, lowest, longest, and shortest: extremes in ecology. Ecology 74:1677-1692.

102. Gardon, J., N. Gardon-Wendel, D. Ngangue, J. Kamgno, J. P. Chippaux, and M. Boussinesq.1997. Serious reactions after mass treatment of onchocerciasis with ivermectin in an area endemic for *Loa loa*infection. Lancet 350:18-22.

103. Garfield, R. M. 1989. War-related changes in health and health services in Nicaragua. Soc. Sci. Med.28:669-676.

104. Garfield, R. M., E. Prado, J. R. Gates, and S. H. Vermund. 1989. Malaria in Nicaragua: community-based control efforts and the impact of war. Int. J. Epidemiol. 18:434-439.

105. Garnham, P. C. C. 1948. The incidence of malaria at high altitudes. J. Natl. Malaria Soc. 7:275-284.

106. Garrett, L. 1996. The return of infectious disease. Foreign Affairs 75:66-79.

107. Georghiou, G. P. 1994. Principles of insecticide resistance management. Phytoprotection75(Suppl.):51-59.

108. Ghebreyesus, T. A., M. Haile, K. H. Witten, A. Getachew, A. Medhin, A. Yohannes, S. W. Lindsay, and P. Byass. 2000. Household risk factors for malaria among children in the Ethiopian Highlands. Trans. R. Soc. Trop. Med. Hyg. 94:17-21.

109. Gillett, J. D. 1989. The maintenance and spread of insect-borne disease by the agency of man, p. 35-46. *In* M. H. Service (ed.), Demography and vector-borne diseases. CRC Press, Inc., Boca Raton, Fla.

110. Githeko, A. K., S. W. Lindsay, U. E. Confalonieri, and J. A. Patz. 2000. Climate change and vector-borne diseases: a regional analysis. Bull. W. H. O. 78:1136-1147.

111. Githeko, A. K., M. W. Service, C. M. Mbogo, and F. K. Atieli. 1996. Resting behaviour, ecology and genetics of malaria vectors in large-scale agricultural areas of western Kenya. Parassitologia 38:481-489.

112. Glantz, M. H. 1991. The use of analogies in forecasting ecological and societal responses to global warming. Environment 33:10-15.

113. Go, V., J. Garey, M. S. Wolff, and B. G. T. Pogo. 1999. Estrogenic potential of certain pyrethroid compounds in the MCF-7 human breast carcinoma cell line. Environ. Health Perspect. 1-7:173-177.

114. Gonidec, G., P. Fauran, and G. Le Gonidec. 1981. Arbovirus diseases of the south-western Pacific. Med. Trop. 41:85-92. (In French.)

115. Gossling, S. 2002. Global environmental consequences of tourism. Global Environ. Change 12:283-302.

116. Gouteux, J., and M. Jarry. 1998. Tsetse flies, biodiversity and the control of sleeping sickness. Structure of a *Glossina* guild in southwest Cote d'Ivoire. Acta Oecol. 19:453-471.

117. Gratz, N. G. 1999. Emerging and resurging vector-borne diseases. Annu. Rev. Entomol. 44:51-75

118. Greenland, D. J., P. J. Gregory, and P. H. Nye. 1998. Land resources and constraints to crop production, p. 39-55. *In* J. C. Waterlow, D. G. Armstrong, L. Fowden, and R. Riley (ed.), Feeding a world population of more than eight billion people: a challenge to science. Oxford University Press, Oxford, United Kingdom.

119. Gregory, P. J., J. S. I. Ingram, B. Campbell, J. Goudriaan, L. A. Hunt, J. J. Landsberg, S. Linder, M. Stafford-Smith, R. W. Sutherst, and C. Valentin. 1999. Managed productions systems, p. 229-

270. *In* B. Walker, W. Steffen, J. Canadell, and J. Ingram (ed.), The terrestrial biosphere and global change. Implications for natural and managed ecosystems. Cambridge University Press, Cambridge, United Kingdom.

120. Gryseels, B. 2000. Schistosomiasis vaccines: a devils' advocate view. Parasitol. Today 16:46-48.

121. Gubler, D. J. 1998. Climate change: implications for human health. Health Environ. Digest 12:54-56.

122. Gubler, D. J. 1998. Dengue and dengue hemorrhagic fever. Clin. Microbiol. Rev. 11:480-496.

123. Gubler, D. J. 1998. Resurgent vector-borne diseases as a global health problem. Emerg. Infect. Dis.4:442-450.

124. Guzman, M. G., and G. Kouri. 2002. Dengue: an update. Lancet Infect. Dis. 2:33-42.

125. Haines, A. 1998. Global warming and vector-borne diseases. Lancet 351:1737-1738.

126. Haines, A., A. J. McMichael, and P. R. Epstein. 2000. Environment and health. 2. Global climate change and health. Can. Med. Assoc. J. 16:729-734.

127. Hales, S., S. Kovats, and A. Woodward. 2000. What El Niño can tell us about human health and global climate change. Global Change Hum. Health 1:66-77.

128. Hales, S., P. Weinstein, Y. Souares, and A. Woodward. 1999. El Niño and the dynamics of vectorborne disease transmission. Environ. Health Perspect. 107:99-102.

129. Hales, S., P. Weinstein, and A. Woodward. 1996. Dengue fever epidemics in the South Pacific: driven by El Niño Southern Oscillation? Lancet 348:1664-1665.

130. Hancock, J., et al. 1996. The Macroeconomic impact of HIV/AIDS, p. 111-128. *In* S. Forsythe and B. Rau (ed.), AIDS in Kenya: socio-economic impact and policy implications. FHI/AIDSCAP, Washington, D.C.

131. Handman, E. 2001. Leishmaniasis: current status of vaccine development. Clin. Microbiol. Rev.14:229-243.

132. Hanna, J. N., S. A. Ritchie, D. A. Phillips, J. Shield, M. C. Bailey, J. S. Mackenzie, M. Poidinger, B. J. McCall, and P. Mills. 1996. An

outbreak of Japanese encephalitis in the Torres Strait, Australia, 1995.Med. J. Aust. 165:256-260.

133. Hargrove, J. W. 2000. A theoretical study of the invasion of cleared areas by tsetse flies Diptera: Glossinidae. Bull. Entomol. Res. 90:201-209.

134. Harvell, C. D., C. E. Mitchell, J. R. Ward, S. Altizer, A. P. Dobson, R. S. Ostfeld, and M. D. Samuel. 2002. Climate warming and disease risks for terrestrial and marine biota. Science 296:2158-2162.

135. Hawley, W. A. 1988. The biology of *Aedes albopictus*. J. Am. Mosq. Control Assoc. 4:1-39.

136. Hay, S. I., J. Cox, D. J. Rogers, S. E. Randolph, D. I. Stern, G. D. Shanks, M. F. Myers, and R. W. Snow. 2002. Climate change and the resurgence of malaria in the East African highlands. Nature415:905-909.

137. Hay, S. I., J. A. Omumbo, M. H. Craig, and R. W. Snow. 2000. Earth observation, geographic information systems and *Plasmodium falciparum* malaria in subSaharan Africa. Adv. Parasitol. 47:173-215.

138. Heilig, G. K., G. Fischer, and H. van Velthuizen. 2000. Can China feed itself? An analysis of China's food prospects with special reference to water resources. Int. J. Sustain. Dev. World Ecol. 7:153-172.

139. Houghton, J. T., L. G. Meira Filho, B. A. Callander, N. Harris, A. Kattenberg, and K. Maskell.1996. Climate change 1995: the science of climate change. Contribution of working group I to the Second Assessment Report of the Intergovernmental Panel on Climate Change. Cambridge University Press, Cambridge, United Kingdom.

140. Huang, C. H. 1982. Studies of Japanese encephalitis in China. Adv. Virus Res. 27:71-101.

141. Hughes, L. 2000. Biological consequences of global warming: is the signal already. TREE 15:56-61.

142. Ijumba, J. N., and S. W. Lindsay. 2001. Impact of irrigation on malaria in Africa: paddies paradox.Med. Vet. Entomol. 15:1-11.

143. Intergovernmental Panel on Climate Change. 2001. Climate change 2001. Third Assessment Report. Cambridge University Press, Cambridge, United Kingdom.

144. Intergovernmental Panel on Climate Change. 2001. Technical summary. Climate change 2001. Impacts, adaptation and vulnerability. A report of working group II of the Intergovernmental Panel on Climate Change. IPCC, World Meteorological Office, Geneva, Switzerland.

145. International Plant Protection Convention. 1997. International Plant Protection Convention 1997: Secretariat of the International Plant Protection Convention. [Online.] Food and Agriculture Organization, Rome, Italy. http://www.fao.org/ag/agp/agpp/pq/default.htm.

146. Jetten, T. H., and D. A. Focks. 1997. Potential changes in the distribution of dengue transmission under climate warming. Am. J. Trop. Med. Hyg. 57:285-297.

147. Jetten, T. H., W. J. M. Martens, and W. Takken. 1996. Model simulations to estimate malaria risk under climate change. J. Med. Entomol. 33:361-371.

148. Jetten, T. H., and W. Takken. 1994. Anophelism without malaria in Europe. A review of the ecology and distribution of the genus *Anopheles* in Europe. Wageningen Agricultural University Papers, Wageningen, The Netherlands.

149. Jobin, W. 1999. Dams and disease: ecological design and health impacts of large dams, canals and irrigation systems. E. and F. N. Spon Ltd., London, United Kingdom.

150. Jones, R. N. 2000. Analysing the risk of climate change using an irrigation demand model. Clim. Res.14:89-100.

151. Kamimura, K. 1998. Studies on the population dynamics of the principal vector mosquito of Japanese encephalitis. Med. Entomol. Zool. 49:181-185.

152. Kanesa-thasan, N. 1998. Development of dengue vaccines: an overview. Indian Pediatr. 35:97-100.

153. Karl, T. R., P. D. Jones, and R. W. Knight. 1993. A new perspective on global warming: asymmetric trends of daily maximum and minimum temperatures. Bull. Am. Meteorol. Soc. 74:1007-1023.

154. Karl, T. R., R. W. Knight, and N. Plummer. 1996. Trends

in high-frequency climate variability in the twentieth century. Nature 377:217-220.

155. Kelly-Hope, L. A., B. H. Kay, D. M. Purdie, and G. M. Williams. 2002. The risk of Ross River and Barmah Forest virus disease in Queensland: implications for New Zealand. Aust. N. Z. J. Public Health26:69-77.

156. Keoleian, G. A., and D. Menerey. 1994. Sustainable development by design: review of life cycle design and related approaches. Air Waste 44:645-668.

157. Kinley, D. H. 1998. Aerial assault on the tsetse fly. Environment 40:14-18, 40-41.

158. Kitron, U. 1998. Landscape ecology and epidemiology of vector-borne diseases—tools for spatial analysis. J. Med. Entomol. 35:435-445.

159. Knols, B. G. J., and W. Takken. 1998. The wide-scale use of impregnated bednets for malaria control in Africa: impact on mosquitoes. Proc. Sect. Exp. Appl. Entomol. Neth. Entomol. Soc. 9:15-22.

160. Knudsen, A. B. 1995. Geographic spread of *Aedes albopictus* in Europe and the concern among public health authorities. Eur. J. Epidemiol. 11:345-348.

161. Kondrachine, A. V., and P. I. Trigg. 1997. Global overview of malaria. Indian J. Med. Res. 106:39-52.

162. Kovats, R. S. 2000. El Niño and human health. Bull. W. H. O. 78:1127-1135.

163. Kovats, R. S., D. H. Campbell-Lendrum, A. J. McMichael, A. Woodward, and J. S. Cox. 2001. Early effects of climate change: do they include changes in vector-borne disease? Philos. Trans. R. Soc. Lond. Ser. B 356:1057-1068.

164. Kovats, R. S., A. Haines, R. Stanwell-Smith, P. Martens, B. Menne, and R. Bertollini. 1999. Climate change and human health in Europe. Br. Med. J. Clin. Res. Ed. 318:1682-1685.

165. Kovats, S., and A. Haines. 1995. The potential health impacts of climate change: an overview. Med. War 11:168-178.

166. Krimsky, S. 2000. Hormonal chaos. The scientific and social origins of the environmental endocrine hypothesis. John Hopkins University Press, Baltimore, Md.

167. Kriticos, D. J., and P. R. Randall. 2001. A comparison of systems to analyse potential weed distributions, p. 61-79. *In* R. H. Groves, F. D. Panetta, and J. G. Virtue (ed.), Weed risk assessment. CSIRO, Melbourne, Australia.

168. Kuhn, K. G. 1999. Global warming and leishmaniasis in Italy. Bull. Trop. Med. Int. Health 7:1-2.

169. Kullman, L. 2002. Rapid recent range-margin rise of tree and shrub species in the Swedish Scandes. J. Ecol. 90:68-77.

170. Lacey, L. A., and C. M. Lacey. 1990. The medical importance of riceland mosquitoes and their control using alternatives to chemical insecticides. J. Am. Mosq. Control Assoc. 2(Suppl.):1-93.

171. Lane, R. S., J. Piesman, and W. Burgdorfer. 1991. Lyme borreliosis: relation of its causative agent to its vectors and hosts in North America and Europe. Annu. Rev. Entomol. 36:587-609.

172. Laurance, W. F. 2001. Future shock: forecasting a grim fate for the earth. TREE 6:531-533.

173. Laventure, S., J. Mouchet, S. Blanchy, L. Marrama, P. Rabarison, L. Andrianaivolambo, E. Rajaonarivelo, I. Rakotoarivony, and J. Roux. 1996. Rice, a source of life and death on the Madagascan plateaux. Cah. Etudes Rech. Francophones/Sante 6:79-86.

174. Lawton, J., and R. May. 1995. Extinction rates. Oxford University Press, Oxford, United Kingdom.

175. Legner, E. F. 1995. Biological control of Diptera of medical and veterinary importance. J. Vector Ecol.20:59-120.

176. Lenorman, T., D. Bourguet, T. Guillemaud, and M. Raymond. 1999. Tracking the evolution of insecticide resistance in the mosquito *Culex pipiens*. Nature 400:861-864.

177. Leveque, C. 1990. The impact of vector control on the aquatic environment. Ann. Parasitol. Hum. Comp. 65(Suppl. 1):119-124.

178. Lewis, W. J., J. C. van Lenteren, S. C. Phatak, and J. H. I. Tumlinson. 1997. A total system approach to sustainable pest management. Proc. Natl. Acad. Sci. USA 94:12243-12248.

179. Li, Y. S., A. C. Sleigh, A. G. P. Ross, G. M. Williams, M. Tanner, and D. P. McManus. 2000. Epidemiology of *Schistosoma japonicum* in China: morbidity and strategies for control in the Dongting Lake region. Int. J. Parasitol. 30:273-281.

180. Lifson, A. R. 1996. Mosquitoes, models, and dengue. Lancet 347:1201-1202.

181. Lim, B. L. 1986. Filariasis in Indonesia: a summary of published information from 1970-1984. Trop. Biomed 3:193-210.

182. Linacre, E. 1992. Climate data and resources: a reference and guide. Routledge, London, United Kingdom.

183. Lindblade, K. A., E. D. Walker, A. W. Onapa, J. Katungu, and M. L. Wilson. 1999. Highland malaria in Uganda: prospective analysis of an epidemic associated with El Niño. Trans. R. Soc. Trop. Med. Hyg. 93:480-487.

184. Lindblade, K. A., E. D. Walker, A. W. Onapa, J. Katungu, and M. L. Wilson. 2000. Land use change alters malaria transmission parameters by modifying temperature in a highland area of Uganda. Trop. Med. Int. Health 5:263-274.

185. Lindgren, E. 1998. Climate change, tick-borne encephalitis and vaccination needs in Sweden—a prediction model. Ecol. Modelling 110:55-63.

186. Lindgren, E., and R. Gustafson. 1998. Climate and tick-borne encephalitis in Sweden. Conserv. Ecol.21:5.

187. Lindgren, E., L. Talleklint, and T. Polfeldt. 2000. Impact of climatic change on the northern latitude limit and population density of the disease-transmitting European tick *Ixodes ricinus*. Environ. Health Perspect. 108:119-123.

188. Lindsay, S. W., and M. H. Birley. 1996. Climate change and malaria transmission. Ann. Trop. Med. Parasitol. 90:573-588.

189. Lindsay, S. W., R. Bodker, R. Malima, H. A. Msangeni, and W. Kisinza. 2000. Effect of 1997-98 El Niño on highland malaria in Tanzania. Lancet 355:989-990.

190. Lindsay, S. W., and A. Joyce. 2000. Climate change and the disappearance of malaria from England. Global Change Hum. Health 1:184-187.

191. Lindsay, S. W., and W. J. M. Martens. 1998. Malaria in the African highlands: past, present and future. Bull. W. H. O. 76:33-45.

192. Lindsay, S. W., L. Parson, and C. J. Thomas. 1998. Mapping the ranges and relative abundance of the two principal African malaria vectors, *Anopheles gambiae sensu stricto* and *An. arabiensis*, using climate data. Proc. R. Soc. London Ser. B 265:847-853.

193. Lindsay, S. W., and C. J. Thomas. 2000. Mapping and estimating the population at risk from lymphatic filariasis in Africa. Trans. R. Soc. Trop. Med. Hyg. 94:37-45.

194. Linthicum, K. J., A. Anyamba, C. J. Tucker, P. W. Kelley, M. F. Myers, and C. J. Peters. 1999. Climate and satellite indicators to forecast Rift Valley fever epidemics in Kenya. Science 285:397-400.

195. Loder, N. 2000. Royal Society warns on hormone disruptors. Nature 406:4.

196. Loevinsohn, M. E. 1994. Climatic warming and increased malaria incidence in Rwanda. Lancet343:714-718.

197. Lortholary, O., J. Robert, and J. Le Bras. 1994. Epidemiology of drug resistant *Plasmodium falciparum* malaria. Ann. Med. Interne 145:429-432.

198. Maciel, A., A. Rocha, K. B. F. Marzochi, Z. Medeiros, A. B. Carvalho, L. Regis, W. Souza, T. Lapa, and A. Furtado. 1996. Epidemiological study of bancroftian filariasis in Recife, northeastern Brazil.Mem. Inst. Oswaldo Cruz 91:449-455.

199. Mackenzie, J., M. Lindsay, and P. Daniels. 2000. The effect of climate on the incidence of vector-borne viral diseases in Australia: the potential value of seasonal forecasting, p. 429-452. *In* G. L. Hammer, N. Nicholls, and C. Mitchell (ed.), Applications of seasonal climate forecasting in agricultural and natural ecosystems. The Australian experience. Kluwer Academic Publishers, Dordrecht, The Netherlands.

200. Maelzer, D., S. Hales, P. Weinstein, M. Zalucki, and A. Woodward. 1999. El Niño and arboviral disease prediction. Environ. Health Perspect. 107:817-818.

201. Maguire, T. 1994. Do Ross River and dengue viruses pose a threat to New Zealand? N. Z. Med. J.107:448-450.

202. Malakooti, M. A., K. Biomndo, and G. D. Shanks. 1998. Re-emergence of epidemic malaria in the highlands of Western Kenya. Emerg. Infect. Dis. 4:671-676.

203. Marco, G. J., R. M. Hollingworth, and W. Durham. 1987. Silent spring revisited. American Chemical Society, Washington, D.C.

204. Martens, P. 1998. Health and climate change: modelling the impacts of global warming and ozone depletion. Earthscan Publications Ltd., London, United Kingdom.

205. Martens, P. 1999. How will climate change affect human health? Am. Sci. 87:534-541.

206. Martens, P., and L. Hall. 2000. Malaria on the move: human population movement and malaria transmission. Emerg. Infect. Dis. 6:7-13.

207. Martens, P., R. S. Kovats, S. Nijhof, P. de. Vries, M. T. J. Livermore, D. J. Bradley, J. Cox, and A. J. McMichael. 1999. Climate change and future populations at risk of malaria. Global Environ. Change9:S89-S107.

208. Martens, W. J. M., T. H. Jetten, and D. A. Focks. 1997. Sensitivity of malaria, schistosomiasis and dengue to global warming. Climate Change 35:145-146.

209. Martens, W. J. M., T. H. Jetten, J. Rotmans, and L. W. Niessen. 1995. Climate change and vector-borne diseases: a global modelling perspective. Global Environ. Change 5:195-209.

210. Martens, W. J. M., L. W. Niessen, J. Rotmans, T. H. Jetten, and A. J. McMichael. 1995. Potential impact of global climate change on malaria risk. Environ. Health Perspect. 103:458-464.

211. Martin, P. H., and M. G. Lefebvre. 1995. Malaria and climate: sensitivity of malaria potential transmission to climate. AMBIO XXIV:200-209.

212. Massad, E., and O. P. Forattini. 1998. Modelling the temperature sensitivity of some physiological parameters of epidemiologic significance. Ecosyst. Health 4:119-129.

213. Matola, Y. G., G. B. White, and S. A. Magayuka. 1987. The changed pattern of malaria endemicity and transmission at Amani in the eastern Usumbara mountains, northeastern Tanzania. J. Trop. Med. Hyg.90:127-134.

214. Matsuoka, Y., and K. Kai. 1994. An estimation of climate change effects on malaria. J. Global Environ. Eng. 1:1-15.

215. Maxwell, C. A., C. F. Curtis, H. Haji, S. Kisumku, A. I. Thalib, and S. A. Yahya. 1990. Control of Bancroftian filariasis by integrating therapy with vector control using polystyrene beads in wet pit latrines.Trans. R. Soc. Trop. Med. Hyg. 84:709-714.

216. Mayer, J. D. 2000. Geography, ecology and emerging infectious diseases. Soc. Sci. Med. 50:937-952.

217. McCarroll, L., M. G. Paton, S. H. P. P. Karunaratne, H. T. R. Jayasuryia, K. S. P. Kalpage, and J. Hemingway. 2000. Insecticides and mosquito-borne disease. Nature 407:961-962.

218. McCarty, J. P. 2001. Ecological consequences of recent climate change. Conserv. Biol. 15:320-331.

219. McMichael, A. J. 1997. Integrated assessment of potential health impact of global environmental change: prospects and limitations. Environ. Model. Assess. 2:129-137.

220. McMichael, A. J. 2000. The urban environment and health in a world of increasing globalization: issues for developing countries. Bull. W. H. O. 78:1117-1126.

221. McMichael, A. J., and A. Haines. 1997. Global climate change: the potential effects on health. Br. Med. J. Clin. Res. Ed. 315:805-809.

222. McMichael, A. J., A. Haines, R. Sloff, and S. Kovats. 1996. Climate change and human health. World Health Organization, Geneva, Switzerland.

223. McMichael, A. J., and R. S. Kovats. 2000. Climate change and climate variability: adaptations to reduce adverse health impacts. Environ. Monit. Assess. 61:49-64.

224. Mellor, P. S. 1998. Climate change and the distribution of vector borne diseases with special reference to African horse sickness virus, p. 439-454. Towards livestock disease diagnosis and control in the 21st century. Proceedings of an International Symposium on Diagnosis and Control of Livestock Diseases Using Nuclear and Related Techniques. International Atomic Energy Agency (IAEA), Vienna, Austria.

225. Mockenhaupt, F. P., J. May, U. Bienzle, and C. G. Meyer. 1997. Drug-resistant malaria. Dtsch. Med. Wochenschr. 122:1293-1297.

226. Modiano, D., V. Petrarca, B. S. Sirima, I. Nebie, G. Luoni, F. Esposito, and M. Coluzzi. 1998. Baseline immunity of the population and impact of insecticide-treated curtains on malaria infection. Am. J. Trop. Med. Hyg. 59:336-340.

227. Molyneux, D. H. 1997. Patterns of change in vector-borne diseases. Ann. Trop. Med. Parasitol.91:827-839.

228. Mouchet, J., and J. Brengues. 1990. Vector-borne diseases and vector control at the public health-agriculture interface. Bull. Soc. Pathol. Exot. 83:376-393.

229. Mouchet, J., and P. Carnevale. 1997. Impact of environmental changes on vector-borne diseases.Cah. Etudes Rech. Francophones/Sante 7:263-269.

230. Mouchet, J., S. Manguin, J. Sircoulon, S. Laventure, O. Faye, A. W. Onapa, P. Carnevale, J. Julvez, and D. Fontenille. 1998. Evolution of malaria in Africa for the past 40 years: impact of climatic and human factors. J. Am. Mosq. Control Assoc. 14:121-130.

231. Mulla, M. S., G. Majori, and A. A. Arata. 1979. Impact of biological and chemical mosquito control agents on nontarget biota in aquatic ecosystems. Residue Rev. 71:121-173.

232. Murray-Smith, S., and P. Weinstein. 1993. A time bomb in north Queensland: a case report of introduced malaria south of the nineteenth parallel. Comm. Disease Intell. 17:211-213.

233. National Oceanic and Atmospheric Administration. 1999. An experiment in the application of climate forecasts: NOAA-OGP activities related to the 1997-98 El Niño event. Office of Global Programs, United States Department of Commerce, Boulder, Colo.

234. New, M., M. Hulme, and P. Jones. 1999. Representing twentieth-century space-time climate variability. I. Development of a 1961-90 mean monthly terrestrial climatology. J. Climate 12:829-856.

235. Newton, P., and N. White. 1999. Malaria: new developments in treatment and prevention. Annu. Rev. Med. Select. Top. Clin. Sci. 50:179-192.

236. Nicholls, N. 1986. A method for predicting Murray Valley encephalitis in southeast Australia using the Southern Oscillation. Aust. J. Exp. Biol. Med. Sci. 64:587-594.

237. Nicholls, N. 1993. El Niño-Southern Oscillation and vector-borne disease. Lancet 342:1284-1285.

238. Omumbo, J. A., S. I. Hay, S. J. Goetz, R. W. Snow, and D. J. Rogers. 2002. Updating historical maps of malaria transmission

intensity in East Africa using remote sensing. Photogramm. Eng. Remote Sens.68:161-166.

239. Ostfeld, R. S., and F. Keesing. 2000. Biodiversity and disease risk: the case of Lyme disease. Conserv. Biol. 14:722-728.

240. Packard, R. M., and P. Gadelha. 1994. A land filled with mosquitoes: Fred L. Soper, the Rockefeller Foundation, and the *Anopheles gambiae* invasion of Brazil. Parassitologia 36:197-213.

241. Pant, C. P., and N. G. Gratz. 1979. Malaria and agricultural development. Outlook Agric. 10:111-115.

242. Parmesan, C., and G. Yohe. 2003. A globally coherent fingerprint of climate change impacts across natural systems. Nature 421:37-42.

243. Parry, M., and T. Carter. 1998. Climate impact and adaptation assessment. Earthscan, London, United Kingdom.

244. Parry, M. L., and M. Livermore. 1999. A new assessment of the global effect of climate change.Global Environ. Change 9(Suppl. Issue).

245. Patz, J. A. 2001. Public health risk assessment linked to climatic and ecological change. Hum. Ecol. Risk Assess. 7:1317-1327.

246. Patz, J. A., M. Hulme, C. Rosenzweig, T. D. Mitchell, R. A. Goldberg, A. K. Githeko, S. Lele, A. J. McMichael, and D. Le Sueur. 2002. Regional warming and malaria resurgence. Nature 420:627-628.

247. Patz, J. A., and S. W. Lindsay. 1999. New challenges, new tools: the impact of climate change on infectious diseases. Curr. Opin. Microbiol. 2:445-451.

248. Patz, J. A., M. A. McGeehin, S. M. Bernard, K. L. Ebi, P. R. Epstein, A. Grambsch, D. J. Gubler, P. Reiter, I. Romieu, J. B. Rose, J. M. Samet, and J. Trtanj. 2000. The potential health impacts of climate variability and change for the United States: executive summary of the report of the health sector of the US National Assessment. Environ. Health Perspect. 108:367-376.

249. Patz, J. A., K. Strzepek, S. Lele, M. Hedden, S. Greene, B. Noden, S. I. Hay, L. Kalkstein, and J. C. Beier. 1998. Predicting key malaria transmission factors, biting and entomological inoculation rates, using modelled soil moisture in Kenya. Trop. Med. Int. Health 3:818-827.

250. Pearce, F. 1990. High and dry in the global greenhouse. New Sci. 128:34-37.
251. Peters, W. 1989. Changing pattern of antimalarial drug resistance. J. R. Soc. Med. 82(Suppl. 17):10-11.
252. Peyton, E. L., S. R. Campbell, T. M. Candeletti, M. Romanowski, and W. J. Crans. 1999. *Aedes Finlaya japonicus japonicus* Theobald, a new introduction into the United States. J. Am. Mosq. Control Assoc. 15:238-241.
253. Phillips, R. S. 2001. Current status of malaria and potential for control. Clin. Microbiol. Rev. 14:208-226.
254. Porter W. P., J. W. Jaeger, and I. H. Carlson. 1999. Endocrine, immune, and behavioral effects of aldicarb (carbamate), atrazine (triazine) and nitrate (fertilizers) mixtures at groundwater concentrations.Toxicol. Ind. Health 15:133-150.
255. Poveda, G., W. Rojas, M. L. Quinones, I. D. Velez, R. I. Mantilla, D. Ruiz, J. S. Zuluaga, and G. L. Rua. 2001. Coupling between annual and ENSO timescales in the malaria-climate association in Colombia. Environ. Health Perspect. 109:489-493.
256. Prasittisuk, C., and C. F. Curtis. 1982. Absence of effects of insecticides on susceptibility of anophelines to *Plasmodium yoelii nigeriensis*. Southeast Asian J. Trop. Med. Public Health 13:127-132.
257. Prothero, R. M. 1977. Disease and mobility: a neglected factor in epidemiology. Int. J. Epidemiol.6:259-267.
258. Prothero, R. M. 2001. Migration and malaria risk. Health Risk Soc. 3:19-38.
259. Pépin, J. 1997. Zaire (Congo): resurgence of trypanosomiasis ("patients within borders"). Lancet349(Suppl. 3):10-11.
260. Ramirez, J. A., and B. Finnerty. 1996. CO_2 and temperature effects on evapotranspiration and irrigated agriculture. J. Irrigation Drainage Eng. 122:155-163.
261. Randolph, S. E., and D. J. Rogers. 1997. A generic population model for the African tick*Rhipicephalus appendiculatus*. Parasitology 115:265-279.
262. Raymond, M., A. Callaghan, P. Fort, and N. Pasteur. 1991. Worldwide migration of amplified insecticide resistance genes in mosquitoes. Nature 350:151-153.

263. Reeves, W. C., J. L. Hardy, W. K. Reisen, and M. M. Milby. 1994. Potential effect of global warming on mosquito-borne arboviruses. J. Med. Entomol. 31:323-332.

264. Reiter, P. 1988. Weather, vector biology, and arboviral recrudescence, p. 245-255. *In* T. P. Monath (ed.), The arboviruses: epidemiology and ecology. CRC Press, Inc., Boca Raton, Fla.

265. Reiter, P. 1996. Global warming and mosquito-borne disease in USA. Lancet 348:622.

266. Reiter, P. 1998. Global-warming and vector-borne disease in temperature regions and at high altitude.Lancet 351:839-840.

267. Reiter, P. 2000. Biting back. New Sci. 167:41-43.

268. Reiter, P. 2000. From Shakespeare to Defoe: malaria in England in the little ice age. Emerg. Infect. Dis. 6:1-11.

269. Reiter, P. 2001. Climate change and mosquito-borne disease. Environ. Health Perspect. 109(Suppl. 1):141-161

270. Remme, J. H. F., F. Binka, and D. Nabarro. 2001. Toward a framework and indicators for monitoring Roll Back Malaria. Am. J. Trop. Med. Hyg. 64:76-84.

271. Richie, T. L., and A. Saul. 2002. Progress and challenges for malaria vaccines. Nature 415:694-701.

272. Ritchie, S. A., and W. Rochester. 2001. Wind-blown mosquitoes and introduction of Japanese encephalitis into Australia. Emerg. Infect. Dis. 7:900-903.

273. Robbins A. H., M. D. Borden, B. S. Windmiller, M. Niezgoda, L. C. Marcus, S. M. O›Brien, S. M. Kreindel, M. W. McGuill, A. Jr. DeMaria, C. E. Rupprecht, and S. Rowell. 1998. Prevention of the spread of rabies to wildlife by oral vaccination of raccoons in Massachusetts. J. Am. Vet. Med. Assoc.213:1407-1412.

274. Rocha e Silva, E. O., D. M. V. Wanderley, and V. L. C. C. Rodrigues. 1998. *Triatoma infestans:*importance, control and elimination of the species in the State of Sao Paulo, Brazil. Rev. Soc. Bras. Med. Trop. 31:73-88.

275. Rodhain, F. 1996. Worldwide situation of dengue. Bull. Soc. Pathol. Exot. 89:87-90.

276. Roger, P. A., I. Simpson, R. Oficial, S. Ardales, and R. Jimenez. 1994. Effects of pesticides on soil and water microflora

and mesofauna in wetland ricefields: a summary of current knowledge and extrapolation to temperate environments. Aust. J. Exp. Agric. 34:1057-1068.

277. Rogers, D. J. 1995. Remote sensing and the changing distribution of tsetse flies in Africa, p. 177-193.*In* R. Harrington and N. E. Stork (ed.), Insects in a changing environment. Academic Press, Ltd., London, United Kingdom.

278. Rogers, D. J., and S. E. Randolph. 1993. Distribution of tsetse and ticks in Africa: past, present and future. Parasitol. Today 9:266-271.

279. Rogers, D. J., and S. E. Randolph. 2000. The global spread of malaria in a future, warmer world.Science 289:1763-1766.

280. Rogers, D. J., and S. E. Randolph. 2002. A response to the aim of eradicating tsetse from Africa.Trends Parasitol. 18:534-536.

281. Root, T. L., J. T. Price, K. R. Hall, S. H. Schneider, C. Rosenzweig, and J. A. Pounds. 2003. Fingerprints of global warming on wild animals and plants. Nature 421:57-60.

282. Rosatte, R. C., C. D. MacInnes, R. T. Williams, and O. Williams. 1997. A proactive prevention strategy for raccoon rabies in Ontario, Canada. Wild. Soc. Bull. 25:110-116.

283. Rosen, L., D. J. Gubler, and P. H. Bennett. 1981. Epidemic polyarthritis (Ross River) virus infection in the Cook Islands. Am. J. Trop. Med. Hyg. 30:1294-1302.

284. Russell, B. M., L. E. Muir, P. Weinstein, and B. H. Kay. 1996. Surveillance of the mosquito *Aedes aegypti* and its biocontrol with the copepod *Mesocyclops aspericornis* in Australian wells and gold mines.Med. Vet. Entomol. 10:155-160.

285. Russell, R. C. 1998. Mosquito-borne arboviruses in Australia: the current scene and implications of climate change for human health. Int. J. Parasitol. 28:955-969.

286. Sabatini, A., V. Raineri, G. Trovato, and M. Coluzzi. 1990. *Aedes albopictus* in Italy and the possible spread of this species in the Mediterranean area. Parassitologia 32:301-304.

287. Schapira, A., P. F. Beales, and M. R. Halloran. 1993. Malaria: living with drug resistance. Parasitol. Today 9:168-174.

288. Schofield, C. J. 1991. Vector population responses to control interventions. Ann. Soc. Belge Med. Trop. 71(Suppl. 1):201-217.

289. Schoute, J. F. T., P. A. Finke, F. R. Veeneklaas, and H. P. Wolfert. 1995. Scenario studies for the rural environment. Kluwer Academic Publishers, Dordrecht, The Netherlands.

290. Serufo, J. C., A. M. Souza, V. A. Tavares, M. C. Jammal, and J. G. Silva. 1993. Dengue in the south-eastern region of Brazil: historical analysis and epidemiology. Rev. Saude Publica 27:157-167.

291. Service, M. H. 1989. Demography and vector-borne diseases. CRC Press Inc., Boca Raton, Fla.

292. Shanks, G. D., and J. J. Karwacki. 1991. Malaria as a military factor in Southeast Asia. Mil. Med.156:684-686.

293. Shanks, G. D., Kiomndo K., S. I. Hay, and R. W. Snow. 2000. Changing patterns of clinical malaria since 1965 among a tea estate population located in the Kenyan highlands. Trans. R. Soc. Trop. Med. Hyg.94:253-255.

294. Snow, K. 1999. Malaria and mosquitoes in Britain: the effect of global climate change. Eur. Mosq. Bull. 4:17-25.

295. Snow, R. W. 2000. The burden of malaria: understanding the balance between immunity, public health and control. J. Med. Microbiol. 49:1053-1055.

296. Southgate, V. R., L. A. T. Tchuente, M. Sene, D. DeClercq, A. Theron, J. Jourdane, B. L. Webster, D. Rollinson, B. Gryseels, and J. Vercruysse. 2001. Studies on the biology of schistosomiasis with emphasis on the Senegal river basin. Mem. Inst. Oswaldo Cruz 96:75-78.

297. Southwood, T. R. E. 1977. Habitat, the templet for ecological strategies? J. Anim. Ecol. 46:337-365.

298. Spielman, A., U. Kitron, and R. J. Pollack. 1993. Time limitation and the role of research in the worldwide attempt to eradicate malaria. J. Med. Entomol. 30:6-19.

299. Stoute, J. A., and W. R. Ballou. 1998. The current status of malaria vaccines. Biodrugs 10:123-136

300. Strobel M., and I. Lamaury. 2001. Dengue fever—a review. Rev. Med. Interne 22:638-647.

301. Sutherst, R. W. 1983. Variation in the numbers of the cattle tick, *Boophilus microplus* (Canestrini), in a moist habitat made

marginal by low temperatures. J. Aust. Entomol. Soc. 22:1-5.

302. Sutherst, R. W. 1993. Arthropods as disease vectors in a changing environment, p. 124-145. *In* J. V. Lake, G. R. Bock, and K. Ackrill (ed.), Environmental change and human health. John Wiley & Sons, Chichester, United Kingdom.

303. Sutherst, R. W. 1998. Implications of global change and climate variability for vector-borne diseases: generic approaches to impact assessments. Int. J. Parasitol. 28:935-945.

304. Sutherst, R. W. 2000. Climate change and invasive species—a conceptual framework, p. 211-240. *In*H. A. Mooney and R. J. Hobbs (ed.), Invasive species in a changing world. Island Press, Washington, D.C.

305. Sutherst, R. W. 2000. Climate variability, seasonal forecasting and invertebrate pests—the need for a synoptic view, p. 381-397. *In* G. L. Hammer, N. Nicholls, and C. Mitchell (ed.), Applications of seasonal climate forecasting in agricultural and natural ecosystems. The Australian experience. Kluwer Academic Publishers, Dordrecht, The Netherlands.

306. Sutherst, R. W. 2001. The vulnerability of animal and human health to parasites under global change.Int. J. Parasitol. 31:933-948.

307. Sutherst, R. W., and H. N. Comins. 1979. The management of acaricide resistance in the cattle tick,*Boophilus microplus* (Canestrini) (Acari: Ixodidae), in Australia. Bull. Entomol. Res. 69:519-540.

308. Sutherst, R. W., J. Ingram, and H. Scherm. 1998. Global change and vector-borne diseases.Parasitol. Today 14:297-299.

309. Sutherst, R. W., J. Ingram, T. Yonow, H. Scherm, and K. Sutton (ed.). 1998. Global change impact assessment approaches for vectors and vector-borne diseases. GCTE Working Document no. 27. GCTE Office, Oxford, United Kingdom.

310. Sutherst, R. W., and G. F. Maywald. 1985. A computerised system for matching climates in ecology.Agric. Ecosyst. Environ. 13:281-299.

311. Sutherst, R. W., G. F. Maywald, and B. L. Russell. 2000. Estimating vulnerability under global change: modular modelling of pests. Agric. Ecosyst. Environ. 82:303-319.

312. Sutherst, R. W., G. F. Maywald, and D. B. Skarratt. 1995. Predicting insect distributions in a changed climate, p. 59-91. *In* R. Harrington and N. E. Stork (ed.), Insects in a changing environment. Academic Press, Ltd., London, United Kingdom.

313. Sutherst, R. W., G. F. Maywald, T. Yonow, and P. M. Stevens. 1999. CLIMEX. Predicting the effects of climate on plants and animals. CD-ROM and user guide. CSIRO Publishing, Melbourne, Australia.

314. Sutherst, R. W., T. Yonow, S. Chakraborty, C. O›Donnell, and N. White. 1996. A generic approach to defining impacts of climate change on pests, weeds and diseases in Australasia, p. 281-307. *In*W. J. Bouma, G. I. Pearman, and M. R. Manning (ed.), Greenhouse: coping with climate change. CSIRO Publishing, Melbourne, Australia.

315. Tadei, W. P., B. D. Thatcher, J. M. M. Santos, V. M. Scarpassa, I. B. Rodri, and M. S. Rafael.1998. Ecologic observations on anopheline vectors of malaria in the Brazilian Amazon. Am. J. Trop. Med. Hyg. 59:325-335.

316. Tauber, M. J., C. A. Tauber, and S. Masaki. 1986. Seasonal adaptations of insects. Oxford University Press, Oxford, United Kingdom.

317. Taubes, G. 1997. Apocalypse not. Science 278:1004-1006.

318. Tellier, X., J. Steffan, and A. Buhlmann. 1991. Mechanisms of resistance to insecticides and acaricides. Practical consequences. Rev. Med. Vet. 142:657-667.

319. Thakare, J. P., S. R. Shenoy, V. S. Padbidri, C. S. Rajput, D. P. Karmarkar, and S. S. Deo.1999. Japanese encephalitis in Sangli district, Maharashtra. Indian J. Med. Res. 109:165-166.

320. Thompson, L. G. 1999. Ice core evidence for climate change in the tropics: implications for our future.Q. Sci. Rev. 19:19-35.

321. Tigertt, W. D., and D. F. Clyde. 1976. Drug resistance in the human malarias. Antibiot. Chemother.20:246-272.

322. Tilman, D., J. Fargione, B. Wolff, C. D›Antonio, A. Dobson, R. Howarth, D. Schindler, W. H. Schlesinger, D. Simberloff, and D. Swackhamer. 2001. Forecasting agriculturally driven global environmental change. Science 292:281-284.

323. Toole, M. J., and R. J. Waldman. 1997. The public health aspects of complex emergencies and refugee situations. Annu. Rev. Public Health 18:288-312.

324. Topouzis, D., and J. de Guerny. 1999. Sustainable agricultural/ rural development and vulnerability to the AIDS epidemic. FAO and UNAIDS. UNAIDS Best Practice Collection, Geneva, Switzerland.

325. United Nations Environment Programme. 1999. Gobal environment outlook 2000. United Nations Environment Programme, Geneva, Switzerland.

326. Utzinger, J., Y. Tozan, and B. H. Singer. 2001. Efficacy and cost-effectiveness of environmental management for malaria control. Trop. Med. Int. Health 6:677-687.

327. van den Hurk, A. F., S. A. Ritchie, A. Ingram, and R. D. Cooper. 1998. The first report of*Anopheles farauti sensu stricto* below the nineteenth parallel at Mackay, Queensland. Med. J. Aust. 169:89-90.

328. van der Hoek, W., Sakthivadivel, R., Renshaw, M., Silver, J. B., Birley, M. H., and Konradsen, F. 2001. Alternate wet/dry irrigation in rice cultivation: a practical way to save water and control malaria and Japanese encephalitis? IWMI research report no. 47. [Online.] International Management Institute, Silverton, South Africa. http://www.cgiar.org/iwmi/pubs/pub 047/RR047.htm.

329. Van Emden, H. F., and D. B. Peakall. 1996. Beyond silent spring: integrated pest management and chemical safety. Chapman and Hall Ltd., London, United Kingdom.

330. Vulule, J. M., R. F. Beach, F. K. Atieli, J. M. Roberts, D. L. Mount, and R. W. Mwangi. 1994. Reduced susceptibility of *Anopheles gambiae* to permethrin associated with the use of permethrin-impregnated bednets and curtains in Kenya. Med. Vet. Entomol. 8:71-75.

331. Walker, J. 1998. Malaria in a changing world: an Australian perspective. Int. J. Parasitol. 28:947-953.

332. Watts, J. 1999. Malaysia-Japanese encephalitis outbreak leads to military intervention. Lancet353:1075.

333. Weidhaas, D. E., and D. A. Focks. 2000. Management of arthropodborne diseases by vector control, p. 539-563. *In* B. F.

Eldridge and J. D. Edman (ed.), Medical entomology: a textbook on public health and veterinary problems caused by arthropods. Kluwer Academic Publishers, Dordrecht, The Netherlands.

334. Weihe, W. H. 1991. Human well-being, diseases, and climate, p. 352-359. *In* J. Jager and H. L. Ferguson (ed.), Climate change: science, impacts and policy. Proceedings of the Second World Climate Conference. Cambridge University Press, Cambridge, United Kingdom.

335. Weintraub, P. 2001. The bitter feud over LYMErix. Big pharma takes on the wrong little osp. [Online.] http://news.bmn.com/hmsbeagle/106/notes/feature3.

336. Weintraub, P. 2001. Tick menagerie [Online.] http://news.bmn.com/hmsbeagle/115/notes/feature2.

337. Wellde, B. T., D. A. Chumo, D. Waema, and M. J. Reardon. 1989. A history of sleeping sickness in Kenya. Ann. Trop. Med. Parasitol. 83(Suppl. 1):1-11.

338. Wernsdorfer, W. H. 1991. The development and spread of drug-resistant malaria. Parasitol. Today7:297-303.

339. Wernsdorfer, W. H. 1994. Epidemiology of drug resistance in malaria. Acta Trop. 56:143-156.

340. Wernsdorfer, W. H., and D. Payne. 1991. The dynamics of drug resistance in *Plasmodium falciparum.* Pharmacol. Ther. 50:95-121.

341. Wery, M., and M. Coosemans. 1980. Drug resistance in malaria. Ann. Soc. Belge Med. Trop.60:137-162.

342. Whitby, M. 1997. Drug resistant *Plasmodium vivax* malaria. J. Antimicrob. Chemother. 40:749-752.

343. White, G. B. 1989. Malaria p. 1-22. *In* Geographical distribution of arthropod-borne diseases and their principal vectors. World Health Organization, Geneva, Switzerland.

344. White, N. J. 1998. Drug resistance in malaria. Br. Med. Bull. 54:703-715.

345. Wigley, T. M. L. 1985. Impact of extreme events. Nature 316:106-107.

346. Wilson, M. E. 1995. Travel and the emergence of infectious diseases. Emerg. Infect. Dis. 1:39-46.

347. Woodward, A., S. Hales, and P. Weinstein. 1998. Climate change and human health in the Asia Pacific region: who will be the most vulnerable? Climate Res. 11:31-38.

348. World Health Organization. 1986. Resistance of vectors and reservoirs of disease to pesticides. 10th report of the WHO Expert Committee on Vector Biology and Control. WHO Tech. Rep. Se. 737:1-87.

349. World Health Organization. 1990. Potential health effects of climatic change. WHO report WHO/PEP/90/10. World Health Organization, Geneva, Switzerland.

350. World Health Organization. 2001. Global water supply and sanitation assessment 2000 report. 1. Water supply statistics. 2. Water resources development. 3. Sanitation statistics. I. WHO/ UNICEF Joint Monitoring Programme for Water Supply and Sanitation. World Health Organization and UNICEF, Geneva, Switzerland.

351. World Resources Institute. 1996. World resources: a guide to the global environment. The urban environment. 1996-97. World Resources Institute, Washington, D.C.

352. Wu, N., L. X. Qin, G. H. Liao, W. M. Zhou, W. K. Geng, Y. M. Shi, Y. Tan, and K. R. Zhao.1993. Field evaluation of bednets impregnated with deltamethrin for malaria control. Southeast Asian J. Trop. Med. Public Health 24:664-671.

353. Wu, Y. C., Y. S. Huang, L. J. Chien, T. L. Lin, Y. Y. Yueh, W. L. Tseng, K. J. Chang, and G. R. Wang. 1999. The epidemiology of Japanese encephalitis on Taiwan during 1966-1997. Am. J. Trop. Med. Hyg. 61:78-84.

354. Ye-ebiyo, Y., R. J. Pollack, and A. Spielman. 2000. Enhanced development in nature of larval*Anopheles arabiensis* mosquitoes feeding on maize pollen. Am. J. Trop. Med. Hyg. 63:90-93.

355. Yu, Z. N., and L. S. Yu. 1990. Large-scale field evaluations of larvicidal preparation of *Bacillus thuringiensis* H-14 for mosquito control in town and rural environment in China. Bull. Soc. Vector Ecol.15:189-195.

356. Zulueta, D. J., C. D. Ramsdale, and M. Coluzzi. 1975. Receptivity to malaria in Europe. Bull. W. H. O. 52:109-111.

Chapter 2

Plant Viruses Alter Insect Behavior to Enhance their Spread

Laura L. Ingwell,[1] Sanford D. Eigenbrode,[1] and Nilsa A. Bosque-Pérez[a,1]

[1]Department of Plant, Soil, and Entomological Sciences, P.O. Box 442339, University of Idaho, Moscow, ID 83844-2339, USA

ABSTRACT

Pathogenic and parasitic organisms interact with their hosts on a variety of cellular and organismal levels that potentially cause changes in host behavior leading to enhanced transmission[1,2,3,4,5]. This phenomenon led to the emergence of the "Host Manipulation Hypothesis" (HMH)[6]. The HMH and its synonyms the adaptive manipulation[7] and behavioral manipulation[8] hypotheses posit that natural selection on the parasite or pathogen has favored the capacity to elicit host behavior that enhances their transmission. Although examination of the HMH has progressed from descriptive studies to investigations of the mechanisms through which parasites affect host behavior and their consequences for parasite spread[9,10], the field remains predominantly focused on animal pathosystems.

Pathogens or parasites can influence the behavior not only of their primary hosts, but also of their vectors. Arthropods are important vectors of both animal and plant pathogens, transmitting thousands of species of pathogens, including viruses, bacteria, phytoplasmas, trypanosomes and Plasmodia[2,11]. The effects of pathogens on vector biology and behavior have been documented in several pathosystems, including those associated with important human diseases such as malaria, leishmaniasis and sleeping sickness[2,5]. The observed changes in vector behavior include those related to pathogen transmission. For example, mosquitoes infected with the malaria parasite exhibit increased biting frequency and increased attraction to humans infected with the gametocytes of the parasite compared to noninfected humans[1,3].

In contrast to animal pathosystems, plant pathosystems have been less well studied for evidence of host or vector manipulation by pathogens[12]. While animal pathogens can alter the behavior of both hosts and vectors in ways that increase frequency of host-host or host-vector encounters[2,4,5], in plant pathosystems the host is sessile, so the potential for behavioral manipulation is restricted to the vector, the mobile component in these systems. Furthermore, unlike animal pathogens most plant pathogens, including the majority of plant viruses, do not replicate within the vector, so these vectors are not pathogen hosts, *sensu stricto*.

We previously demonstrated that *Barley yellow dwarf virus* (BYDV) infecting wheat and *Potato leafroll virus* (PLRV) infecting potato indirectly induce changes in the host selection behavior of their respective principal aphid vectors, *Rhopalosiphum padi* and *Myzus persicae*[13,14,15,16]. We also have shown that plants infected with these viruses have altered volatile organic compound profiles that elicit greater settling of or arrestment by their noninfective vectors[13,14,16,17]. Luteoviruses (viruses in the family Luteoviridae), including BYDV and PLRV are persistently transmitted. They are ingested and pass through the midgut or hindgut into the hemocoel, eventually associating with the accessory salivary glands of the vector[18]. These viruses rely almost exclusively on insect vectors for transmission and require sustained feeding by a vector for their successful acquisition and transmission[19]. After acquisition, the insect remains a vector for life. Although they do not replicate within the vector, persistently-transmitted viruses interact with the vector at the cellular level during movement among tissues and organs[20], with the potential to directly alter vector physiology and behavior.

Preferential settling by vectors onto infected plants, as occurs for BYDV and PLRV, could contribute to enhanced pathogen spread. Models indicate that a preference for infected plants will accelerate pathogen spread, but only when infected plants are rare, not when they are prevalent in a plant population[21]. Conditional vector preference, however, could enhance pathogen spread regardless of the prevalence of infected plants. Specifically, if noninfective vectors prefer infected plants thereby promoting acquisition, and infective vectors prefer noninfected hosts promoting transmission, overall spread would be accelerated. The possibility of conditional vector preference for pathogen-infected plants has hardly been examined despite its potential importance. Changes in vector behavior that occur after feeding on virus-infected plants could be attributed to direct effects of the acquired virus on the vector, but such direct effects are difficult to distinguish from indirect ones associated with feeding on virus-infected plants. Here we test the hypothesis that a change in host plant selection behavior by an insect vector is the direct result of virus acquisition by the vector. We provide the first experimental evidence that acquisition of a plant virus through *in vitro* feeding, which eliminates indirect effects of an infected plant host, directly alters subsequent host plant selection behavior of its vector. These findings enhance our understanding of how plant viruses spread to new hosts, with implications for disease and vector management.

RESULTS

We first examined host plant selection preferences of infective (reared on virus-infected plants) and noninfective (reared on virus-free plants) *R. padi.* In dual-choice bioassays using an arena in a platform[22] (Fig. 1) infective or noninfective insects were allowed to select BYDV-infected or sham-inoculated wheat plants as their hosts. Sham-inoculated plants are noninfected plants previously fed upon by noninfective aphids and are utilized in our bioassays to account for potential aphid feeding-induced changes in plants[23]. Infective and noninfective insects were tested simultaneously in separate platforms. Each platform contained a leaf from each plant treatment, BYDV-infected or sham-inoculated, onto which aphids could settle and feed throughout the bioassay. We compared the responses of infective and noninfective aphids by examining the proportion of aphids that settled on BYDV-infected or sham-inoculated plants every 12 h for 72 h. A 72-h time period is sufficiently long for virus acquisition by noninfective aphids to occur when exposed to BYDV-infected plants, while a 12-h time period is unlikely to result in noninfective aphids becoming infective due to the latent period of the virus[24,25]. We therefore compared aphid responses at the first 12-h observation, and after 72 h when responses were pooled over time. The 12-h observation occurs before additional virus acquisition was expected while the 72-h comparison is more powerful statistically and incorporates a time period more meaningful for transmission dynamics in the field. Noninfective aphids significantly preferred to settle on BYDV-infected wheat compared to infective aphids at the first 12-h observation point (generalized linear model; $\chi^2 = 3.12$, $p = 0.0774$, marginally significant) (Fig. 2a,Supplementary Table S1a) and throughout the duration of the experiment (generalized linear model; $\chi^2 = 19.33$, $p < 0.0001$) (Fig. 2b, Supplementary Table S2a). In contrast, infective aphids significantly preferred to settle on sham-inoculated wheat compared to noninfective aphids at the first observation point (generalized linear model; $\chi^2 = 3.12$, $p = 0.0774$, marginally significant) (Fig. 2a, Supplementary Table S1b) and throughout the duration of the experiment (generalized linear model; $\chi^2 = 20.14$, $p < 0.0001$) (Fig. 2b,Supplementary Table S2b). The time at which the observations were made was not a significant factor when examining the response to BYDV-infected wheat (generalized linear model; $\chi^2 = 4.96$, $p = 0.4203$) (Supplementary Table S2a) or sham-inoculated wheat (generalized linear model; $\chi^2 = 2.15$, $p = 0.8282$) (Supplementary Table S2b). The results suggest that virus acquisition changes vector host plant selection behavior to favor noninfected plants rather than infected plants.

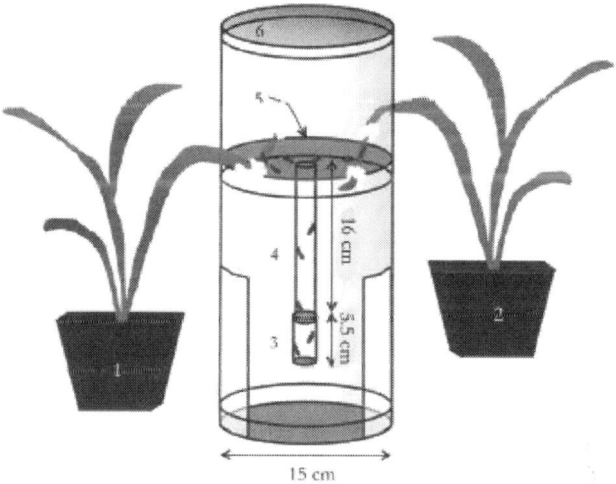

Figure 1: Diagrammatic illustration of the dual-choice bioassay arena used in experiments.

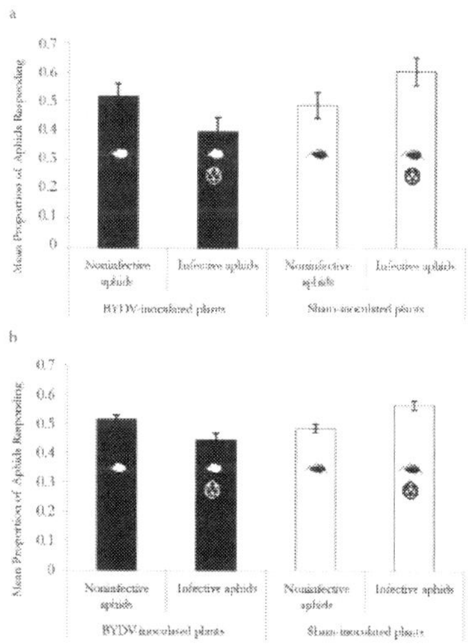

Figure 2: Mean proportion of infective and noninfective aphids responding in a dual-choice bioassay examining host plant selection preferences to BYDV-infected and sham-inoculated wheat (noninfected plants previously fed upon by noninfective aphids) as influenced by indirect effects of feeding on virus-infected plants.

Each replicate (n = 12) consisted of one arena with noninfective aphids paired with one arena of infective aphids, randomized in a complete block design over time. Statistical analyses compared the response of infective and noninfective aphids to the BYDV-infected or sham-inoculated plant treatment. (a) Aphid responses at the first observation point made 12 h after release. Noninfective aphids preferred BYDV-infected wheat compared to infective aphids (generalized linear model; $\chi^2 = 3.12$, $p = 0.0774$, marginally significant). Infective aphids preferred sham-inoculated plants compared to noninfective aphids (generalized linear model; $\chi^2 = 3.12$, $p = 0.0774$, marginally significant). (b) Aphid responses pooled over time (6 observations). Noninfective aphids significantly preferred BYDV-infected wheat compared to infective aphids (generalized linear model; $\chi^2 = 19.33$, $p < 0.0001$). Infective aphids significantly preferred sham-inoculated plants compared to noninfective aphids (generalized linear model; $\chi^2 = 20.14$, $p < 0.0001$). Data are means ± SE following logit transformation. Errors bars are s.e.m.

These behavioral changes could result either from direct effects of acquired virus particles on the aphid, or from insect exposure to cues from virus-infected host plants. To isolate potential direct effects of virus acquisition on the vector we conducted a similar experiment using *in vitro* feeding to obtain infective and noninfective aphids. Insects were first reared on virus-free plants and subsequently transferred to membrane feeding chambers[26] (Fig. 3) that contained artificial phloem with either purified BYDV particles or no virus. Host plant selection preferences of infective and noninfective insects were examined every 12 h for 72 h using an arena as described above. Observation time was not a significant factor when examining the response to BYDV-infected wheat (generalized linear model; $\chi^2 = 2.41$, $p = 0.7906$) (Supplementary Table S2c) or sham-inoculated wheat (generalized linear model; $\chi^2 = 3.66$, $p = 0.5995$) (Supplementary Table S2d). We present the results of the aphid responses at the first 12-h observation point as well as the responses pooled over time. Noninfective aphids significantly preferred BYDV-infected wheat compared to infective aphids at the first observation point (generalized linear model; $\chi^2 = 4.24$, $p = 0.0394$) (Fig. 4a, Supplementary Table S1c), and throughout the duration of the experiment (generalized linear model; $\chi^2 = 16.18$, $p < 0.0001$) (Fig. 4b, Supplementary Table S2c). Similar to the patterns obtained using aphids that acquired virus from plants, infective aphids significantly preferred sham-inoculated wheat compared to noninfective aphids at the first observation point (generalized linear model; $\chi^2 = 5.64$, $p = 0.0176$) (Fig. 4a, Supplementary Table S1d), and throughout the duration of the experiment (generalized linear model; $\chi^2 = 16.32$, $p < 0.0001$) (Fig. 4b,Supplementary Table S2d).

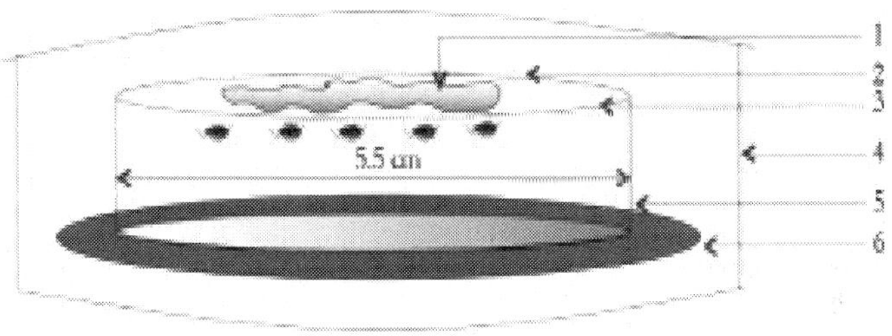

Figure 3: Diagrammatic illustration of a membrane feeding chamber.

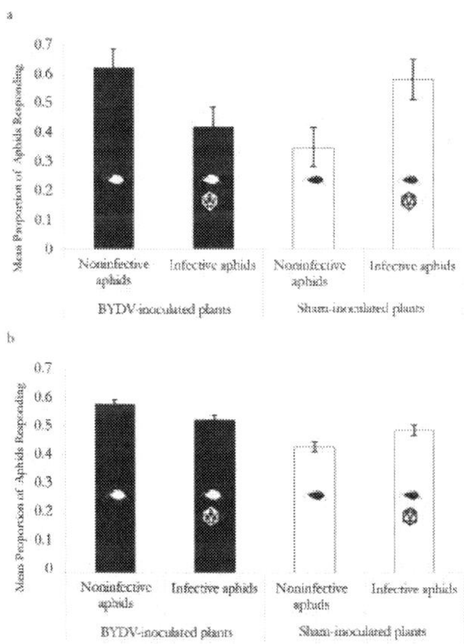

Figure 4: Mean proportion of infective and noninfective aphids responding in a dual-choice bioassay examining host plant selection preferences to BYDV-infected and sham-inoculated wheat plants as influenced by direct effects of virus acquisition following membrane feeding.

Each replicate (n = 12) consisted of one arena with noninfective aphids paired with one arena of infective aphids, randomized in a complete block design over time. Statistical analyses compared the response of infective and noninfective aphids to the BYDV-infected or sham-inoculated plant treatment. (a) Aphid responses at the first observation point made 12 h after release. Noninfective aphids significantly preferred BYDV-infected wheat compared to infective aphids (generalized linear model; $\chi^2 = 4.24$, $p = 0.0394$). Infective aphids significantly preferred sham-inoculated wheat compared to noninfective aphids (generalized linear model; $\chi^2 = 5.64$, $p = 0.0176$). (b) Aphid responses pooled over time (6 observations). Noninfective aphids significantly preferred BYDV-infected wheat compared to infective aphids (generalized linear model; $\chi^2 = 16.18$, $p < 0.0001$). Infective aphids significantly preferred sham-inoculated wheat compared to noninfective aphids (generalized linear model; $\chi^2 = 16.32$, $p < 0.0001$). Data are means ± SE following logit transformation. Errors bars are s.e.m.

Results from RT-PCR tests verified that our inoculation and acquisition methods were successful. All plants used in the dual choice tests were tested via RT-PCR immediately after the bioassays. Sham-inoculated plants remained virus-free and infected plants remained BYDV-infected, indicating that during the bioassays (72 h) the plant treatments were stable, despite being exposed to potential feeding by infective aphids. Tests of aphids using RT-PCR revealed that infective aphids remained BYDV-infective subsequent to the bioassay, while 25% of noninfective aphids acquired BYDV during the 72-h bioassay when they had access to BYDV-infected plants in the bioassay arena. Although the bioassay design unavoidably results in virus acquisition by some noninfective aphids, the result is a more conservative test of our hypothesis since within-bioassay virus acquisition should tend to diminish detectable differences between the aphid treatments. Furthermore, the aphid responses after 72 h in the bioassay arena are consistent with the preferences observed after 12 h, during which time noninfective aphids almost certainly remained noninfective[24,25]. The lack of BYDV infection of the sham-inoculated plants after 72 h of exposure to initially noninfective aphids in an arena with BYDV-infected plants also indicates that these aphids did not become infective during the bioassay.

DISCUSSION

Assays utilizing membrane-fed infective aphids yielded results similar to those obtained using aphids that acquired BYDV from infected plants, confirming our hypothesis that changes in host plant selection by the vector are mediated by direct effects of virus acquisition, rather than indirect effects of feeding on infected host plants. Direct effects of virus acquisition on the vector host plant selection behavior in a manner that will promote the spread of the virus is consistent with an evolved strategy in the pathogen of manipulation of its vector. We propose the "Vector Manipulation Hypothesis" (VMH) to explain the evolution of strategies in plant pathogens that enhance their spread to new hosts through their effects on mobile vectors. Selection should favor both direct and indirect mechanisms producing such effects. Vectors that feed on virus-infected host plants exhibit faster growth rates, higher fecundity, greater longevity and/or enhanced production of alate forms of the vector[27,28,29,30,31,32,33], which can lead to increased virus spread and are typically attributed to indirect effects of virus infection on host quality. Virus- infection-mediated alterations of the host plant's secondary chemistry can affect vector behavior. Evidence for such indirect effects of pathogens on vector behavior continues to accumulate and is consistent with the VMH[13,14,15,16,34,35,36]. We provide the first evidence for a direct effect of a plant virus on its vector consistent with the VMH, specifically by influencing the vector's host selection behavior to maximize pathogen spread. In our model pathosystem, noninfective vectors are attracted to virus-infected host plants, which is beneficial as it increases vector fitness[23]. After virus acquisition virus vector preferences shift to noninfected hosts, maximizing pathogen transmission potential by promoting the movement of infective aphids onto noninfected host plants. Our results offer a specific example of a plant virus directly manipulating its vector in a manner that is likely to maximize pathogen transmission potential between hosts, providing support for the VMH.

Results supportive of the VMH also have been reported from work on nonpersistently-transmitted plant viruses examining effects on noninfective vector behavior. Non-persistently transmitted viruses bind transiently to insect mouthparts[20] and interactions in these pathosystems are likely limited to indirect effects on vectors. Recent work with the non-persistently transmitted *Cucumber mosaic virus* (CMV), which is acquired rapidly during aphid feeding and benefits from rapid vector dispersal, showed that aphids are initially attracted to volatile organic compounds from CMV-infected squash plants, but subsequently prefer to colonize noninfected plants[34]. Attraction to CMV-infected plants appears to be mediated by their increased emission of volatile organic compounds similar to those from healthy plants. Since CMV can be acquired within a few seconds by an aphid probing on an infected plant, these behaviors can act to enhance virus spread[34] and illustrate manipulation of an insect vector by the virus. Interestingly, in addition to manipulating vectors, CMV also may manipulate defensive signaling pathways in plants that could result in enhanced vector survival[37].

Our findings highlight the ecological and evolutionary significance of vector manipulation by pathogens and parasites. Effects like those we document for a plant virus, consistent with the VMH, may be widespread since direct and indirect mechanisms that enhance the spread of plant viruses should be favored by natural selection. Furthermore, similar patterns in behavioral changes among vectors of other plant pathogens, such as bacteria and phytoplasmas, which are limited to sessile plant hosts, might also occur. Although our results do not address the specific cellular and molecular mechanisms mediating direct plant virus effects on their vectors, they offer strong quantitative evidence for the VMH, providing a foundation upon which to base further studies of pathogen-mediated manipulation of their vectors and the identification of underlying mechanisms. The evolution of host-vector interactions has recently been suggested to be in part, mediated by virus transmission mechanisms[38] underlying the importance of studying such interactions. Greater understanding of host plant-virus-vector interactions has the potential to improve management of vectors and plant diseases in agricultural settings and enhance our understanding of the role plant viruses play in natural settings[39], including their effects on ecological processes at the community and ecosystem levels[38].

Virus Maintenance and Insect Rearing

The model system for our study was the wheat-*R. padi*-BYDV pathosystem. BYDV is exclusively transmitted among *Poaceae* hosts by aphids, including *R. padi,* in a persistent circulative manner and the virus does not replicate within the vector[40,41]. A Washington State isolate of BYDV-PAV maintained by mass transfer of *R. padi,* the bird-cherry oat aphid, on cv. Sprinter barley plants was used to inoculate wheat plants[23]. *Rophalosiphum padi* is the most efficient vector of the BYDV PAV serotype[40]. Both the virus and an infective colony of *R. padi* are maintained at the University of Idaho (UI) Agricultural Biotechnology Laboratory. Aphids were originally obtained from Washington State University and are kept virus-infective through serial transfer[23]. A noninfective colony of *R. padi* was derived from the infective colony and is maintained at the UI Manis Entomological Laboratory. Infective and noninfective aphid colonies are reared on Sprinter barley in environmental chambers (20±2°C; 16 h light photoperiod). Aphids from each colony are examined on a regular basis using RT-PCR tests to ensure that the respective colonies remain virus-free or BYDV-PAV infected (see Supplementary Methods).

Plant Rearing and Inoculation

Winter wheat cv. Lambert was used for all bioassays. Seeds were planted at a density of one per pot in 10.2 cm^2 plastic pots. Pots were filled with a mixture of 6:1:0.02 ratio of Sunshine mix #1: sand: Osmocote®, placed on trays in an environmental chamber (20±2°C; 16 h light photoperiod) and bottom watered. After germination, plants were fertilized using a soluble N-P-K fertilizer (15:30:15) biweekly.

Plant inoculations were done at the 2–3 leaf stage (14–16 days after planting). BYDV-infected plants were obtained by caging 10 adult aphids from the infective colony per plant for a 72 h virus inoculation access period[23]. Cages consisted of a 4-cm long piece of 23 mm dialysis tubing (14.6 mm D, Spectra/Por®) sealed on both ends with a foam stopper. Since BYDV is exclusively insect-transmitted, all BYDV-infected plants are fed-upon by aphids. Insect feeding may induce resistance in plants and potentially affect the response of insects subsequently exposed to such plants[23]. To account for such potential confounding effects sham-inoculated plants were produced and served as virus-free controls. Sham-inoculation was conducted by caging 10 adult aphids from the noninfective colony per plant for 72 h[23].

Infective and Noninfective Aphid Handling

To examine effects of plant virus acquisition from infected plants on host selection behavior, apterous aphids (fourth nymphal stage to early adults) originated from the respective infective and noninfective colonies. Previous research in this pathosystem has focused on aptera[14,15,23,25]. While alates are important vectors for long-distance dispersal events, apterous aphid behavior can be used to predict severity of epidemics within a field once the virus and vector are established[21]. Future studies will examine alate behavior in response to BYDV-infection. Aphids for each treatment were individually removed from plants using a number 3 camel's hair brush and placed into vials (2.3x5.5 cm; DxH). Fifty aphids were placed per vial. Vials were capped and aphids starved for one hour prior to the bioassay. A total of 600 aphids of each treatment (infective and noninfective) were tested among 12 replicates of the dual-choice bioassay described below.

Aphids for the experiment to assess the direct effects of virus acquisition originated from the noninfective *R. padi* colony. Tests were conducted using membrane feeding chambers modified after Trebicki et al.[26] (Fig. 3), containing artificial diet as described by Ramsey and Jander[42]. After preparation the diet solution was sieved using a bacteria-proof filter (0.2 µm cellulose acetate). To set up membrane feeding chambers, the bottom halves of glass petri dishes (5.5 cm; D) were first sterilized under UV light for 10 min. Aphids (fourth nymphal stage to early adults) were collected from colony plants using a number 3 camel's hair brush and placed in the petri dishes, 35 aphids per dish. Parafilm®, sterilized with 70% ethanol, was used as membrane material. After placing the aphids in the petri dish, the dish was immediately sealed with a layer of Parafilm® stretched tightly across the dish top. After all dishes were sealed with the first Parafilm® layer 100 µL of artificial diet was pipetted onto the membrane and a second layer of Parafilm® was stretched tightly to sandwich the diet[26]. The diet was then spread across the surface of the membrane by applying pressure to the top layer with a fingertip. Dishes were placed in a tray with moistened filter paper and the tray covered with cling wrap and placed inside an environmental chamber (20±2°C; 16 h light photoperiod) for 24 h. Non-infective aphids were fed on an amino acid and sucrose diet solution. To obtain infective aphids, insects were fed on the same diet solution that was infused with purified BYDV at a concentration of 100 μg/mL. Virus was purified following a method adapted from Hammond et al.[43], and obtained from Dr. Alex Karasev, UI PSES Department. After a 24-h feeding period, aphids were transferred into a vial as described above, starved for one hour and released in a bioassay arena (see below). A total of 840 aphids of each treatment were placed in membrane chambers, 600 were tested among 12 replicates of the dual-choice bioassay described below. The remaining aphids were stored in 70% ethanol at −20°C to verify their status (infective vs. noninfective). Virus-infection status of plants and aphids was determined using RT-PCR

We recognize that purified virus may contain phloem proteins. Such proteins have been reported to occur *in vivo*, and were recently reported to play a role in virus transmission[44]. Additional studies are required to determine if a virus-plant protein complex is present *in vitro* and if such a complex could contribute to behavioral changes in vectors.

Bioassays to Assess Aphid Preferences

Dual-choice bioassays were performed 40–46 days after plant inoculation, utilizing an arena adapted from Castle et al.[22] (Fig. 1). The base of the arena was glued into the lid portion of a 15 cm D petri dish. The platform of the arena consisted of the inverted bottom of the petri dish with a 2.5 cm D hole cut in the center. A clear plastic tube (16x2.5 cm; LxD) was inserted into the bottom of the dish and secured with glue. The arena was wrapped in a heavy weight mylar frame (30.5x46.1 cm; WxL) to add stability to the structure. Holes were cut in the mylar, four (2 cm; D) equally spaced around the top and two (8x8 cm^2) in the bottom to access the arena. One leaf still attached to the plant from each treatment (BYDV-infected and sham-inoculated) was inserted through holes on either side of the arena and held in place with a cotton seal. A vial (5.5x2.5 cm; LxD) containing 50 aphids, starved for one hour, was inserted into the bottom of the plastic tube leading to the arena. Apterous infective and noninfective aphids were released simultaneously into separate arenas. Aphids crawled up the tube and emerged onto a platform with one leaf from each treatment on either side (3 cm on either side of where aphids entered the arena). Aphids were able to settle on, feed and move between the two leaves. Aphids were released at the start of a dark period and monitored every 12 h (alternating dark and light times) for a 72-h period. The number of aphids on each leaf was counted at each observation, using a red light when monitoring during the dark cycles[14]. Assays were conducted in a growth room (14±3°C; 12 h light photoperiod). One replicate consisted of an arena containing infective aphids paired with another arena containing noninfective aphids, constituting a single block. Twelve replicates were performed across time in a randomized complete block repeated measures design.

Data Analysis

The proportion of aphids responding to either the BYDV-infected or sham-inoculated plant treatment was compared using a generalized linear model assuming a binomial distribution and logit transformation (SAS, Proc Genmod). Logit transformation was performed to stabilize the variance and meet the assumptions of normality for analysis. Aphids not located on either plant leaf in an arena were considered non responsive and excluded from the analysis. The partial model examined the main effects of replicate (block; n = 12) and aphid treatment (infective or noninfective). The analysis was conducted separately four times, once for each plant treatment (BYDV-infected or sham-inoculated) for the indirect effects experiment (aphids reared on noninfected plants or virus-infected plants) (Supplemental Table S1a-b) and the direct effects experiment (aphids fed on membrane chambers with or without virus) (Supplemental Table S1c-d). The full model examined the main effects of replicate, aphid treatment and time (n = 6) assuming a compound symmetric correlation. The time variable examined observations made at 12, 24, 36, 48, 60 and 72 h after release using a repeated measures design. Observations made at 12, 36, and 60 h were recorded in the dark. Light and dark observations were examined with the model separately and no significant interactions were observed, thus results were pooled in the overall analysis (Supplemental Table S2). All statistical tests (likelihood ratio χ^2) were carried out at the alpha = 0.05 level of significance.

AUTHOR CONTRIBUTIONS

N.B.P., L.L.I., and S.D.E. conceived and designed research; L.L.I. performed research and analyzed data; L.L.I., N.B.P., and S.D.E. interpreted results and wrote the paper.

ACKNOWLEDGMENTS

Our research was supported by USDA-AFRI award 2009-6510405730. We thank A. Busch, S. Eid, E. Kmieciak, J. Knerr, A. Poplawsky, P. Trębicki, and L. Unger for technical assistance, A. Karasev for providing purified BYDV, and B. Price for input on statistical analysis.

REFERENCES

1. Koella J. C., Sorensen F. L. & Anderson R. A. The malaria parasite, *Plasmodium falciparum*, increases the frequency of multiple feeding of its mosquito vector, *Anopheles gambiae*. Proc. R. Soc. Lond. Ser. B. Biol. Sci. 265, 763–768 (1998).
2. Hurd H. Manipulation of medically important insect vectors by their parasites. Annu. Rev. Entomol.48, 141–161 (2003).
3. Lacroix R., Mukabana W. R., Gouagna L. C. & Koella J. C. Malaria infection increases attractiveness of humans to mosquitoes. PLoS Biol 3, e298 (2005).
4. Vyas A., Kim S. K., Giacomini N., Boothroyd J. C. & Sapolsky R. M. Behavioral changes induced by Toxoplasma infection of rodents are highly specific to aversion of cat odors. Proc. Natl. Acad. Sci. U. S. A. 104, 6442–6447 (2007).
5. Lefèvre T. & Thomas F. Behind the scene, something else is pulling the strings: Emphasizing parasitic manipulation in vector-borne diseases. Infect., Genet. Evol. 8, 504–519 (2008).
6. Holmes J. C. & Bethel W. M. in Behavioral Aspects of Parasite Transmission (eds Canning E. U., & Wright C. A.) 123–149.149– (Academic Press, 1972).

7. Poulin R. Manipulation of host behaviour by parasites: a weakening paradigm? Proc. R. Soc. Lond. Ser. B. Biol. Sci. 267, 787–792 (2000).

8. Thomas F., Adamo S. & Moore J. Parasitic manipulation: where are we and where should we go?Behav. Processes 68, 185–199 (2005).

9. Poulin R. "Adaptive" changes in the behaviour of parasitized animals: A critical review. Int. J. Parasitol. 25, 1371–1383 (1995).

10. Moore J. & Gotelli N. J. in Parasitism and Host Behaviour (eds Barnard C. J., & Behnke J. M.) 193–233 (Taylor & Francis Ltd., 1990).

11. Gray S. M. & Banerjee N. Mechanisms of arthropod transmission of plant and animal viruses.Microbiol. Mol. Biol. Rev. 63, 128–148 (1999).

12. Bosque-Pérez N. A. & Eigenbrode S. The influence of virus-induced changes in plants on aphid vectors: Insights from luteovirus pathosystems. Virus Res 159, 201–205 (2011).

13. Eigenbrode S. D., Ding H., Shiel P. & Berger P. H. Volatiles from potato plants infected with potato leafroll virus attract and arrest the virus vector, *Myzus persicae* (Homoptera: Aphididae).Proc. R. Soc. Lond. Ser. B. Biol. Sci. 269, 455–460 (2002).

14. Jiménez-Martínez E. S. *et al.* Volatile cues influence the response of *Rhopalosiphum padi*(Homoptera: Aphididae) to *Barley yellow dwarf virus*-infected transgenic and untransformed wheat. Environ. Entomol. 33, 1207–1216 (2004).

15. Medina Ortega K. J., Bosque-Pérez N. A., Ngumbi E., Jiménez-Martínez E. S. & Eigenbrode S. D.*Rhopalosiphum padi* (Hemiptera: Aphididae) responses to volatile cues from *Barley yellow dwarf virus*-infected wheat. Environ. Entomol. 38, 836–845 (2009).

16. Werner B. J., Mowry T. M., Bosque-Pérez N. A., Ding H. & Eigenbrode S. Changes in green peach aphid responses to potato leafroll virus-induced volatiles emitted during disease progression.Environ. Entomol. 38, 1429–1438 (2009).

17. Ngumbi E., Eigenbrode S. D., Bosque-Pérez N. A., Ding H. & Rodriguez A. *Myzus persicae* is arrested more by blends than by individual compounds elevated in headspace of PLRV-infected potato. J. Chem. Ecol. 33, 1733–1747 (2007).

18. Gildow F. Evidence for receptor-mediated endocytosis regulating luteovirus acquisition by aphids.Phytopathology 83, 270–277 (1993).
19. Sylvester E. S. Circulative and propagative virus transmission by aphids. Annu. Rev. Entomol. 25, 257–286 (1980).
20. Nault L. R. Arthropod transmission of plant viruses: A new synthesis. Ann. Entomol. Soc. Am. 90, 521–541 (1997).
21. McElhany P., Real L. A. & Power A. G. Vector preference and disease dynamics: A study of*Barley yellow dwarf virus*. Ecology 76, 444–457 (1995).
22. Castle S. J., Mowry T. M. & Berger P. H. Differential settling by *Myzus persicae* (Homoptera: Aphididae) on various virus infected host plants. Ann. Entomol. Soc. Am. 91, 661–667 (1998).
23. Jiménez-Martínez E. S., Bosque-Pérez N. A., Berger P. H. & Zemetra R. S. Life history of the bird cherry-oat aphid, *Rhopalosiphum padi* (Homoptera: Aphididae) on transgenic and untransformed wheat challenged with *Barley yellow dwarf virus*. J. Econ. Entomol. 97, 203–212 (2004).
24. Gray S. M., Power A. G., Smith D. M., Seaman A. J. & Altman N. S. Aphid transmission of *Barley yellow dwarf virus*: acquisition access periods and virus concentration requirements. Phytopathology81, 539–545 (1991).
25. Jiménez- Martínez E. S. & Bosque-Pérez N. A. Variation in *Barley yellow dwarf virus* transmission efficiency by *Rhopalosiphum padi* (Homoptera: Aphididae) after acquisition from transgenic and non-transformed wheat genotypes. J. Econ. Entomol. 97, 1790–1796 (2004).
26. Trębicki P., Harding R. M. & Powell K. S. Anti-metabolic effects of *Galanthus nivalis* agglutinin and wheat germ agglutinin on nymphal stages of the common brown leafhopper using a novel artificial diet system. Entomol. Exp. Appl. 131, 99–105 (2009).
27. Kennedy J. S. Benefits to aphids from feeding on galled and virus-infected leaves. Nature 168, 825–826 (1951).
28. Baker P. F. Aphid behavior on healthy and on yellow virus infected sugar beet. Ann. Appl. Biol.48, 384–391 (1960).
29. Gildow F. E. Increased production of alatae by aphids reared on

oats infected with *Barley yellow dwarf virus*. Ann. Entomol. Soc. Am. 73, 343–347 (1980).

30. Hodgson C. J. Effects of infection with the cabbage black ringspot strain of turnip mosaic virus on turnip as a host to *Myzus persicae* and *Brevicoryne brassicae*. Ann. Appl. Biol. 98, 1–14 (1981).
31. Ajayi O. & Dewar A. M. The effect of *Barley yellow dwarf virus* on field populations of the cereal aphids, *Sitobion avenae* and *Metopolophium dirhodum*. Ann. Appl. Biol. 103, 1–11 (1983).
32. Araya J. E. & Foster J. E. Laboratory study on the effects of *Barley yellow dwarf virus* on the life cycle of *Rhopalosiphum padi* (L.). J. Plant Dis. Protect. 94, 195–198 (1987).
33. Fereres A. & Moreno A. Behavioural aspects influencing plant virus transmission by homopteran insects. Virus Res. 141, 158–168 (2009).
34. Mauck K. E., De Moraes C. M. & Mescher M. C. Deceptive chemical signals induced by a plant virus attract insect vectors to inferior hosts. Proc. Natl. Acad. Sci. U. S. A. 107, 3600–3605 (2010).
35. Mann R. S. *et al.* Induced release of a plant-defense volatile 'deceptively' attracts insect vectors to plants infected with a bacterial pathogen. PLoS Path. 8, e1002610 (2012).
36. Stafford C. A., Walker G. P. & Ullman D. E. Infection with a plant virus modifies vector feeding behavior. Proc. Natl. Acad. Sci. U. S. A. 108, 9350–9355 (2011).
37. Ziebell H. *et al.* Cucumber mosaic virus and its 2b RNA silencing suppressor modify plant-aphid interactions in tobacco. Sci. Rep. 1, 187; 10.1038/srep00187 (2011)
38. Mauck K. E., Bosque-Pérez N. A., Eigenbrode S., De Moraes C. M. & Mescher M. C. Transmission mechanisms shape pathogen effects on host-vector interactions: evidence from plant viruses. Funct. Ecol. 10.1111/j.1365–2435.2012.02026.x. (2012).
39. Malmstrom C., Melcher U. & Bosque-Pérez N. A. The expanding field of plant virus ecology: Historical foundations, knowledge gaps, and research directions. Virus Res. 159, 84–94 (2011).

40. Gildow F. E., Frank J., Bingham D. & Powell C. Barley yellow dwarf viruses in small grains in Pennsylvania: isolate identification, distribution, and vector efficiency. Plant Dis. 71, 922–926 (1987).
41. Power A. G. Virus spread and vector dynamics in genetically diverse plant populations. Ecology72, 232–241 (1991).
42. Ramsey J. S. & Jander G. Testing nicotine tolerance in aphids using an artificial diet experiment.JoVE, e701 (2008).
43. Hammond J., Lister R. M. & Foster J. E. Purification, identity and some properties of an isolate of*Barley yellow dwarf virus* from Indiana. J. Gen. Virol. 64, 667–676 (1983).
44. Bencharki B. *et al.* Phloem protein partners of *Cucurbit aphid borne yellows virus*: Possible involvement of phloem proteins in virus transmission by aphids. Mol. Plant. Microbe Interact. 23, 799–810 (2010).

Chapter 3

Impact of Anthropogenic Environmental Alterations on Vector-Borne Diseases

Neil Vora, MS4

University of California at San Francisco, California

ABSTRACT

The spread of infectious vector-borne diseases involves at least 3 organisms: a parasite, a vector, and a host. Alterations to the natural environment may change the context within which these entities interact, thus potentially affecting vector-borne disease epidemiology. In this review, examples are presented in which human-driven ecological changes may be contributing to the spread of vector-borne diseases. Such changes include deforestation, agriculture and animal husbandry, water control projects, urbanization, loss of biodiversity, introduction of alien species, and climate change. The global environment is currently being degraded at an alarming pace, potentially placing human populations at increasing risk for unnecessary and preventable outbreaks of vector-borne diseases. Further research is needed to improve our ability to predict and prevent emergence and reemergence of vector-borne diseases from environmental alterations.

INTRODUCTION

Over the past several decades, a number of vector-borne diseases have reemerged in locations in which they were declining or have emerged in areas in which the disease was previously not known.[1] Understanding the factors contributing to these alarming observations is vital to preventing further spread of vector-borne diseases. Vector-borne diseases are unique among human diseases because of the extent to which they depend on the natural environment. Ecological alterations directly or indirectly affecting populations of the pathogen, the vector, or the nonhuman hosts of the pathogen may culminate in altered epidemiology of vector-borne diseases afflicting humans.[2]

This paper reviews human-driven ecosystem alterations that may increase the transmission of vector-borne diseases. The term "vector" refers to organisms that transfer a pathogen from one host to another.[3] The environmental disturbances to be discussed include: (1) deforestation, (2) agriculture and animal husbandry, (3) water control projects, (4) urbanization, (5) loss of biodiversity, (6) introduction of alien species, and (7) climate change. These alterations are diverse but are often interrelated.[2] While some have primarily local effects (such as water control projects) and others global (such as climate change), all of these disturbances are exacerbated by a rapidly expanding human population.[4–6]

The inherent complexities of the global environment and infectious disease transmission make predictions regarding the impact of the former on the latter at times uncertain and imprecise.[6] Nonetheless, through an interdisciplinary approach, the major ecological variables and patterns affecting transmission of vector-borne diseases can be identified.[2,4,7,8]

DEFORESTATION

Deforestation may bring about whole-scale ecosystem reconstitution. This in turn may influence vector-borne disease transmission through altered vegetation, introduction of livestock, development of human settlements, and loss of biodiversity. Forest-related activities, such as mining and logging, have been associated with increased exposure to the vectors of yellow fever, malaria, and leishmaniasis.[2,8,9]

Deforestation may create ecological niches favoring proliferation of vectors and parasites.[9] For example, water puddles in deforested areas tend to have lower salinity and acidity than puddles in forests. Such deforested water puddles may be more conducive for the larval development of certain *Anopheles* mosquito species (the vectors of malaria), particularly *A darlingi*, the most effective vector of malaria in the Amazon.[1,2,9]

The blackfly vectors of onchocerciasis found in savannahs preferentially transmit the more severe form of the disease compared with forest blackflies. Reports from several African countries show that the geographical distribution of savannah blackflies has increased after deforestation.[10] Loiasis is another vector-borne disease (transmitted by tabanid flies) in which deforestation has contributed to the emergence of more efficient vector species.[2]

Increased malaria transmission has coincided with deforestation in Africa, Asia, and Latin America.[1,9] In a study of the human biting rate and distribution of *A darlingi* in relation to deforestation and ecological alteration in the Amazon, it was reported that the *A darlingi* biting rate increased in deforested areas compared with predominantly forested areas after controlling for the presence of humans.[11] In another study of *Anopheles* distribution, areas that were both altered and unaltered by human activity were surveyed, and *A darlingi* was found in all of the altered sites but in none of the unaltered sites.[12]

Agriculture and Animal Husbandry

The growing worldwide demand for food has increased the conversion of natural ecosystems into agrarian ones that suit the raising of both plants and animals.[6] The ecosystem disturbances caused by farming may favor vector-borne disease transmission through a variety of mechanisms.

Land cover changes due to agriculture can alter local microclimates. In a study conducted at high altitudes in Uganda, areas in which natural swamp vegetation were replaced by agricultural crops experienced higher temperatures. This microenvironmental change was thought to be a contributing factor to the increased risk for malaria in those cultivated areas.[13]

Animal husbandry may also increase the transmission of some vector-borne diseases. Vector populations may grow with the additional feeding options livestock offer; a larger vector population may in turn result in increased frequency of feeding on humans. Furthermore, farm animals are potential reservoir hosts, thus making pathogens more widespread.[9] When grazing extends into recently altered natural habitats, livestock may contribute to the emergence of vector-borne disease by facilitating the exchange of a pathogen from nonhuman reservoirs to humans.[2,8,9]

Transmission of Japanese encephalitis is increasing in parts of Southeast Asia and the western Pacific, largely because of increased irrigated agriculture (especially rice paddies) and pig husbandry (an important natural host of the virus). Furthermore, breeding sites within human-made structures are deemed more important for the mosquito vectors of Japanese encephalitis than natural sites.[14,15]

Water Control Projects

There are numerous examples of artificial bodies of water contributing to vector and parasite proliferation. Dams and canals form breeding sites for mosquitoes.[2,9] Smaller water impoundments are especially conducive to vector proliferation given the expansive aggregate surface area they occupy and shallow depth they provide for larval breeding.[8]

The emergence of *Plasmodium falciparum* malaria, the most deadly form of malaria, in the Thar Desert of India coincided with the construction of irrigation canals.[1] In addition, while there was just one anopheline mosquito species before the construction of the canals, several anopheline mosquito species have since been established.[16]

In another damaging example, an outbreak of schistosomiasis affecting thousands of people occurred after the construction of the Diama Dam on the Senegal River.[1,2,17] In Egypt, the prevalence of *Schistosoma mansoni* infection nearly doubled in a desert that was altered by construction of irrigation projects. Several factors are thought to have contributed to the increased prevalence of this parasite. The irrigation water originated from the Nile River and may have introduced snail vectors to the irrigated area. Furthermore, some settlers to the irrigated area may have been infected when they arrived and inadvertently contaminated the local water supply due to inadequate treatment of sewage. In contrast, other settlers may have had little or no immunity to schistosomiasis if they were not previously exposed and thus were highly susceptible to infection.[18,19]

Urbanization

Urbanization represents an ecosystem disturbance directly through the conversion of natural habitat into human settlements and indirectly through waste generation. The concentration of new urbanization in developing countries, which often lack the infrastructure to support a large, dense urban population, will present many challenges to public health.[1,4,20]

Vector-borne diseases may flourish with rapid urbanization. Expanding cities encroaching upon neighboring environments may increase exposure to some vectors and nonhuman hosts of vector-borne diseases, as has occurred with yellow fever, trypanosomiasis, and Kyasanur Forest disease.[2,4,8,9] Furthermore, migrants to new areas may lack immunity to the prevalent endemic vector-borne diseases, thus increasing their susceptibility to illness; alternatively, migrants may introduce new pathogens and vectors to their resettled locations.[1,2,9, 21–23]

Drainage of waste water is another important determinant of vector-borne disease transmission in urban locales. In resource-limited settings undergoing rapid urbanization, there is often inadequate clearance of standing water collected in used containers and tires, thus facilitating mosquito vector reproduction, a problem particularly evident for dengue and yellow fever.[2,4]

An example of disease proliferation arising from urbanization includes outbreaks of leishmaniasis in Brazil. Formerly, visceral leishmaniasis was predominantly a rural disease. However, outbreaks of the disease have recently occurred in several Brazilian cities due to massive population movement from rural areas to cities.[19,24,25] Also, some forms of cutaneous leishmaniasis typically occur as epidemics in densely populated cities in central and western Asia.[21]

LOSS OF BIODIVERSITY

In simple terms, biodiversity refers to the variety of species on Earth.[5] The threats to biodiversity from human activities are many, including stratospheric ozone depletion; pollution; introduction of invasive species; global warming; and most important, habitat degradation.[5] The rate of species loss today is the highest it has been since the dinosaurs went extinct.[4]

Reduction in global biodiversity is likely to contribute to vector-borne disease transmission. One theory of how biodiversity protects against vector-borne diseases is termed the "dilution effect." Locales with few species capable of sustaining vectors will have higher disease risk because vectors feed more frequently on the species that serve as hosts of the pathogen. In contrast, "dilution" occurs in areas with high biodiversity because more species (not all of which harbor parasites) are available to sustain vectors.[2,26] This model seems consistent with observations of the epidemiology of several vector-borne diseases, including leishmaniasis, African trypanosomiasis, Chagas› disease, West Nile virus, and Rocky Mountain spotted fever.[2,5]

Lyme disease is a bacterial infection passed through the bite of the *Ixodes* tick and is the most common vector-borne disease in the United States. The risk for Lyme disease is lower in areas with higher vertebrate-species diversity because not all vertebrates transmit the bacteria to the tick vector equally well, thus breaking the disease cycle. Furthermore, the population of the main reservoir host of Lyme disease, the white-footed mouse, is lower in ecosystems with more biodiversity due to the presence of mouse predators, thus lowering disease risk.[5,26] Similarly, in Lake Malawi, over-fishing has disrupted the foodweb such that snail populations have blossomed, thus increasing the prevalence of schistosomiasis.[2]

INTRODUCTION OF ALIEN SPECIES

Human introduction of alien species to an ecosystem occurs for a variety of reasons, from the accidental escape of an offending species to the intentional release for pest control. A nonindigenous species becomes invasive when, after establishing itself in a new environment, it subsequently begins to spread.[3] The environmental impact of invasive species can be great; invasive species are the second largest cause of biodiversity loss after habitat degradation.[27]

Nonindigenous species impact vector-borne disease epidemiology in several ways. Through their role in biodiversity loss, invasive species indirectly contribute to vector-borne disease risk. Nonindigenous species introduced by humans play a direct role in vector-borne disease transmission when the introduced species is itself a vector. This is increasingly a concern with widespread use of modern technology, such as air and sea travel, which remove the geographic barriers that previously limited vector migration.[22,28]

The Asian tiger mosquito, *Aedes albopictus*, is the most invasive mosquito in the world.[29] It has spread in the past 2 decades from the western Pacific and Southeast Asia to Africa, the Middle East, North and South America, and Europe.[30] This spread has occurred largely due to the international trade of used tires in which mosquito eggs have been laid. In addition to the inherent ecological problems associated with this rapid mosquito invasion, the global expansion of *A albopictus* poses a threat to human health. This mosquito is a potential vector for at least 22 viruses.[29,30]

A albopictus was implicated as a vector of the chikungunya virus on several Indian Ocean islands involved in a 2006 chikungunya fever outbreak. *A albopictus* is not the vector typically associated with chikungunya fever, but it is thought that a new variant of the chikungunya virus better adapted to *A albopictus* was partially responsible for the outbreak.[22,28,31] This example highlights the role shifting vector populations may play in the emergence of vector-borne diseases. More recently, in 2007 there was an outbreak of chikungunya fever in Italy by the virus variant adapted to *A albopictus*. This was the first-ever reported outbreak in a temperate country. This mosquito was first introduced in Italy in 1990 through tires imported from the United States; it is now widespread in Italy.[31,32]

Climate Change

There is a wealth of evidence that human activities, in particular the emission of greenhouse gases, are causing climate change.[33,34] Climate change will have a wide-ranging impact, from warmer global temperatures to altered hydrological patterns.[9,35] Vector-borne disease epidemiology is inherently dependent on climate, as the life cycles of many vectors are affected by ambient meteorologic conditions.[34]

The overall effect of anthropogenic climate change on vector-borne diseases remains debated, and the outcome may vary regionally.[4,8,9, 34–38] Nonetheless, there appears to be an overall expansion of the global distributions of malaria, various mosquito- and tick-borne encephalitides, and yellow fever that is at least partially attributable to rising global temperatures.[2]

Modeling serves an important role in predicting the impact of anthropogenic climate change on vector-borne disease epidemiology. One such model predicts that transmission of schistosomiasis may be increasing in nonendemic areas of China due to climate change.[33] Another model anticipates that dengue fever incidence will increase worldwide secondary to climate change.[39]

Warmer temperatures are associated with altered rates at which mosquitoes reach sexual maturity, frequency of mosquito blood meals, and rates at which parasites are acquired, as well as shortened incubation time of parasites within mosquitoes. These factors together can favor transmission of mosquito-borne diseases.[2,4,9,13,23,35, 37–39] Similarly, increased precipitation associated with global warming may benefit mosquito populations by increasing the number of breeding sites.[1,9]

The impact of climate change on malaria is of special concern given its high global distribution.[4] Although in the past the lower temperatures at high altitudes in Africa have limited the expansion of malaria vectors, there are recent reports of malaria epidemics occurring in these previously unaffected areas, perhaps in part due to higher temperatures and increased precipitation.[4,34] The International Panel on Climate Change has warned that climate change may continue to increase the incidence of malaria in areas of high altitude.[36,40]

Climate change may alter the distribution of vector-borne disease by affecting nonhuman hosts. Plague is a bacterial disease transmitted to humans typically by fleas from rodents. In a study of the incidence of human plague in New Mexico in relation to precipitation, the number of human plague cases was positively associated with higher-than-normal winter-spring precipitation, perhaps because the wetter conditions favored rodent breeding.[41]

The El Niño weather cycle provides further evidence of the importance of climate on vector-borne disease transmission. While differences exist in the changes effected by anthropogenic climate change and El Niño and the time scale over which they occur, El Niño is a helpful model to investigate the impact of climate on infectious diseases given the short period over which it exerts its effects.[4] El Niño has driven heat waves and drought in parts of Africa and Asia as well as heavy rains and floods in South America.[4] In the Asia-Pacific region, El Niño has impacted dengue fever outbreaks.[23] In South America, Asia, and Africa, malaria transmission is sensitive to the climate variability from El Niño. Additionally, the frequency and severity of El Niño events is expected to increase with anthropogenic climate change.[34,35]

CONCLUSION

The pace at which we are degrading the global environment is accelerating. Under these circumstances, vector-borne diseases represent a significant risk to public health due to their inherent dependence on the global environment. The evidence reviewed here indicates that in many instances the transmission of vector-borne diseases will increase with human-driven environmental alteration. We must remain cautious in our interactions with the biosphere to ensure that we do not bring about unnecessary outbreaks of serious vector-borne diseases. Further research is necessary so that we can predict and prevent emerging and reemerging vector-borne diseases due to environmental damage.

ACKNOWLEDGMENTS

I would like to thank Grant Dorsey and Aaron Bernstein for their comments on this manuscript.

REFERENCES

1. Harrus S, Baneth G. Drivers for the emergence and re-emergence of vector-borne protozoal and bacterial diseases. Int J Parasitol. 2005;35:1309–1318.
2. Chivian E, editor. Biodiversity: Its importance to human health. Interim executive summary. Available at:http://chge.med.harvard.edu/publications/documents/Biodiversity_v2_screen.pdf Accessed August 31, 2008.
3. Lounibos LP. Invasions by insect vectors of human disease. Annu Rev Entomol. 2002;47:233–266.
4. Sutherst RW. Global change and human vulnerability to vector-borne diseases. Clin Microbiol Rev.2004;17:136–173.
5. Chivian E, Bernstein AS. Embedded in nature: human health and biodiversity. Environ Health Perspect.2004;112:A12–A13.
6. Tilman D, Fargione J, Wolff B, et al. Forecasting agriculturally driven global environmental change.Science. 2001;292:281–284.
7. Louria DB. Undernutrition can affect the invading microorganism. Clin Infect Dis. 2007;45:470–474.
8. Molyneux DH. Common themes in changing vector-borne disease scenarios. Trans R Soc Trop Med Hyg.2003;97:129–132.
9. Patz JA, Graczyk TK, Geller N, Vittor AY. Effects of environmental change on emerging parasitic diseases. Int J Parasitol. 2000;30:1395–1405.
10. Wilson MD, Cheke RA, Flasse SP, et al. Deforestation and the spatio-temporal distribution of savannah and forest members of the Simulium damnosum complex in southern Ghana and south-western Togo. Trans R Soc Trop Med Hyg. 2002;96:632–639.
11. Vittor AY, Gilman RH, Tielsch J, et al. The effect of deforestation on the human-biting rate of Anopheles darlingi, the primary

vector of Falciparum malaria in the Peruvian Amazon. Am J Trop Med Hyg.2006;74:3–11.

12. Tadei WP, Thatcher BD, Santos JM, Scarpassa VM, Rodrigues IB, Rafael MS. Ecologic observations on anopheline vectors of malaria in the Brazilian Amazon. Am J Trop Med Hyg. 1998;59:325–335.
13. Lindblade KA, Walker ED, Onapa AW, Katungu J, Wilson ML. Land use change alters malaria transmission parameters by modifying temperature in a highland area of Uganda. Trop Med Int Health.2000;5:263–274.
14. Keiser J, Maltese MF, Erlanger TE, et al. Effect of irrigated rice agriculture on Japanese encephalitis, including challenges and opportunities for integrated vector management. Acta Trop. 2005;95:40–57.
15. Chatterjee P. Japanese encephalitis outbreak in India. Lancet Neurol. 2005;4:700.
16. Tyagi BK. A review of the emergence of Plasmodium falciparum-dominated malaria in irrigated areas of the Thar Desert, India. Acta Trop. 2004;89:227–239.
17. Southgate V, Tchuem Tchuente LA, Sene M, et al. Studies on the biology of schistosomiasis with emphasis on the Senegal river basin. Mem Inst Oswaldo Cruz. 2001;96(Suppl):75–78.
18. el-Sayed HF, Rizkalla NH, Mehanna S, Abaza SM, Winch PJ. Prevalence and epidemiology of Schistosoma mansoni and S. haematobium infection in two areas of Egypt recently reclaimed from the desert.Am J Trop Med Hyg. 1995;52:194–198.
19. Cohen J, Powderly WG, editors. Infectious Diseases. 2nd ed. Edinburgh: Elsevier Limited; 2004.
20. UNFPA. State of World Population 2007: Unleashing the Potential of Urban Growth. 2007.
21. Ashford RW. The leishmaniases as emerging and re-emerging zoonoses. Int J Parasitol. 2000;30:1269–1281.
22. Charrel RN, de Lamballerie X, Raoult D. Chikungunya outbreaks–the globalization of vectorborne diseases. N Engl J Med. 2007;356:769–771.
23. McMichael AJ, Woodruff RE, Hales S. Climate change and human health: present and future risks.Lancet. 2006;367:859–869.

24. Werneck GL, Rodrigues L, Santos MV, et al. The burden of Leishmania chagasi infection during an urban outbreak of visceral leishmaniasis in Brazil. Acta Trop. 2002;83:13–18.
25. Jeronimo SM, Oliveira RM, Mackay S, et al. An urban outbreak of visceral leishmaniasis in Natal, Brazil. Trans R Soc Trop Med Hyg. 1994;88:386–388.
26. Keesing F, Holt RD, Ostfeld RS. Effects of species diversity on disease risk. Ecol Lett. 2006;9:485–498.
27. Shirley SM, Kark S. Amassing efforts against alien invasive species in Europe. PLoS Biol. 2006;4:e279.
28. Reiter P, Fontenille D, Paupy C. Aedes albopictus as an epidemic vector of chikungunya virus: another emerging problem? Lancet Infect Dis. 2006;6:463–464.
29. Benedict MQ, Levine RS, Hawley WA, Lounibos LP. Spread of the tiger: global risk of invasion by the mosquito Aedes albopictus. Vector Borne Zoonotic Dis. 2007;7:76–85.
30. Gratz NG. Critical review of the vector status of Aedes albopictus. Med Vet Entomol. 2004;18:215–227.
31. Chretien JP, Linthicum KJ. Chikungunya in Europe: what›s next? Lancet. 2007;370:1805–1806.
32. Rezza G, Nicoletti L, Angelini R, et al. Infection with chikungunya virus in Italy: an outbreak in a temperate region. Lancet. 2007;370:1840–1846.
33. Zhou XN, Yang GJ, Yang K, et al. Potential impact of climate change on schistosomiasis transmission in China. Am J Trop Med Hyg. 2008;78:188–194.
34. Patz JA, Kovats RS. Hotspots in climate change and human health. BMJ. 2002;325:1094–1098.
35. Khasnis AA, Nettleman MD. Global warming and infectious disease. Arch Med Res. 2005;36:689–696
36. Hay SI, Cox J, Rogers DJ, et al. Climate change and the resurgence of malaria in the East African highlands. Nature. 2002;415:905–909.
37. Rogers DJ, Randolph SE, Snow RW, Hay SI. Satellite imagery in the study and forecast of malaria.Nature. 2002;415:710–715.

38. Patz JA, Campbell-Lendrum D, Holloway T, Foley JA. Impact of regional climate change on human health. Nature. 2005;438:310–317.

39. Hales S, de Wet N, Maindonald J, Woodward A. Potential effect of population and climate changes on global distribution of dengue fever: an empirical model. Lancet. 2002;360:830–834.

40. McCarthy JJ, Canziani OF, Leary NA, Dokken DJ, White KS, editors. Climate Change 2001: Impacts, Adaptation and Vulnerability–Contribution of Working Group II to the Third Assessment Report of the Intergovernmental Panel on Climate Change. Cambridge: Cambridge University Press; 2001.

41. Parmenter RR, Yadav EP, Parmenter CA, Ettestad P, Gage KL. Incidence of plague associated with increased winter-spring precipitation in New Mexico. Am J Trop Med Hyg. 1999;61:814–821.

Chapter 4

Genetically Modified Plants and Human Health

Suzie Key, Julian K-C Ma, and Pascal MW Drake

Molecular Immunology Unit, Centre for Infection, Department of Cellular and Molecular Medicine, St George's University of London, Cranmer Terrace, London SW17 0RE, UK.

SUMMARY

Genetically modified (or GM) plants have attracted a large amount of media attention in recent years and continue to do so. Despite this, the general public remains largely unaware of what a GM plant actually is or what advantages and disadvantages the technology has to offer, particularly with regard to the range of applications for which they can be used. From the first generation of GM crops, two main areas of concern have emerged, namely risk to the environment and risk to human health. As GM plants are gradually being introduced into the European Union there is likely to be increasing public concern regarding potential health issues. Although it is now commonplace for the press to adopt 'health campaigns', the information they publish is often unreliable and unrepresentative of the available scientific evidence. We consider it important that the medical profession should be aware of the state of the art, and, as they are often the first port of call for a concerned patient, be in a position to provide an informed opinion.

This review will examine how GM plants may impact on human health both directly – through applications targeted at nutrition and enhancement of recombinant medicine production – but also indirectly, through potential effects on the environment. Finally, it will examine the most important opposition currently facing the worldwide adoption of this technology: public opinion.

INTRODUCTION

Plants with favourable characteristics have been produced for thousands of years by conventional breeding methods. Desirable traits are selected, combined and propagated by repeated sexual crossings over numerous generations. This is a long process, taking up to 15 years to produce new varieties.[1] Genetic engineering not only allows this process to be dramatically accelerated in a highly targeted manner by introducing a small number of genes, it can also overcome the barrier of sexual incompatibility between plant species and vastly increase the size of the available gene pool.[1]

Transgenic (GM) plants are those that have been genetically modified using recombinant DNA technology. This may be to express a gene that is not native to the plant or to modify endogenous genes. The protein encoded by the gene will confer a particular trait or characteristic to that plant. The technology can be utilized in a number of ways, for example to engineer resistance to abiotic stresses, such as drought, extreme temperature or salinity, and biotic stresses, such as insects and pathogens, that would normally prove detrimental to plant growth or survival. The technology can also be used to improve the nutritional content of the plant, an application that could be of particular use in the developing world. New-generation GM crops are now also being developed for the production of recombinant medicines and industrial products, such as monoclonal antibodies, vaccines, plastics and biofuels.[2–4]

In 2007, for the twelfth consecutive year, the global area of biotech crops planted continued to increase, with a growth rate of 12% across 23 countries.[5] The principle crops grown are soybean and maize, although cotton, canola and rice are also on the increase. However, genetically modified crops grown in the EU amount to only a few thousand hectares (~0.03% of the world production),[6] which is probably a reflection of European opposition to this technology. In contrast, food derived from GM plants is ubiquitous in the USA. Indeed, many animal feeds used in Europe derived from imported plant material contain GM products. Similarly, GM cotton is widely used in clothing and other products.

Genetically Modifying a Plant

A number of techniques exist for the production of GM plants. The two most commonly employed are the bacterium *Agrobacterium tumefaciens*, which is naturally able to transfer DNA to plants, and the 'gene gun', which shoots microscopic particles coated with DNA into the plant cell.[1] Generally, individual plant cells are targeted and these are regenerated into whole GM plants using tissue culture techniques. Three aspects of this procedure have raised debate with regard to human health.

- The use of selectable markers to identify transformed cells
- Transfer of extraneous DNA into the plant genome (i.e. genes other than those being studied)
- The possibility of increased mutations in GM plants compared to non-GM counterparts due to tissue culture processes used in their production and the rearrangement of DNA around the insertion site of foreign genes.

To facilitate the transformation process, a selectable marker gene conferring, for example, resistance to an antibiotic (e.g. kanamycin, which will kill a normal non-GM plant cell), is often co-transferred with the gene of interest to allow discrimination of GM tissue and regeneration of GM plants. Critics of the technology have stated that there is a risk of the spread of antibiotic resistance to the bacterial population either in the soil or in the human gut after ingestion of GM food. However, these antibiotic resistance genes were initially isolated from bacteria and are already widespread in the bacterial population. In addition, kanamycin itself has GRAS status (Generally Regarded As Safe) and has been used for over 13 years without any known problems. Studies have concluded that the probability of transmission of antibiotic resistance from plants to bacteria is extremely low and that the hazard occurring from any such transfer is, at worst, slight.[7,8]Nevertheless, other selection strategies that do not rely on antibiotic resistance have been developed,[9] and procedures to eliminate the selectable marker from the plant genome once its purpose has been fulfilled have also been designed.[10]

The second aspect of the plant transformation procedure that has been criticized is that unnecessary DNA is transferred into the plant genome as a consequence of the engineering and transfer process.[11] Of course, there is no reason that DNA *per se* should be harmful, as it is consumed by humans in all foods, but again plant technologists have responded to the criticism by designing 'minimal cassettes' in which only the gene of interest is transferred into the plant.[12]

Finally, it has been claimed that GM plants carry more mutations than their untransformed counterparts as a result of the production method.[13] Genome-wide mutations may be produced by the tissue culture process, generating so called somaclonal variation, and endogenous DNA rearrangements may occur around the integrated transgene.[13] Theoretically, this may mean that plants may be produced with, for example, reduced levels of nutrients or increased levels of allergens or toxins[13] (although the alternative must also hold true, that positive traits may be expressed). Latham *et al.*[13] have stated that mutations around foreign gene insertion sites have not been fully characterized in either experimental or commercialized GM plants. Consequently, these authors have proposed several recommendations involving improved molecular analysis prior to the future commercialization of GM crops.[13]

However, as described in this report, it must be emphasized that GM crops grown to date have been produced under rigorous regulatory frameworks, and have been extensively safety tested prior to commercialization.

Food Applications for GM Plants

In the developing world, 840 million people are chronically undernourished, surviving on fewer than 8000 kJ/day (2000 Kcal/day).[14,15] Approximately 1.3 billion people are living on less than US$1/day[16,17] and do not have secure access to food. Many of these are also rural farmers in developing countries, depending entirely on small-scale agriculture for their own subsistence and to make their living.[18] They generally cannot afford to irrigate their crops or purchase herbicides or pesticides, leading to a vicious circle of poor crop growth, falling yields and pest susceptibility.[18] In addition, the world's population is predicted to double over the next 40 years, with over 95% of individuals being born in developing countries.[19] It is estimated that to meet these increased demands, food production must increase by at least 40% in the face of decreasing fertile lands and water resources.[20,21] GM plant technologies are one of a number of different approaches that are being developed to combat these problems. Specifically, studies are under way to genetically modify plants to increase crop yields, or to directly improve nutritional content.

Increasing Nutritional Content

In the developed world the nutritional content of food items is not of major concern, as individuals have access to a wide variety of foods that will meet all of their nutritional needs. In the developing world, however, this is often not the case, with people often relying on a single staple food crop for their energy intake.[18] GM technology offers a way to alleviate some of these problems by engineering plants to express additional products that can combat malnutrition. An important example of the potential of this technology is the 'Golden Rice Project'. Vitamin A deficiency is widespread in the developing world and is estimated to account for the deaths of approximately 2 million children per year.[18] In surviving children it has been identified as the leading cause of blindness.[22] Humans can synthesize vitamin A from its precursor -carotene, which is commonly found in many plants but not in cereal grains.[18] The strategy of the Golden Rice Project was to introduce the correct metabolic steps into rice endosperm to allow -carotene synthesis. In 2000, Ye *et al.*[23] engineered rice that contained moderate levels of -carotene and since then researchers have produced the much higher yielding 'Golden Rice 2'.[24] It is estimated that 72 g of dry Golden Rice 2 will provide 50% of the RDA of vitamin A for a 1–3-year-old child.[24]

Golden Rice was developed for farmers in the poorest countries, and from the beginning, the aim of the scientists was to provide the technology free of charge, which required the negotiation of more than 100 intellectual and technical property licenses.[25] Golden Rice will be given to subsistence farmers with no additional conditions[18] and is an impressive example of a health solution that can be offered by plant biotechnology.

Increasing Food Production

Crop yields worldwide are significantly reduced by the action of pathogens, parasites and herbivorous insects.[26] Two examples of commercial GM crop growth in this area are the insect-resistant crops expressing the *bt* gene (from the bacterium *Bacillus thuringiensis*) and virus-resistant GM papaya.[27] The first of these has been particularly successful; in the USA, for example, insect resistant GM maize is grown over an area of 10.6 million hectares and comprises 35% of all maize (GM and non-GM) grown in the country.[28] At the laboratory level, resistance has also been engineered to bacterial and fungal plant pathogens.[29,30]

A primary cause of plant loss worldwide is abiotic stress, particularly salinity, drought, and temperature extremes.[31] In the future, these losses will increase as water resources decline and desertification intensifies. Drought and salinity are expected to cause serious salinization of all arable lands by 2050,[32] requiring the implementation of new technologies to ensure crop survival. Although a number of promising targets have been identified in the production of abiotic stress tolerant GM plants, research remains at the laboratory-based level. An example is the study by Shou *et al.*[33] demonstrating that expression of an enzyme in GM maize activates an oxidative signal cascade that confers cold, heat and salinity tolerance.

Are GM foods Safe to Eat?

GM crops are tightly regulated by several government bodies. The European Food Safety Authority and each individual member state have detailed the requirements for a full risk assessment of GM plants and derived food and feed.[34] In the USA, the Food and Drug Agency, the Environmental Protection Agency and the US Department of Agriculture, Animal and Plant Health Inspection Service are all involved in the regulatory process for GM crop approval.[35] Consequently, GM plants undergo extensive safety testing prior to commercialization (for an example see http://www.efsa.europa.eu/EFSA/KeyTopics/efsa_locale-1178620753812_GMO.htm).

Foods derived from GM crops have been consumed by hundreds of millions of people across the world for more than 15 years, with no reported ill effects (or legal cases related to human health), despite many of the consumers coming from that most litigious of countries, the USA.

There is little documented evidence that GM crops are potentially toxic. A notorious study claiming that rats fed with GM potatoes expressing the gene for the lectin *Galanthus nivalis* agglutinin suffered damage to gut mucosa was published in 1999.[36] Unusually, the paper was only published after one of the authors, Arpad Pusztai, announced this apparent finding on television.[37] The Royal Society has since stated that the study 'is flawed in many aspects of design, execution and analysis' and that 'no conclusions should be drawn from it': for example the authors used too few rats per test group to derive meaningful, statistically significant data.

Is there any *a priori* reason to believe that GM crops might be harmful when consumed? The presence of foreign DNA sequences in food *per se* poses no intrinsic risk to human health.[38] All foods contain significant amounts of DNA and RNA, consumed in the range of 0.1–1.0 g/day.[39] Of potential concern is the possibility that the protein produced by the transgene may be toxic. This would occur if the transgene coded for a toxin that was subsequently absorbed systemically by the host. However, the potential toxicity of the protein expressed in a GM food is an essential component of the safety assessment that has to be performed.[40] Potential allergenicity to the novel gene product is another commonly expressed concern. Allergies to non-GM foods such as soft fleshed fruit, potatoes and soy are widespread. Clearly, new varieties of crops produced by either GM techniques or conventional breeding both have the potential to be allergenic. Concern surrounding this topic relates to two factors; the possibility that genes from known allergens may be inserted into crops not typically associated with allergenicity and the possibility of creating new, unknown allergens by either inserting novel genes into crops or changing the expression of endogenous proteins.

Assessment of the allergenic potential of compounds is problematic and a number of different bodies have produced guidelines and decision trees to experimentally evaluate allergenic potential.[41–43] These are effective at assessing compounds which may prove to be hazardous through a hierarchical approach which includes determining whether the source of the introduced gene is from an allergenic plant, whether GM foods react with antibodies in the sera of patients with known allergies and whether the product encoded by the new gene has similar properties to known allergens. In addition, animal models are used to screen GM foods.[40] Tests are not performed to formally assess any risk posed by inhalation of pollens and dusts; however, this is not assessed for conventionally grown foods and feeds either, and no allergies have been attributed to commercially grown GM pollen to date. Two examples are frequently quoted regarding GM crop allergenicity:

- A project to develop genetically modified peas by adding a protein from beans that conferred resistance to weevils was abandoned after it was shown that the GM peas caused a lung allergy in mice[44]
- Soya bean engineered to express a Brazil nut protein was withdrawn from production after it was also found to be allergenic in tests.[45]

Opponents of GM technology often cite these examples as proof that it is inherently unpredictable and dangerous, although another interpretation would be to say that safety testing of GM plants was effective in both cases, having identified allergenic potential before either product was released to market. It is perhaps a sobering thought, that if conventional plant breeding techniques had been used to achieve the same aims, there would have been no legal requirement for the assessment of allergenicity and the plant varieties could have been commercialized without *in vivo* testing. However, GM technology might also be used to *decrease* the levels of allergens present in plants by reducing expression levels of the relevant genes. For example, research was recently undertaken to identify an allergen in soybeans and remove it using GM technology.[46]

Non-food Applications for GM Plants

There are also a number of uses for plants outside of the food industry, for example in the timber, paper and chemical sectors and increasingly for biofuels. In all cases, non-GM and GM approaches are both being developed. Of significance to the medical field is the use of GM plants for production of recombinant pharmaceuticals. Molecular farming to produce GM plant-derived pharmaceutical proteins (PDPs) is currently being studied by academic and industrial groups across the world[4]. The first full-size native human recombinant PDP, human serum albumin, was demonstrated in 1990,[47] and since then antibodies, blood products, hormones and vaccines have all been expressed in plants.[48] Protein pharmaceuticals can be harvested and purified from GM plants, or alternatively, plant tissue in a processed form expressing a pharmaceutical could potentially be consumed as an 'edible vaccine'. As the molecular farming industry is still in its infancy, only one product has been approved for use so far – recombinant human intrinsic factor for use in vitamin B12 deficiency (http://www.cobento.dk). However, a number of molecular farming candidates are in clinical trials, including hepatitis B vaccine produced in potatoes and lettuce,[49] vaccines for heat labile toxin produced by *E. coli* and Norwalk virus,[50,51] human pro-insulin[52] and several monoclonal antibodies.[53–57]

Using GM plants as a platform for producing pharmaceuticals has many potential advantages over traditional systems. For example, GM plants can produce complex multimeric proteins such as antibodies that cannot be readily expressed by microbial systems. In addition, pharmaceutical production can potentially be on a vast agricultural scale.[4,58] The latter point is particularly important as it opens the way for many new applications that require administration of large amounts of proteins. These include topical application of antibodies and microbicides on mucosal surfaces for the prevention of infection. Not all applications need be on such a large scale; the hepatitis B vaccine is currently produced in genetically modified yeast, but not enough can be made at an affordable price to meet the demands of developing countries.[58] It has been estimated that 250 acres of greenhouse space would be enough to grow the amount of GM potatoes required to meet the annual demand for hepatitis B vaccine in the whole of South East Asia.[58]

Currently, over three million people die every year from vaccine-preventable diseases, the vast majority in the developing world. The current model of profit-motivated pharmaceutical production by companies in the developed world is ineffective in ridding the developing world of disease. GM plant technology may provide an alternative, as it is relatively low-tech and can be applied locally in the developing world by scientists working in partnership with governments and not-for-profit research funding agencies.

As with all aspects of GM crops, objections have been raised to the use of plants for manufacturing recombinant pharmaceuticals. Of greatest concern is that the pharmaceutical could inadvertently enter the human food chain. Theoretically, this might happen by uncontrolled dispersal of GM seed or by hybridization with a sexually compatible food crop following escape of GM pollen. In 2002, a company called Prodigene was fined and was severely censured for breaches in safety regulation when, due to inappropriate removal procedures, GM maize expressing a PDP was found to be growing in a soybean crop destined for human food consumption in the next growing cycle.[59] Although rare, incidents such as these demonstrate the potential risks of the technology. One proposal is to limit molecular farming to non-food crops, such as tobacco. Whilst feasible, there are significant advantages to the use of food crops for recombinant pharmaceutical production, such as attainment of GRAS status and utilizing well-established agricultural techniques for production. In the next section, the development of techniques to minimize GM gene flow are discussed.

GM Plants and the Environment

Any adverse effects on the environment through the large-scale growth of GM plants may indirectly affect human health. The following concerns have been expressed with regard to GM plants and the environment:

- That GM plants will sexually hybridize with non-GM plants through the transfer of pollen
- That GM plants may themselves become invasive weeds
- That the conditions required to grow GM plants will affect local wildlife populations.

In 2001, in a highly publicized study, evidence was presented that GM genes from GM maize had, by cross-pollination, contaminated wild maize in Mexico, the global centre for biodiversity of this species.[60] The validity of this work was disputed at the time of publication,[61,62] and later studies have also failed to detect any evidence of transgene spread to Mexican maize growing in the wild.[63] More recently, it has been reported that GM herbicide-resistant creeping bentgrass (*Agrostis stolonifera* L) planted in Oregon, USA, was found up to 3.8 km outside the designated area of cultivation.[64] The authors of the study postulated that this dispersal was a result of both pollen-mediated sexual crossing with plants in the wild, and GM crop seed dispersal.

In 1999, a scientific paper was published which claimed that maize engineered to express the insecticidal Bt toxin was harmful to the larvae of the Monarch butterfly, an iconic species in American culture.[65] It was claimed that larvae reared on their staple diet of milkweed, dusted with pollen from Bt maize, ate less, grew more slowly and suffered higher mortality rates.[65] A number of longer term studies have since investigated the likelihood of Monarch butterfly larvae being exposed to sufficient quantities of Bt maize pollen in nature to illicit a toxic response, and this was found to be insignificant.[66–68]

It is difficult to evaluate the effect of GM crops, or probably more importantly the regime required to grow them, on surrounding wildlife, particularly when considering long-term effects. The UK Farm-Scale Evaluations[69] were the biggest study of the potential environmental impact of GM crops conducted anywhere in the world. In a four-year programme, researchers studied the effect of management practices associated with 'genetically modified herbicide tolerance' on farm wildlife, compared with conventional weed control.[69] The study reported that for three of the four crops tested, the wildlife was reduced in the GM fields compared to non-GM, but in the final crop (maize) the opposite occurred. The researchers stated that this difference did not occur because the crops were genetically modified, but because the farmer was able to employ a different herbicide regime to that used on conventional crops. The study has provided a platform for the government to objectively evaluate the effect of these crops, and even though the results were portrayed by critics of the technology as evidence for environmental hazards of GM, they resulted in government approval for the commercial growth of a herbicide-resistant GM maize in the UK.[69]

GM plants are also being assessed for how they might have a positive role to play in the environment by selective removal of pollutants – a process known as phytoremediation. For example, plants have already been genetically engineered to accumulate heavy metal soil contaminants such as mercury and selenium to higher levels than would be possible for non-GM plants,[70,71] so not only can they grow on contaminated sites but they can also remediate contamination. These plants can be harvested and destroyed, the heavy metals disposed of or recycled, and the decontaminated field re-used.

Gene Transfer in the Environment

A number of strategies have been proposed to prevent gene flow from GM plants to the wider environment. The transfer of a gene to wild or non-GM crops is a particular concern when it is expressing a protein that is designed for use in industry or pharmaceuticals. It is widely agreed that food should not contain products that have been specifically designed for these applications.[72] Two strategies to prevent this happening are physical isolation and genetic containment. Physical isolation can be difficult and costly and must be carried out at every stage of production. The crop must be bred in isolation and both small- and large-scale field trials should also be carried out in isolated areas.[72] The seed and commercial crops themselves could be grown either in contained greenhouse conditions, or in areas where no weed or food crop relatives are grown.[72] In addition, the ground where the GM crop has been grown and the surrounding fields should be left to 'lie fallow' for a time to ensure no seeds remain and grow in the next crop cycle.[72] In practice, the most likely approach will be to have specified farms where dedicated planting and harvesting equipment, transport, grain-handling, drying and storage systems would be used.[72]

Genetic containment can be achieved at a number of levels by technological means. Existing sterility and incompatibility systems to limit the transfer of pollen can be utilized,[72] as can Genetic Use Restriction Technologies (GURTS) which interfere with fertility or seed formation.[72] Transfer of the foreign genes into the chloroplast genome is another strategy, as in many plant species chloroplasts are maternally inherited and not contained in pollen.[73]

The co-existence of crops for human consumption alongside related varieties grown for industrial products, that would be harmful if consumed by people, is not a new phenomenon, nor one that is confined to GM plants. For example, farmers in Canada grow two varieties of (non-GM) rapeseed – high and low erucic acid producers. The erucic acid extracted from the high producing variety is used as an industrial lubricant and is toxic to humans if consumed, whilst the low producing rapeseed variety, called canola, is used to make cooking oil. Canadian farmers have developed systems to routinely keep the two apart during growth and processing.

GM Plants and Public Opinion

Several NGO and media organizations are implacably opposed to GM plants. Crops that have been designed to help relieve malnutrition in the developing world, such as Golden Rice, are attacked on the basis that it 'tastes awful'[25] and that 'to be of any benefit a child would have to eat approximately 7kg of cooked Golden Rice',[74] an over-estimation by more than 15 times according to the founder of the product.[75] Insect-resistant cotton engineered to produce the Bt toxin requires far less pesticide application and produces higher crop yields than the non-GM counterpart,[76] generating savings of up to $500 per hectare for farmers.[77] Despite this, the crop has been criticized on the unsubstantiated grounds that it 'is killing the natural parasitic enemies of the cotton bollworm and increasing a number of other pests' and that 'its success will be short-lived as the bollworm will become resistant to the insecticide'.[74] These allegations have been made in spite of the fact that Bt bacteria have been widely used as a spray on organic crops by farmers for decades without any resistance developing in insects, in addition to no evidence of any emerging resistance after eight years of growing the GM crop.[76]

In some quarters, GM food is cited as being 'unnatural', although this accusation could be levelled at all of our food, which has been produced over millennia by artificial breeding. Very few commercialized crops would be able to survive unaided in nature. When considering 'natural' food production, it should be recognized that technology has always played an important part in the food industry. For example, antibiotics are widely used in feed in the poultry industry, and modern varieties of wheat were produced with the aid of radiation-induced mutation.[78] Scientists were greeted with expressions of outrage in many quarters when they genetically engineered frost-resistant plants with a gene from a cold water fish[79] – and yet fish and plants have a large proportion of genes in common, as do all living creatures.

Opposition to GM crops is perceived to be greater in the EU compared with other countries such as the USA, where food from GM crops has become part of the normal diet.[37] However, the situation is complex and UK public opinion is perhaps not so set against GM crops as is generally believed. Surveys have reported findings in which only 13% of consumers said they actively avoid GM foods, while 74% were not sufficiently concerned to actively avoid it.[80] This seems surprising considering the amount of anti-GM media coverage. From many of these articles it would seem appropriate to assume that the public as a whole are adamantly opposed to GM foods, but this is not substantiated by the surveys conducted.[80–82]

Nevertheless, considerable opposition to GM crops does exist and scientists must engage with the public to a much greater extent to ensure that the subject is debated rationally. This opposition is having many serious effects, not least because many developing countries that could benefit from the technology will not take it up as long as they believe that there remain significant areas of concern and that they will not be able to export produce to the EU market.[83] The implementation of the improvements to the design of GM crops discussed in this report would also further reassure the general public and pave the way for widespread acceptance of a technology that will be crucial in helping to alleviate current and future challenges in food and medicine supply.

ACKNOWLEDGEMENTS

None

REFERENCES

1. Southgate EM, Davey MR, Power JB, Merchant R. Factors affecting the genetic engineering of plants by microprojectile bombardment. Biotechnol Adv. 1995;13:631–57.
2. Sticklen M. Plant genetic engineering to improve biomass characteristics for biofuels. Curr Opin Biotechnol. 2005;17:315–9.
3. Conrad U. Polymers from plants to develop biodegradable plastics. Trends Plant Sci. 2005;10:511–2.
4. Ma JKC, Drake PMW, Christou P. The production of recombinant pharmaceutical proteins in plants.Nature. 2003;4:794–805.
5. ISAAA Briefs No. 37. Ithaca, NY: ISAAA; 2007. Executive summary of Global Status of Commercialised Biotech/GM crops: 2007.
6. Brandt P. Overview of the current status of genetically modified plants in Europe as compared to the USA. J Plant Physiol. 2003;160:735–40.
7. Gay PB, Gillespie SH. Antibiotic resistance markers in genetically modified plants; a risk to human health.Lancet Infect Dis. 2005;5:637–46.
8. Bennett PM, Livesey CT, Nathwani D, Reeves DS, Saunders JR, Wise R. An assessment of the risks associated with the use of antibiotic resistance genes in genetically modified plants: report of the Working Party of the British Society for Antimicrobial Chemotherapy. J Antimicrob Chemother. 2004;53:418–31.
9. Goldstein DA, Tinland B, Gilbertson LA, et al. Human safety and genetically modified plants: a review of antibiotic resistance markers and future transformation selection technologies. J App Microbiol. 2005;99:7–23.
10. Hare PD, Chua NH. Excision of selectable marker genes from GM plants. Nat Biotech. 2002;20:575–80.
11. Wu HX, Sparks CA, Jones HD. Characterisation of T-DNA loci and vector backbone sequences in GM wheat produced by *Agrobacterium*-mediated transformation. Mol Breed. 2006;18:195–208.
12. Fu XD, Duc LT, Fontana S, et al. Linear transgene constructs

lacking vector backbone sequences generate low-copy-number GM plants with simple integration patterns. Transgenic Res. 2000;9:11–9.

13. Latham JR, Wilson AK, Steinbrecher RA. The mutational consequences of plant transformation. J Biomed Biotech. 2006:1–7. Article ID 25376.
14. Pinstrup-Anderson P, Pandra-Lorch R, Rosegrant MW. World food prospects: critical issues for the early twenty-first century. 1999 Food policy report. Washington DC: International Food Policy Research Institute; 1999.
15. Food and Agriculture Organisation. The State of Food Insecurity in the World. Rome: FAO; 2001.
16. Smith LC, El Obeid AE, Jensen HH. The geography and causes of food insecurity in developing countries. Agriculture Economics. 2000;22:199–215.
17. World Bank. World Development report 2000/2001. Attacking poverty. Washington DC: World Bank; 2000.
18. Christou P, Twyman RM. The potential of genetically enhanced plants to address food insecurity. Nut Research Rev. 2004;17:23–42.
19. Byrnes BH, Bumb BL. Population growth, food production and nutrient requirements. J Crop Prod.1998;1:1–27.
20. Byerlee D, Helsey P, Pingali PL. Realising yield gains for food staples in developing countries in the early 21st century: prospects and challenges. In: Chang BM, Colombo M, Soronolo M, editors. Food Needs of the Developing World in the 21st Century. Vatican City: Political Academy of Sciences; 2000. pp. 207–50.
21. Rosegrant MW, Paisner MS, Mejer S, Witcover J. 2020 Global Food Outlook Trends, Alternatives and Choices. A 2020 Vision for Food Agriculture and the Environment Initiative. Washington DC: IFPRI; 2001.
22. World Health Organisation. Combating vitamin A deficiency. Geneva: WHO; 2001.www.who.int/nut/vad.htm.
23. Ye XD, Al-Babili S, Kloti A, et al. Engineering the provitamin A (-carotene) biosynthetic pathway into (carotenoid-free) rice endosperm. Science. 2000;287:303–5.

24. Paine JA, Shipton CA, Chaggar S, et al. Improving the nutritional content of Golden Rice through increased provitamin A content. Nat Biotechnol. 2005;23:482–7.
25. Potrykus I. Golden Rice and beyond. Plant Physiol. 2001;125:1157–61.
26. Anderson PK, Cunningham AA, Patel NG, Morales FJ, Epstein PR, Daszak P. Emerging infectious diseases of plants: pathogen, pollution, climate change and agrotechnology drivers. Trends Eco Evol.2004;19:535–44.
27. Gurr SJ, Rushton PJ. Engineering plants with increased disease resistance: what are we going to express?Trends Biotech. 2005;23:275–82.
28. Brookes G, Barfoot P. ISAAA briefs. ISAAA; 2006. http://www.isaaa.org.
29. Peschen D, Li HP, Fischer R, Kreuzaler F, Liao YC. Fusion protein comprising a *Fusarium*- specific antibody linked to antifungal peptides protect plants against a fungal pathogen. Nat Biotech. 2004;22:732–8.
30. Tai TH, Dahlbeck D, Clark ET, et al. Expression of Bs2 pepper gene confers resistance to bacterial spot disease in tomatoes. Proc Natl Acad Sci USA. 1999;96:14153–8.
31. Vinocur B, Altman A. Recent advances in engineering plant tolerance to abiotic stress: achievements and limitations. Curr Op Biotech. 2005;16:123–32.
32. Ashraf M. Breeding for salinity tolerance in plants. Crit Rev Plant Sci. 1994;13:17–42.
33. Shou H, Bordallo P, Fan FB, et al. Expression of an active tobacco mitogen activated protein kinase kinase kinase enhances freezing tolerance in GM maize. Proc Natl Acad Sci USA. 2004;101:3298–303.
34. Guidance document of the genetically modified organisms for the risk assessment of genetically modified plants and derived food and feed. EFSA J. 2004;99:1–94.
35. McKeon TA. Genetically modified crops for industrial products and processes and their effects on human health. Trends Food Sci Tech. 2003;14:229–41.

36. Ewen SWB, Pusztai A. Effects of diets containing genetically modified potatoes expressing *Galanthus Nivalis* lectin on rat small intestine. Lancet. 1999;354:1353–4.
37. Burke DM. GM Food and Crops: what went wrong in the UK? EMBO Reports. 2004;5:432–6.
38. FAO/WHO. Evaluation of Allergenicity of Genetically Modified Foods, Report of a joint FAO/WHO Expert Consultation on Allergenicity of Foods derived from Biotechnology. Geneva: FAO/WHO; 2001.
39. DoerflerW, SchubbertR, FremdeDNAimSciugersystem. Deutsches Arzteblatt. 1997;94:51–2.
40. Malarkey T. Human Health concerns with GM crops. Mut Res. 2003;544:217–22.
41. WHO/FAO. Strategies for assessing the safety of foods produced by biotechnology. Report of the Joint WHO/FAO Consultation. Geneva: FAO/WHO; 1991.
42. FDA Statement of policy, foods derived from new plant varieties. Fed Reg. 1992;57
43. OECD. Food Safety Evaluation. Paris: OECD Documents; 1996.
44. Prescott VE, Campbell PM, Moore A, et al. Transgenic expression of bean -amylase inhibitor in peas results in altered structure and immunogenicity. J Agric Food Chem. 2005;53:9023–30.
45. Nordlee JA, Taylor SL, Townsend JA, Thomas LA, Bush RK. Identification of a brazil-nut allergen in GM soybeans. NEJM. 1996;334:688–92.
46. Herman E. Soybean allergenicity and suppression of the immunodominant allergen. Crop Sci.2005;45:462–7.
47. Sijmons PC, Dekker BM, Schranmeijer B, Verwoerd TC, van den Elzen PJ, Hoekema A. Production of correctly processed human serum albumin in GM plants. Biotechnology. 1990;8:217–21.
48. Twyman RM, Schillberg S, Fischer R. Transgenic plants in the biopharmaceutical market. Expert Opin Emerg Drugs. 2005;10:185–218.
49. Kapusta J, Modelska A, Figlerowicz M, et al. A plant-derived edible vaccine against hepatitis B virus.FASED J. 1999;13:1796–9.

50. Tacket CO, Mason HS, Losonsky G, Clements JD, Levine MM, Arntzen CJ. Immunogenicity in humans of a recombinant bacterial antigen delivered in GM potato. Nature Med. 1998;4:607–9.
51. Tacket CO, Mason HS, Losonsky G, Estes MK, Levine MM, Arntzen CJ. Human responses to a novel Norwalk virus vaccine delivered in GM potatoes. J Infect Dis. 2000;182:302–5.
52. http://www.i-sis.org.uk/gmSafflowеHumanPro-Insulin.php
53. Hiatt A, Cafferkey R, Bowdish K. Production of antibodies in GM plants. Nature. 1998;342:76–8.
54. During K, Hippe S, Kreuzaler F, Schell J. Synthesis and self assembly of a functional monoclonal antibody in GM *Nicotiana tabacum*. Plant Mol Biol. 1990;15:281–93.
55. Ma JK-C, Hiatt A, Hein M, et al. Generation and assembly of secretory antibodies in plants. Science.1995;268:716–9.
56. Francisco JA, Gawlak SL, Miller M, et al. Expression and characterisation of bryodin 1 and a bryodin-based single-chain immunotoxin from tobacco cell culture. Bioconjug Chem. 1997;8:708–13.
57. Mayfield SP, Franklin SE, Lerner RA. Expression and assembly of a fully active antibody in algae. Proc Natl Acad Sci USA. 2003;100:438–42.
58. EMBO Reports. Molecular farming for new drugs and vaccines. EMBO Reports. 2005;6:593–9.
59. Fox JL. Puzzling industry response to Prodigene fiasco. Nat Biotech. 2003;21:3–4.
60. Quist D, Chapela JH. Transgenic DNA introgressed into traditional maize landraces in Oaxaca, Mexico.Nature. 2001;414:541–3.
61. Kaplinsky N, Braun D, Lisch D, Hay A, Hake S, Freeling M. Biodiversity (communications arising): maize transgene results in Mexico are artefacts. 2002. p. 601.
62. Metz M, Fulterer J. Biodiversity (communications arising): suspect evidence of GM contamination.Nature. 2002;416:600–1.
63. Ortiz-Garcia S, Ezcurra E, Schoel B, Acevedo F, Soberon J, Snow AA. Absence of detectable transgenes in local landacres of maize in Oaxaca, Mexico (2003–2004) Proc Natl Acad Sci USA.2005;102:12338–43.

64. Reichman JR, Watrud LS, Lee EH, et al. Establishment of GM herbicide-resistance creeping bentgrass (*Agrostis Stolonifera L.)* in nonagronomic habitats. Mol Ecol. 2006;15:4243–55.

65. Losey JE, Rayor LS, Carter ME. Transgenic pollen harms monarch larvae. Nature. 1999;399:214.

66. Sears MK, Hellmich RL, Stanley-Horn DE, et al. Impact of *Bt* corn pollen on monarch butterfly populations: a risk assessment. Proc Natl Acad Sci USA. 2001;98:11937–42.

67. Pleasants JM, Hellmich RL, Dively GP, et al. Corn pollen deposition on milkweeds in and near cornfields. Proc Natl Acad Sci USA. 2001;98:11919–24.

68. Stanley-Horn DE. Assessing the impact of Cry1Ab expressing corn pollen on monarch larvae in field studies. Proc Natl Acad Sci USA. 2001;119:31–36.

69. www.defra.gov.uk/environment/gm/fse

70. Sasaki Y, Hayakawa T, Inoue C, Miyazaki A, Silver S, Kusano T. Generation of mercury hyper-accumulating plants through GM expression of the bacterial mercury membrane transport protein MerC.Transgenic Res. 2006;15:615–25.

71. Banuelos G, Leduc DL, Pilon-Smits EAH, Terry N. Transgenic Indian mustard overexpressing selenocysteine lyase or seloncystiene methyltransferase exhibit enhanced potential for selenium phytoremediation under field conditions. Environ Sci Tech. 2007;41:599–605.

72. Mascia PN, Flovell RB. Safe and acceptable strategies for producing foreign materials in plants. Curr Opin Plant Biol. 2004;7:189–95.

73. Daniell H. GM Crops: public perception and scientific solutions. Trends Plant Sci. 1999;4:467–9.

74. Five Year Freeze Campaign. Why a Five Year Freeze? http://www.fiveyearfreeze.org/indexb.htm.

75. Zhang HX, Blumwald E. Transgenic salt-tolerant tomato plants accumulate salt in foliage but not in fruit.Nat Biotechnol. 2001;19:765–8.

76. Taverne D. The new fundamentalism. Nat Biotechnol. 2005;23:415–6.

77. Von Emden HF, Gray A, editors. GMOs – Ecological Dimensions. Wellsbourne, UK: Association of Applied Biologists;

78. Bradford KJ, Deynze AV, Gutterson N, Parrott W, Strauss SH. Regulating GM crops sensibly: lessons from plant breeding biotechnology and genomics. Nat Biotechnol. 2005;23:439–44.
79. Kenward KD, Altshuler M, Davies PL. Accumulation of type 1 fish antifreeze protein in GM tobacco is cold specific. Plant Mol Biol. 1993;23:377–85.
80. Consumer Watch. GM Food and Farming: What are Consumer›s latest views? Watford, UK: IGD; 2003.
81. Poortinga W, Pidgeon NF. Public perceptions of Genetically Modified Food and Crops, and the GM nation? Norfolk, UK: Centre for Environmental Risk, Norwich; 2004. (Understanding risk, working paper 04–01.)
82. Gorden G. GM Crops opposition may have been 'over-estimated' Scotsman. 2004 Feb 19;
83. Better dead than GM feed? Economist. 2002 Mar 13;31

Chapter 5

The Virulence–Transmission Trade-Off in Vector-Borne Plant Viruses: A Review of (Non-) Existing Studies

R. Froissart[1,2], J. Doumayrou[1,2], F. Vuillaume[2] S. Alizon[1] and Y. Michalakis[1]

[1]laboratoire génétique & évolution des maladies infectieuses (gemi), umr 2724 cnrs ird, 911 avenue agropolis, 34394 montpellier, France

[2]laboratoire biologie & génétique des interactions plantes-parasites (bgpi), umr 385 inra-cirad-supagro, campus international de baillarguet, 34398 montpellier, France

ABSTRACT

The adaptive hypothesis invoked to explain why parasites harm their hosts is known as the trade-off hypothesis, which states that increased parasite transmission comes at the cost of shorter infection duration.

This correlation arises because both transmission and disease-induced mortality (i.e. virulence) are increasing functions of parasite within-host density. There is, however, a glaring lack of empirical data to support this hypothesis. Here, we review empirical investigations reporting to what extent within-host viral accumulation determines the transmission rate and the virulence of vector-borne plant viruses. Studies suggest that the correlation between within-plant viral accumulation and transmission rate of natural isolates is positive. Unfortunately, results on the correlation between viral accumulation and virulence are very scarce. We found only very few appropriate studies testing such a correlation, themselves limited by the fact that they use symptoms as a proxy for virulence and are based on very few viral genotypes. Overall, the available evidence does not allow us to confirm or refute the existence of a transmission–virulence trade-off for vector-borne plant viruses. We discuss the type of data that should be collected and how theoretical models can help us refine testable predictions of virulence evolution.

INTRODUCTION

Although the availability of genomic and molecular details about specific host–parasite interactions is increasing exponentially owing to new molecular biotechnologies, our understanding of the evolution of virulence (i.e. decrease in host fitness due to parasite infection) remains fragmentary. Some pathogens cause noticeable damage to their host, and understanding the parameters underlying virulence evolution is critical for controlling human pathogens and agricultural pests and for the conservation of biodiversity. Moreover, determining the key parameters involved in virulence evolution becomes a priority when ecosystems are submitted to profound modifications such as global climatic change or increased commercial exchanges that spread parasites rapidly to new environments. More simply put, a long-standing question in evolutionary biology is 'Why do parasites harm their hosts?' An adaptive answer to this question states that while a high level of parasite replication increases the possibilities for between-host transmission, rapid replication is also likely to be detrimental to the host (i.e. to be associated with high virulence) owing to, for instance, over-exploitation of host resources by the parasite. Many models thus predict the existence of an optimal level of virulence that integrates the benefits of transmission and the cost of killing the host, which is known as the 'trade-off' hypothesis (Anderson & May 1982; Ewald 1983; Frank 1996). Although much debated, this hypothesis still awaits sufficient empirical data in order to be properly evaluated (Alizon *et al.* 2009). Here, we discuss the evolution of virulence of plant viruses, a group of parasites ignored by most reviews on the subject.

Viruses represent one of the most threatening types of parasites for human health and agriculture because they tend to exhibit high evolutionary rates (Froissart *et al.* 2005; Duffy *et al.* 2008). This rapid evolution, combined with large-scale dispersal, largely explains our limited success in controlling and eradicating viruses, with a few notable exceptions (e.g. small pox virus). Despite their importance in crop yield losses and ecosystem modification, few empirical studies have focused explicitly on the virulence of plant viruses from an evolutionary point of view. Notable exceptions are two recent reviews that address this question but put more emphasis on the evolution of parasite infectivity, i.e. the ability to cause disease (Jarosz 2002;Sacristan & Garcia-Arenal 2008). We focus on the evolution of virulence, which, following the conventions adopted by the American Phytopathological Society (D'Arcy *et al.* 2001), is defined as the degree of damage caused to a host and is usually assumed to correlate negatively with host fitness.

The biological cycles of plant viruses, whose evolution was reviewed by Garcia-Arenal *et al.* (2001), are subject to two specific peculiarities: (i) hosts are not mobile during their vegetative stage and (ii) contact between hosts is rare. Since plant viruses cannot penetrate the intact plant cuticle and the cellulose cell wall, they are transmitted either vertically, or horizontally by vectors (Hull 2001). The latter is by far the most common transmission mode, thus our focus is on vector-borne viruses. The question we ask is the following: 'To what extent does the level of virus replication within a plant determine the virus transmission rate and the virulence to the host?' This question is important because it underlies most of the transmission–virulence trade-off hypothesis.

THEORETICAL PREDICTION OF EVOLUTION OF VIRULENCE IN VECTOR-BORNE DISEASES

Natural selection operates on the rate of parasite spread within and between hosts. In most cases, natural selection thus tends to maximize the so-called parasitic basic reproduction ratio, R_0, which corresponds to the number of new infections generated by a single infected individual in a wholly susceptible population over the duration of the infection (but see Roberts (2007) for exceptions). In other words, R_0 is an expression of the fitness of a pathogen. In the classical Susceptible-Infected model for directly transmitted pathogens, it is given by $R_0 = \beta S/(\mu + \alpha)$, where S is the number of susceptible individuals, β is the transmission rate of the parasite from host to host, μ is the natural host mortality rate and α is the additional host mortality rate caused by the infection—usually called virulence (Anderson & May 1982; Frank 1996; Levin 1996).

In the case of a vector-borne disease, however, the expression of R_0 is slightly different. If we assume that the population dynamics of the vector are rapid and at equilibrium, and if we ignore clearance from the host, we have (Anderson & May 1991; Mideo & Day 2008):

$$R_0 = pb(y)^2 \frac{e^{-\mu v T(y)}}{\mu_v + \alpha_v(y)} \frac{\beta_{p\to v}(x)\beta_{v\to p}(y)}{\mu_p + \alpha_p(x)} \qquad (2.1)$$

where p is the average number of vectors per plant in the population, b is the vector feeding rate (or probing rate in the case of vectors of plant viruses) per day, T is the incubation time of the parasite in the vector (i.e. the time between vector infection and the time the vector becomes infective), μ_p and μ_v are the baseline mortality of the plant and of the vector, respectively, α_p and α_v are the extra mortality (i.e. the virulence) induced by the parasite on the plant and on the vector, respectively, $\beta_{p\to v}$ is the transmission rate from the infected plant to the vector and $\beta_{v\to p}$ is the transmission rate from the viruliferous (i.e. carrying virus) vector to a healthy plant. Finally, y is viral accumulation in the vector and x the viral accumulation in the plant. We present a relatively general case where many components of R_0 depend on viral accumulation, but this is not necessarily the case. This is summarized in figure 1. In this formalism it is assumed that viral accumulation is at least partly determined by viral genotype.

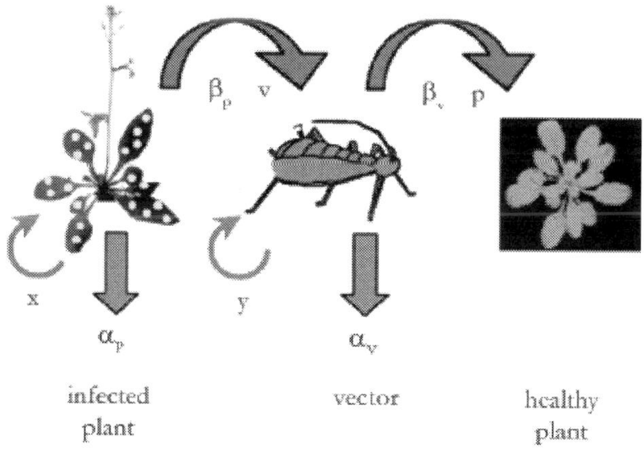

Figure 1: Effect of within-host viral accumulation on transmission rate and virulence of vector-borne plant viruses. The transmission rate can be decomposed into two steps: from infected plant to vector ($\beta_{p\rightarrow v}$) and from viruliferous vector to healthy plant ($\beta_{v\rightarrow p}$). Within-plant (x) and within-vector (y) viral accumulation are thought to have an effect on mortality of the plant (α_p) and vector (α_v), respectively.

The trade-off hypothesis rests on two key assumptions: (i) that increasing viral accumulation increases virulence and (ii) that increasing viral accumulation increases virus transmission to another host. This dependency is indicated in equation (2.1) with an x or a y in brackets. The direct consequence of these two assumptions is that a virus genotype with high accumulation rates will benefit from increased transmission ($\beta_{p\rightarrow v} \times \beta_{v\rightarrow p}$), but will suffer from a shorter infection period owing to rapid host and vector death (α_p and α_v). In other words, the pleiotropic effect of the accumulation rate generates a transmission–virulence trade-off such that it is not possible to maximize transmission rate and the duration of the infection simultaneously. In the following, we present the evidence for such correlations between accumulation rate and virulence and transmission.

If we assume that parasite strains vary with respect to their accumulation rates (*x* and *y*), then this implies that these strains will also have different R_0, i.e. different fitnesses at the between-host level. Theory predicts that the strain with the highest R_0 is evolutionarily stable and will invade the population (Anderson & May 1982). It can be shown mathematically that an optimal strategy associated with a finite non-zero virulence exists if virulence increases more rapidly than transmission with viral accumulation (Anderson & May 1982; Ewald 1983; Alizon *et al.* 2009). Note that, in the case of vector-borne diseases, other components of R_0, such as the vector feeding rate or the incubation time, may depend on viral accumulation in the vector. This means that the trade-off and the existence of an optimal strategy could also occur through other pleiotropic effects of the viral accumulation rate. More generally, the optimal level of virulence is determined by how the variables affecting R_0 depend on the accumulation rate.

Notwithstanding that the trade-off hypothesis is a cornerstone of the theory of virulence evolution, empirical data are scarce. Arguably the major difficulty that could explain the lack of evidence originates from the estimation of the transmission rate. This is maybe why several of the studies that manage to measure the correlation between parasite density and virulence and parasite density and transmission are based on vector-borne diseases, because transmission success to the vector can be estimated experimentally. Studies on rodent malaria (Mackinnon & Read 1999) or on myxoma virus in rabbits (Dwyer *et al.* 1990) found that parasite density was positively correlated to both virulence and transmission. Analyses by Dwyer *et al.* (1990) andBolker *et al.* (2010) also indicate that there is an optimal level of virulence for the myxoma virus. However, studies on rodent malaria have failed to go beyond a mere correlation between virulence and transmission and find an optimal virulence (see Mackinnon & Read 1999 for a review). Maybe this is because the second part of the parasite life cycle (in the vector) plays an important role. Another possibility to bypass the difficulty to estimate transmission is to consider spore-producing pathogens. De Roode *et al.* (2008) studied a protozoa infecting the monarch butterfly and showed that parasite load was positively correlated with transmission to the offspring and with virulence. They also showed that there is a spore load that maximizes the infection fitness (or R_0), which indicates an optimal virulence. Jensen *et al.* (2006) showed that the total number of spores produced during an infection of *Daphnia magna* by the bacteria *Pasteuria ramosa* is maximized by intermediate virulence. However, because they did not explicitly investigate the correlations between parasite load and virulence or transmission, their result cannot be viewed as a direct test of the trade-off hypothesis. Finally, as far as we are aware, the only directly transmitted parasite for which these relationships have been addressed is HIV: Fraser *et al.* (2007) found that set-point viral load was positively correlated with virulence and with transmission and that there was an optimal virulence (which corresponds to what is observed *in vivo*). Several reasons can explain that some studies 'only' showed that virulent genotypes tend to be more transmissible but were unable to reach a conclusion regarding the existence of an optimal virulence (e.g. Mackinnon & Read 1999). For instance, even if variation in virulence is obtained by considering different parasite genotypes, host variability can blur the trade-off relationship making it difficult to determine the optimal virulence. Also, important variations in virulence can occur during the growing phase of an epidemic, which further contributes to blur the trade-off relationship for emerging pathogens (Bolker *et al.* 2010). Finally, the trade-off hypothesis is often criticized through some cases where virulence is clearly not adaptive for the parasite (Levin & Bull 1994). However, these cases can usually be understood through within-host competition (a virulent strain is favoured within a host but disfavoured between hosts). The fact that other processes, in addition to the trade-off, govern virulence evolution does not invalidate the trade-off hypothesis in itself. Overall, the scarcity of empirical data seems to be the main problem and it should be taken as a motivation for the collection of further evidence.

VIRAL ACCUMULATION VERSUS TRANSMISSION RATE

Transmission rate is measured as the percentage of plants that become infected after inoculation of viral particles by vector(s) that have fed previously on infected plants. Typically, experimentalists measuring transmission rates allow vectors to acquire viruses from an infected plant before placing one (or a group) of viruliferous vectors on healthy plants. Viral accumulation is measured as viral load in infected leaf extracts, quantified mainly through techniques involving (i) antibodies targeting viral proteins (ELISA, western blot, etc) or (ii) detection of viral nucleic acids (real-time PCR, northern or Southern blot, etc). In order to obtain a correlation between viral accumulation and transmission rate, researchers need to vary the viral quantity acquired by vectors. To our knowledge, this has been achieved by four procedures. In a first procedure (denoted *'in vitro'* in table 2), virions are purified from infected plants and diluted in an artificial diet medium. Vectors trapped in a feeding cage covered at one end by a stretched parafilm membrane are then fed with different dilutions of virions (Pirone & Megahed 1966; Gera *et al.* 1979; Pirone 1981; van den Heuvel *et al.* 1991; Ng *et al.* 2004; Ng & Falk 2006). Following acquisition feeding, vectors are transferred to uninfected plants for subsequent inoculation. The remaining procedures are denoted as *'in planta'* in table 2. In a second procedure, vectors are allowed to acquire viral particles on different host genotypes varying in their resistance levels to the virus (Romanow *et al.* 1986; Gray *et al.* 1993, 1994; Lapidot *et al.* 2001; Wintermantel *et al.* 2008). A third procedure consists of allowing vectors to feed on infected leaves of different ages harboring different levels of virus accumulation (Gray *et al.* 1991; van den Heuvel *et al.* 1991). In a fourth procedure, vectors are allowed to acquire viral particles on plants harboring different levels of viruses owing to differential growth conditions (De Bokx *et al.* 1978; Dusi & Peters 1999) or viral genotypes differing in their accumulation (Banik & Zitter 1990).

Table 2: Correlation between viral accumulation and transmission rate of vector-borne plant viruses

		transmission rate[b]					
virus	**mode of transmission**[a]	$\beta_{p \to v}$	$\beta_{v \to p}$	$(\beta_{p \to v} \times \beta_{v \to p})$	**assay**	**origin of variation**	**references**
CMV	NC		+		*in vitro*	dilution	Pirone & Megahed (1966); Gera *et al.* (1979)
CMV	NC			+	*in planta*	differential viral accumulation *in planta*	Banik & Zitter (1990)
PVY^N	NC			+	*in planta*	growing conditions	De Bokx *et al.* (1978)
PVY	NC		+		*in vitro*	dilution	Pirone (1981)
WMV2	NC	+			*in planta*	levels of host resistance	Romanow *et al.* (1986)
BtMV	NC			+	*in planta*	season	Dusi & Peters (1999)
LIYV	NC		+		*in vitro*	dilution	Ng & Falk 2006; Ng *et al.* (2004)
TICV or ToCV	NC			+	*in planta*	levels of host resistance	Wintermantel *et al.* (2008)
PLRV	C		+	+	*in vitro*	dilution	van den Heuvel *et al.* (1991)
PLRV	C		+	+	*in planta*	leaf age	van den Heuvel *et al.* (1991)
BYDV	C	+	+		*in planta*	levels of host resistance	Gray *et al.* (1991, 1993, 1994)
TSWV	P		+		*in planta*	accumulation in vector	Rotenberg *et al.* (2009)
TYLCV	P			+	*in planta*	levels of host resistance	Lapidot *et al.* (2001)

[a]Viruses transmitted in a non-circulative (NC), circulative (C) or propagative (P) manner.

[b]A (+) indicates a positive correlation between the measured trait and viral accumulation. Empty cells indicate that the relationship has not been measured.

A substantial part of the phytopathological literature deals with studies on the phenotypic expression of point mutation(s) introduced *in vitro* into infectious viral clones or isolated randomly from a viral population (for a review, see Blanc 2008). Results from such 'engineered' viruses provide us mostly with information concerning molecular mechanisms involved in transmission. They also reveal the phenotypic effects of mutations prior to any action of natural selection in the wild. They can thus inform us on whether a particular type of relationship between, e.g. viral accumulation and transmission is 'hardwired' and arises necessarily owing to genomic constraints. Interestingly, studies reporting the effect of one or few mutation(s) do not show a positive correlation between transmission and viral accumulation. For instance, different mutations induce a loss of transmission associated with a decrease, an increase or no modification in viral accumulation (Gera *et al.* 1979; Bruyère *et al.* 1997; Escriu *et al.* 2000*a,b*; Gal-On 2007). We now turn to studies based on viral populations collected in the field.

Transmission of vector-borne plant viruses is achieved through different routes depending on virus genera. Modes of transmission are briefly summarized below and in table 1 and figure 2 (for reviews, see Gray & Banerjee 1999; Ng & Falk 2006; Hogenhout *et al.* 2008). The studies reviewed here on the relationship between viral accumulation and transmission are summarized in table 2. We discuss modes of transmission because these are likely to impact the overall transmission rate ($\beta_{p\rightarrow v}$ and $\beta_{v\rightarrow p}$) and thus potentially affect the evolution of virulence.

Table 1: Mode of transmission of plant viruses

mode of transmission	interaction with the vector	viral genera examples	transmission from infected plant to vector ($\beta_{p \to v}$)	transmission from viruliferous vector to healthy plant ($\beta_{v \to p}$)	time during which vectors are viruliferous	example references
non-circulative	restricted to mouth parts	*Potyvirus*, *Cucumovirus*	minutes	minutes to hours[a]	minutes to hours[a]	Palacios *et al.* (2002); Kalleshwaraswamy & Kumar (2008)
circulative	interaction with haemocoel	*Luteovirus*	minutes to a few hours	days to weeks	days to weeks	Gray *et al.* (1991)
propagative	replication within the vector	*Tospovirus*, *Tenuivirus*	minutes to a few hours	days to weeks	vector lifespan	Mehta *et al.* (1994)

[a]Exception: *Nepovirus*.

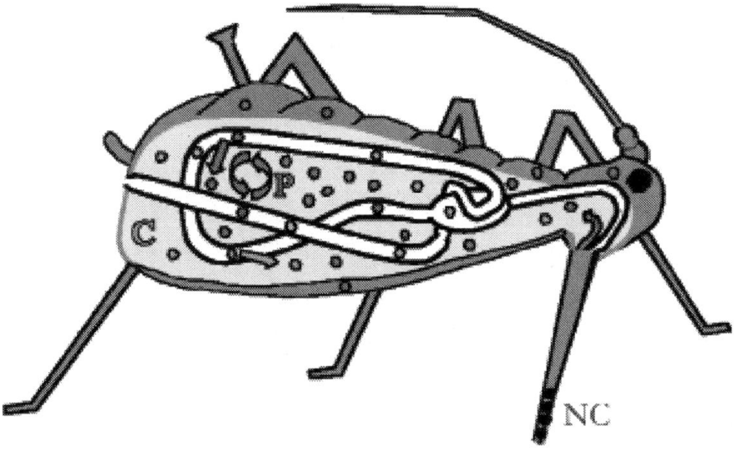

Figure 2: Schematic representation of modes of transmission by vectors. Viruses transmitted in a non-circulative (NC) manner (black) are restricted to the mouth parts. Viruses transmitted in a circulative (C) manner (green) enter the haemocoel (yellow) by endocytosis–exocytosis from the gut, do not replicate in the vector and usually enter the salivary glands from the haemolymph. Viruses transmitted in a propagative (P) manner (red) replicate in different organs of the vectors and may enter the salivary glands either from the haemolymph or from other connecting tissues, e.g. the nervous system or trachea (reviewed in Ng & Falk 2006; Hogenhout *et al.* 2008). Figure modified from Brault *et al.* (in press).

Some viruses interact only with the vector's exterior mouth parts (e.g. stylets—the outermost needle-like mouth parts of aphids and other piercing–sucking insects); in such cases, transmission is termed 'non-circulative' (Harris 1977). The time between the acquisition of such a virus by a vector from an infected plant and inoculation to another plant ranges from minutes (e.g. CMV) to hours (e.g. BtMV) and even, exceptionally, years (nepoviruses are retained in nematode mouth parts; Demangeat *et al.* 2005). No transmission occurs after viruliferous vectors have transmitted all the viral particles retained in their mouth parts (Yuan & Ullman 1996; Kalleshwaraswamy & Kumar 2008). The period during which vectors remain viruliferous is very short. This is due partly to the fact that most viral particles are lost (and thus never transmitted) a few minutes after the acquisition period even without feeding behaviour (Palacios *et al.* 2002;Kalleshwaraswamy

& Kumar 2008). These findings also indicate that few viral particles are retained and inoculated by vectors in the case of non-circulating viruses (Ali *et al.* 2006; Moury *et al.* 2007; Betancourt *et al.* 2008).

Another group of viruses 'circulate' through the insect haemocoel and reach the salivary glands, allowing them to be inoculated to new plants without reproducing within the vector. Such viruses seem to hijack a constitutive endocytosis–exocytosis mechanism without greatly perturbing cell metabolism (Hogenhout *et al.* 2008; Brault *et al.* 2010). To be transmitted, these viruses require a relatively long acquisition time compared with non-circulative viruses (ranging from hours to days) and a latent time, i.e. the time necessary for viral particles to enter the haemocoel from the gut and migrate to the salivary glands, ranging from hours to days. Contrary to viruses transmitted in a non-circulative manner, the time period during which vectors remain viruliferous depends on the vector lifespan and on the amount of viral particles ingested, which is positively correlated to acquisition time (van den Heuvel *et al.* 1991; Reynaud & Peterschmitt 1992) and viral accumulation *in planta* (Chen & Gilbertson 2008).

Finally, a variant of the previous mode of transmission is 'circulative–propagative' transmission, where the virus replicates in the vector (e.g. TSWV). For some of these viruses, transovarial transmission to vector offspring has been described (e.g. MStV; Ammar *et al.* 1995). Acquisition of viral particles by vectors can be achieved after a few minutes of feeding on an infected host plant (TYLCV; Mehta *et al.* 1994; Czosnek *et al.* 2001). However, inoculation of ingested viruses to another plant will occur only after a latent period, which, depending on virus genus, varies from 24 h (TYLCV; Mehta *et al.* 1994) to more than one week (MStV;Ammar *et al.* 1995). As with viruses transmitted in a circulative manner, the period during which vectors remain viruliferous depends on vector lifespan. The main difference between circulative and propagative viruses is that, in the latter case, virus load in the vector increases during the first weeks following infection because of virus replication in the vector. Finally, the transmission rate tends to decrease as vectors get older, probably owing to modification of their feeding behaviour (TYLCV; Czosnek *et al.* 2001). Notably, TYLCV represents a special case in classification, since it is usually considered to be transmitted in a circulative manner (Hogenhout *et al.* 2008) but has been shown to replicate within its vector (Czosnek *et al.* 2001).

Inspection of table 2 shows that, in all cases, the correlation between viral accumulation and transmission, be it $\beta_{p \to v}$, $\beta_{v \to p}$ or the overall transmission rate ($\beta_{p \to v} \times \beta_{v \to p}$), is positive. This contrasts with the results on 'engineered' viruses where no correlation between viral accumulation and transmission rate arises, indicating that the positive correlation observed in field samples does not result from genomic constraints. Clearly more relevant studies are needed, especially for the circulative and propagative transmission modes.

VIRAL ACCUMULATION VERSUS VIRULENCE

In the case of vector-borne diseases, parasite density can affect virulence in both the host $\alpha_p(x)$ and the vector$\alpha_v(y)$. In the following section, we report empirical evidence on the correlation between viral accumulation and virulence in both plant and vector. Note that virulence here is estimated through disease-induced mortality. In this, we follow the majority of studies, because fitness components other than survival do not directly affect the R_0 of a horizontally transmitted parasite. Some of the studies we discuss report the effects of virus infection on a host fitness component that might be correlated with host survival, and therefore these studies should be interpreted with caution.

(a) Effect of Viral Accumulation on Components of Plant Fitness

We searched for empirical studies reporting both viral accumulation and accurate measures of components of virulence (i.e. related to survival rate) for several viral genotypes infecting (at least) one host genotype. As for transmission phenotypes, a large number of studies consider the phenotype resulting from point mutation(s) introduced *in vitro* or isolated randomly from viral populations. Reports yield conflicting results. Viral clones differing by only one point mutation present contrasting phenotypes: some studies report a negative correlation between viral accumulation and the dry weight of the host plant (Poulicard *et al.* 2010). For some other viral mutants, higher accumulation is associated with phenotypes with more attenuated symptoms (Rodriguez-Cerezo *et al.* 1991), or with symptoms similar to (Bruyère *et al.* 1997) or more severe than (Gal-On 2007) those of the wild-type. Note that scientists and plant breeders often use symptoms as an indicator of the effect of viruses on host fitness. Although this can actually be the case when infections provoke host stunting, or nanism or other leaf disorders (Jarosz & Davelos 1995; Zaitlin & Hull 2003), it should be remembered that symptoms might not always be a good proxy, especially when host species harbour genes involved in parasite tolerance (Hoffman & Kolb 1998). Even if no general trend arises from results concerning viral mutant genotypes, such studies demonstrate the existence of variation in the relationships between viral accumulation and virulence or symptom severity.

Unfortunately, studies that reported the phenotype of natural isolates often measured only virulence (Yahara & Oyama 1993; Lapidot *et al.* 1997; Maskell *et al.* 1999; Funayama-Noguchi 2001; Malmstrom *et al.* 2005,2006) or viral accumulation (Fargette *et al.* 1987; Llamas-Llamas *et al.* 1998; Thurston *et al.* 2001; Untiveros*et al.* 2007; Wintermantel *et al.* 2008) of one viral isolate in one or several host genotypes in different environments. To our knowledge, only a handful of studies have measured both phenotypes concomitantly for several viral natural isolates after individual inoculation of one host genotype. These studies estimated within-host viral accumulation induced by several natural isolates, some inducing mild, some intermediate and some severe symptoms. Several host–virus interactions exhibited positive correlations: PNRSV–*Rosa indica* (Moury *et al.* 2001), RYMV–*Oryza sativa japonica* cv Azucena (Fargette *et al.* 2002), CMV infecting *Nicotiana glutinosa* or *N. tabacum* (Shi *et al.* 2002) or *Cucumis sativus* (Banik & Zitter 1990), PRSV infecting *Cucurbita pepo* or *Citrullus lanatus* (Pacheco *et al.* 2003), BSV–*Musa accuminata* (Dahal*et al.* 1998). The relative limitation of these studies comes from the fact that only a few isolates are tested, and, as mentioned previously, symptoms may not be a good proxy for host survival. One of the reasons explaining the scarcity of suitable studies is that sometimes the relationship was not investigated at the level of the relevant virulence components for horizontally transmitted parasites, e.g. those linked to duration of infection. For instance, several studies looked at the relationship between fecundity and viral accumulation.

Moreover, the relationship between viral accumulation and virulence may be obscured by potential heterogeneity of the hosts with respect to interactions with pathogens. Indeed, plants can be resistant, tolerant and/or susceptible to parasite infection. Resistance is the ability of the host to limit parasite burden, and tolerance is the ability to limit the harm caused by a given burden (Cooper & Jones 1983). Heterogeneity in host plants with respect to tolerance/resistance may blur the correlations between viral accumulation and either virulence or transmission. For instance, interactions between PNRSV–*Prunus* spp. (Moury *et al.* 2001) and PRSV–*Cucurbita mochata* (Pacheco *et al.* 2003) did not lead to any correlation, probably because some viral isolates accumulated to a high titre in plants, but induced only few or no symptoms. This poses an important methodological problem, as discussed further in the last section.

Empirical data supporting the existence of a correlation between within-host viral accumulation and virulence are scarce. The few studies mentioned above indicate the existence of a positive correlation between virulence and viral accumulation, but of course many more studies, as well as studies looking more directly at the relevant virulence parameters, are needed before a general conclusion can be reached. The effect of host heterogeneity on resistance/tolerance mechanisms and the nature of the observed relationship between viral accumulation and virulence deserve further study.

(b) Effect of Viral Infection on the Vector

The only studies we found on this subject report the qualitative effects of viral infection on transmission through modification of vector behavior/physiology.

Vector mobility certainly plays a role in the variation of the contact rate between vector and host, thus affecting the probability of virus transmission (Fereres & Moreno 2009). Such variation in mobility has been reported for vectors infected by a circulative virus: these insects exhibit more movement around experimental arenas than uninfected controls, causing a slight increase in the number of infected host plants (Hodge & Powell 2008). Interestingly, enhanced plant penetration by aphid stylets was observed on symptomatic virus-infected plants compared with healthy plants (Alvarez *et al.* 2007). Moreover, it has long been known that aphids are significantly attracted by yellow (Doring *et al.* 2009) and that some plant viruses induce symptoms resulting in chlorosis, mosaics or other modifications that lead to yellowing of the leaves. Aphids have been shown to prefer to land and settle on virus-infected plants with yellowing leaves, possibly owing to the fact that insect vectors use visual cues to choose suitable plants (Fereres *et al.* 1999; Hodge & Powell 2008). Insect vectors also choose plants in response to olfactory cues, and the composition of the volatile organic compounds emitted by the leaves of some plants has been shown to change when the plant is infected by viruses (Ngumbi *et al.* 2007; Medina-Ortega *et al.* 2009). These changes can be more or less pronounced. For instance, plants infected by a circulative virus tend to attract their aphid vectors more than plants infected either by non-circulative viruses or by non-vectored viruses or healthy plants (Eigen brode *et al.* 2002). However, this pattern seems to depend on the host–virus interaction, since no such differences were observed on other plants and virus species (Castle *et al.* 1998; Hodge & Powell 2008).

For several plant virus vectors reared on infected plants, studies have shown an increase in components of vector fitness such as survival or fecundity (Hunt & Nault 1990; Blua *et al.* 1994; Mayer *et al.* 2002; Belliure*et al.* 2005; Maris *et al.* 2007; Sisterson 2008). Such increases result from various mechanisms. In one case, they were due to reduced developmental time of larvae reared on infected plants, which resulted in a shorter period of vulnerability to predation (Belliure *et al.* 2008). In other cases, the increase was due to the fact that infected plants had increased amino acid contents in phloem sap and decreased honeydew production compared with healthy plants (BYDV, Ajayi 1986; ZYMV, Blua *et al.* 1994). The latter interpretation is reinforced by the fact that vectors exhibited increased fitness when reared on plants infected by non-vector-borne viruses compared with when reared on healthy plants (Hare & Dodds 1987; Musser *et al.* 2003). Increased performance of insects reared on some virus-infected plants might thus be due to better availability of nutrients in infected plants. Such effects, however, are not universal, and decreases in vector fitness owing to infection have also been reported (Ellsbury *et al.* 1985; Power 1992; Sinisterra *et al.* 2005; Inoue & Sakurai 2006; Hodge & Powell 2008; Matsuura & Hoshino 2009).

Previous studies indicate that vectors settle preferentially on infected plants because of visual or olfactory cues expressed by these plants. Some virus–host interactions lead to an increase in some components of vector fitness. Moreover, infected vectors tend to exhibit increased mobility, which should lead to increase feeding rates. All these processes enhance vector-borne virus transmission, leading to the modification of the basic reproduction ratio R_0 (see McElhany *et al.* (1995) for discussion). Unfortunately, data currently available do not allow us to detect the potential differential effects of viral transmission modes.

CONCLUDING REMARKS

Understanding why parasites harm their hosts is an old question in evolutionary biology. Arguably, one of the most appealing answers comes from the trade-off hypothesis, which states that parasite transmission and virulence are correlated, such that increased transmission leads to shorter infection times (Anderson & May 1982; Ewald 1983). This correlation arises because both transmission and virulence are increasing functions of parasite within-host density.

In the present review, our aim was to investigate whether existing empirical evidence supports the hypothesis that virulence and transmission of vector-borne plant viruses are linked through a common variable, i.e. within-plant viral accumulation. On the one hand, all studies that have looked at the correlation between within-plant viral accumulation and transmission rate, or one of its components, found a positive relationship (table 2). Undoubtedly, more studies are needed on this issue, especially on circulative and propagative viruses; however, the unanimity of positive correlations suggests that this relationship will most probably be confirmed. We were surprised by the paucity of studies on the relationship between viral accumulation and virulence components relevant for testing the trade-off hypothesis. The few studies we identified suffer from their own limitations: disease symptoms were used as a proxy for virulence, and the number of isolates studied was small. The existence, or not, of this correlation thus remains unresolved. At present, we can say only that the existing evidence supports the first part of the trade-off hypothesis, i.e. the correlation between transmission and within-host accumulation, but is inconclusive as to the second part, the virulence–within-host accumulation correlation. Consequently, we cannot conclude whether the trade-off hypothesis holds or not in plant viruses.

It is important to realize that testing the trade-off hypothesis implies more than 'simply' establishing the two correlations discussed throughout this paper. One must also show that an optimal virulence level indeed exists. Theory predicts that if both virulence and transmission increase linearly with viral accumulation, virus populations should evolve towards ever higher levels of virulence. As mentioned in §2, an optimal virulence level is evolutionarily stable only if the rate of increase of virulence with viral accumulation is faster than the rate of increase of transmission with viral accumulation. This is difficult to validate in most host–parasite systems (Alizon *et al.* 2009). In the case of vector-borne plant viruses, a promising option would be to try to show that the transmission rate saturates for high virus accumulation rates within the plant because of the limitation introduced by the vector (Alizon & van Baalen 2008). Such a saturating transmission function combined with, for example, linearly increasing virulence would lead to an intermediate optimal level of viral accumulation.

When addressing this issue, it is thus important to measure all three key parameters (viral accumulation, virulence and transmission) concomitantly for several viral isolates on the same host plant genotype. We feel it is important to clarify two points. The first relates to the relevant virulence components one needs to measure, and the second to the potential effects of host heterogeneity.

Virulence components relevant for testing the trade-off hypothesis are components that directly affect parasite fitness. For horizontally transmitted parasites, such components should typically be related to the duration of the infection, as this determines the time during which the parasite can be transmitted. Host survival is an obvious trait relevant to the duration of infection. In contrast, host fecundity is, *a priori*, not directly relevant, except if it is linked to survival through a survival–reproduction trade-off. Obviously, fecundity would be a trait directly relevant for vertically transmitted parasites.

Host heterogeneity for tolerance/resistance may strongly affect the virulence–accumulation correlation. Resistance (by definition) affects viral accumulation: if a parasite replicates less in one host genotype than in another, then the former can be said to be more resistant. Tolerance affects the relationship between virulence and accumulation:

one host genotype is said to be more tolerant than another if it suffers less from infection, i.e. if virulence is lower, for a given parasite load (Raberg *et al.* 2009). Comparisons of the correlations between virulence, accumulation and transmission across hosts differing in resistance do not pose any specific problem for testing the trade-off hypothesis: resistance should affect directly only accumulation, and, if the trade-off hypothesis holds, more resistant plants should have lower viral loads, lower transmission and lower virulence than less resistant plants. Variation in tolerance across plants would not pose a problem in measuring the accumulation–transmission correlation, assuming that transmission depends only on accumulation (and not on virulence, for example). It would pose a problem for measuring the accumulation–virulence correlation, however, since, by definition, tolerance affects this relationship. Thus, ignoring such variations in tolerance may mask positive correlations. Therefore, it should be realized that measuring this correlation across plants of different tolerance levels would not be an appropriate test of the trade-off hypothesis. The existence of resistance/tolerance presents no challenge to the trade-off hypothesis *per se*. When such variation exists, it should be acknowledged. The trade-off could be tested by controlling for the level of resistance/tolerance. For example, one could compare the virulence of different viral isolates that reach different accumulation levels on hosts with a known level of tolerance.

The correlation between viral accumulation, transmission rate and virulence also calls for more theoretical approaches. One possibility would be to investigate how the mode of vector-borne transmission (propagative, circulative or non-circulative) can affect the evolution of virulence. For instance, a key difference would be that, in the case of a virus transmitted in a propagative manner, once a vector is infected, it remains viruliferous until it dies. In the case of a virus transmitted in a circulative manner, however, the period during which a vector remains infected is likely to be correlated with the amount of virus it ingests. Finally, for viruses transmitted in a non-circulative manner, very few viral particles are retained in vector mouth parts, and particles are lost very quickly. These biological facts can be expressed mathematically by varying the transmission function. We believe that such differences in life cycles should lead to different expressions of R_0 and thus to different predictions in terms of optimal virulence levels.

Transmission modes of vector-borne animal viruses share some similarities with plant viruses. In fact, vector transmission of animal viruses falls into two classes: 'mechanical' and 'biological'. Mechanical transmission docs not involve any replication inside the vector and is exemplified by, for instance, myxoma virus (Barcena*et al.* 2000) or lumpy skin disease virus (Chihota *et al.* 2003). Transmission success seems to be vector-specific as some vector species failed to transmit lumpy skin disease virus in recent studies (Chihota *et al.* 2003), although they were able to transmit other pox viruses (Mellor *et al.* 1987). This specificity for successful transmission strikingly resembles the case of non-circulative transmission in plant viruses. Biological transmission implies reproduction inside the vector, which applies to the vast majority of vector-borne vertebrate-infecting viruses (arboviruses), which are responsible for a number of severe diseases in humans (yellow fever, dengue, various encephalitides, etc.) and livestock (West Nile encephalomyelitis, Rift Valley fever, vesicular stomatitis, etc.). When the characteristics of these viruses are compared with those of plant viruses, several common features appear between all the latter viruses and plant viruses with a circulative–propagative mode of transmission. Further investigations of the parallels between vector-borne animal and plant viruses concerning the correlation between viral accumulation, transmission rate and virulence could be particularly helpful in revealing general patterns for such diseases. Finally, the circulative transmission mode seems to be a distinctive feature of plant viruses. Understanding why this is the case may help us understand how viruses colonize and exploit vectors to increase their transmission.

List of viral acronyms: banana streak virus (BSV, *Badnavirus*), barley yellow dwarf virus (BYDV,*Luteovirus*), beet mild curly top virus (BMCTV, *Curtovirus*), beet mosaic virus (BtMV, *Potyvirus*), beet severe curly top virus (BSCTV, *Curtovirus*), cucumber mosaic virus (CMV, *Cucumovirus*), lettuce infectious yellows virus (LIYV, *Crinivirus*), maize streak virus (MSV, Mastrevirus), maize stripe virus (MStV, *Tenuivirus*), papaya ringspot virus (PRSV, *Potyvirus*), potato leafroll virus (PLRV, *Polerovirus*), potato virus Y (PVY, *Potyvirus*), prunus necrotic ringspot virus (PNRSV, *Ilarvirus*), ribgrass mosaic virus (RMV, *Tobamovirus*), rice yellow mottle virus (RYMV, *Sobemovirus*), tomato chlorosis virus (ToCV,*Crinivirus*), ryegrass mosaic virus (RMV, *Rymovirus*), tomato infectious chlorosis virus (TiCV, *Crinivirus*), tomato spotted wild virus (TSWV, *Tospovirus*), tomato yellow leaf curl virus (TYLCV, *Begomovirus*), turnip mosaic virus (TuMV, *Potyvirus*), watermelon mosaic virus (WMV2, *Potyvirus*).

FOOTNOTES

One contribution of 14 to a Theme Issue 'New experimental and theoretical approaches towards the understanding of the emergence of viral infections'

REFERENCES

1. Ajayi O. 1986. The effect of *Barley yellow dwarf virus* on the amino acid composition of spring wheat.Ann. Appl. Biol. 108, 145–149 (doi:10.1111/j.1744-7348.1986.tb01975.x)
2. Ali A., Li H., Schneider W. L., Sherman D. J., Gray S., Smith D., Roossinck M. J. 2006. Analysis of genetic bottlenecks during horizontal transmission of *Cucumber mosaic virus*. J. Virol. 80, 8345–8350 (doi:10.1128/JVI.00568-06)
3. Alizon S., Van Baalen M. 2008. Transmission–virulence trade-offs in vector-borne diseases. Theor. Popul. Biol. 74, 6–15 (doi:10.1016/j.tpb.2008.04.003)
4. Alizon S., Hurford A., Mideo N., Van Baalen M. 2009. Virulence evolution and the trade-off hypothesis: history, current state of affairs and the future. J. Evol. Biol. 22, 245–259 (doi:10.1111/j.1420-9101.2008.01658.x)
5. Alvarez A. E., Garzo E., Verbeek M., Volman B., Dicke M., Tjallingii W. F. 2007. Infection of potato plants with *Potato leafroll virus* changes attraction and feeding behaviour of *Myzus persicae*. Entomol. Exp. Appl. 125, 135–144 (doi:10.1111/j.1570-7458.2007.00607.x)
6. Ammar E. D., Gingery R. E., Madden L. V. 1995. Transmission efficiency of three isolates of *Maize stripe tenuivirus* in relation to virus titer in the planthopper vector. Plant Pathol. 44, 239–243 (doi:10.1111/j.1365-3059.1995.tb02774.x)

7. Anderson R. M., May R. M. 1982. Coevolution of hosts and parasites. Parasitology 85, 411–426 (doi:10.1017/S0031182000055360) [PubMed]
8. Anderson R. M., May R. M. 1991. Infectious diseases of humans: dynamics and control. Oxford, UK: Oxford University Press
9. Banik M. T., Zitter T. A. 1990. Determination of *Cucumber mosaic virus* titer in muskmelon by enzyme-linked immunosorbent assay and correlation with aphid transmission. Plant Dis. 74, 857–859 (doi:10.1094/PD-74-0857)
10. Barcena J., et al. 2000. Horizontal transmissible protection against myxomatosis and rabbit hemorrhagic disease by using a recombinant myxoma virus. J. Virol. 74, 1114–1123 (doi:10.1128/JVI.74.3.1114-1123.2000)
11. Belliure B., Janssen A., Maris P. C., Peters D., Sabelis M. W. 2005. Herbivore arthropods benefit from vectoring plant viruses. Ecol. Lett. 8, 70–79 (doi:10.1111/j.1461-0248.2004.00699.x)
12. Belliure B., Janssen A., Sabelis M. 2008. Herbivore benefits from vectoring plant virus through reduction of period of vulnerability to predation. Oecologia 156, 797–806 (doi:10.1007/s00442-008-1027-9)
13. Betancourt M., Fereres A., Fraile A., Garcia-Arenal F. 2008. Estimation of the effective number of founders that initiate an infection after aphid transmission of a multipartite plant virus. J. Virol. 82, 12 416–12 421
14. Blanc S. 2008. Vector transmission of plant viruses. In Encyclopedia of virology (eds Mahy B. W. J., Regenmortel M. H. V. V., editors.). New York, NY: Academic Press
15. Blua M. J., Perring T. M., Madore M. A. 1994. Plant virus-induced changes in aphid population development and temporal fluctuations in plant nutrients. J. Chem. Ecol. 20, 691–707 (doi:10.1007/BF02059607)
16. Bolker B. M., Nanda A., Shah D. 2010. Transient virulence of emerging pathogens. J. R. Soc. Interface 7, 811–822 (doi:10.1098/rsif.2009.0384)
17. Brault V., Tanguy S., Reinbold C., Le Trionnaire G., Arneodo J., Jaubert-Possamai S., Guernec G., Tagu D. 2010. Transcriptomic

analysis of intestinal genes following acquisition of *Pea enation mosaic virus*by the pea aphid *Acyrthosiphon pisum*. J. Gen. Virol. 91, 802–808 (doi:10.1099/vir.0.012856-0)

18. BraultV., Uzest M., Monsion B., Jacquot E., Blanc S. In press Aphids as transport devices for plant viruses. C. R. Acad. Sci. Biologie.
19. Bruyère A., Brault V., Ziegler-Graff V., Simonis M. T., Van Den Heuvel J. F. J. M., Richards K., Guilley H., Jonard G., Herrbach E. 1997. Effects of mutations in the *Beet western yellows virus* readthrough protein on its expression and packaging and on virus accumulation, symptoms, and aphid transmission. Virology 230, 323–334 (doi:10.1006/viro.1997.8476)
20. Castle S. J., Mowry T. M., Berger P. H. 1998. Differential settling by *Myzus persicae* (Homoptera: Aphididae) on various virus infected host plants. Ann. Entomol. Soc. Am. 91, 661–667
21. Chen L.-F., Gilbertson R. L. 2008. Curtovirus–Cucurbit interaction: acquisition host plays a role in leafhopper transmission in a host-dependent manner. Phytopathology 99, 101–108 (doi:10.1094/PHYTO-99-1-0101)
22. Chihota C. M., Rennie L. F., Kitching R. P., Mellor P. S. 2003. Attempted mechanical transmission of lumpy skin disease virus by biting insects. Med. Vet. Entomol. 17, 294–300 (doi:10.1046/j.1365-2915.2003.00445.x)
23. Cooper J. I., Jones A. T. 1983. Responses of plants to viruses: proposals for the use of terms.Phytopathology 73, 127–128 (doi:10.1094/Phyto-73-127)
24. Czosnek H., Ghanim M., Morin S., Rubinstein G., Fridman V., Zeidan M. 2001. Whiteflies: vectors, and victims (?), of geminiviruses. Adv. Virus Res. 57, 291–322 (doi:10.1016/S0065-3527(01)57006-2)
25. Dahal G., Pasberg-Gauhl C., Gauhl F., Thottappilly G., Hughes J. D. A. 1998. Studies on a Nigerian isolate of *Banana streak badnavirus*: II. Effect of intraplant variation on virus accumulation and reliability of diagnosis by ELISA. Ann. Appl. Biol. 132, 263–275 (doi:10.1111/j.1744-7348.1998.tb05202.x)
26. D'arcy C. J., Eastburn D. M., Schumann G. L. 2001. Illustrated glossary of plant pathology. The plant health instructor. http://www.apsnet.org/education/IllustratedGlossary/ (doi:10.1094/PHI-I-2001-0219-01)

27. De Bokx J. A., Van Hoof H. A., Piron P. G. M. 1978. Relation between concentration of potato virus Y(N) and its availability to *Myzus persicae*. Eur. J. Plant Pathol. 84, 95–100 (doi:10.1007/BF01981535)

28. Demangeat G., Voisin R., Minot J.-C., Bosselut N., Fuchs M., Esmenjaud D. 2005. Survival of*Xiphinema index* in vineyard soil and retention of *Grapevine fanleaf virus* over extended time in the absence of host plants. Phytopathology 95, 1151–1156 (doi:10.1094/PHYTO-95-1151)

29. De Roode J. C., Yates A. J., Altizer S. 2008. Virulence–transmission trade-offs and population divergence in virulence in a naturally occurring butterfly parasite. Proc. Natl Acad. Sci. USA 105, 7489–7494 (doi:10.1073/pnas.0710909105)

30. Doring T. F., Archetti M., Hardie J. 2009. Autumn leaves seen through herbivore eyes. Proc. Biol. Sci.276, 121–127 (doi:10.1098/rspb.2008.0858)

31. Duffy S., Shackelton L. A., Holmes E. C. 2008. Rates of evolutionary change in viruses: patterns and determinants. Nat. Rev. Genet. 9, 267–276 (doi:10.1038/nrg2323)

32. Dusi A. N., Peters D. 1999. *Beet mosaic virus*: its vector and host relationships. J. Phytopathol. 147, 293–298 (doi:10.1111/j.1439-0434.1999.tb03833.x)

33. Dwyer G., Levin S. A., Buttel L. 1990. A simulation model of the population dynamics and evolution of myxomatosis. Ecol. Monogr. 60, 423–447 (doi:10.2307/1943014)

34. Eigenbrode S. D., Ding H., Shiel P., Berger P. H. 2002. Volatiles from potato plants infected with potato leafroll virus attract and arrest the virus vector, *Myzus persicae* (Homoptera: Aphididae). Proc. R. Soc. B 269, 455–460 (doi:10.1098/rspb.2001.1909)

35. Ellsbury M. M., Pratt R. G., Knight W. E. 1985. Effects of single and combined infection of arrowleaf clover with *Bean yellow mosaic virus* and a *Phytophthora* sp. on reproduction and colonization by pea aphids (Homoptera: Aphididae). Environ. Entomol. 14, 356–359

36. Escrlu F., Fraile A., Garcia-Arenal F. 2000. *a*Evolution of virulence in natural populations of the satellite RNA of *Cucumber mosaic virus*.. Phytopathology 90, 480–485 (doi:10.1094/PHYTO.2000.90.5.480)

37. Escriu F., Perry K. L., Garcia-Arenal F. 2000. *b*Transmissibility of *Cucumber mosaic virus* by *Aphis gossypii* correlates with viral accumulation and is affected by the presence of its satellite RNA.Phytopathology 90, 1068–1072 (doi:10.1094/PHYTO.2000.90.10.1068)
38. Ewald P. W. 1983. Host–parasite relations, vectors, and the evolution of disease severity. Annu. Rev. Ecol. Evol. Syst. 14, 465–485 (doi:10.1146/annurev.es.14.110183.002341)
39. Fargette D., Thouvenel J.-C., Fauquet C. 1987. Virus content of leaves of cassava infected by African cassava mosaic virus. Ann. Appl. Biol. 110, 65–73 (doi:org/10.1111/j.1744-7348.1987.tb03233.x)
40. Fargette D., Pinel A., Traoré O., Ghesquière A., Konaté G. 2002. Emergence of resistance-breaking isolates of Rice yellow mottle virus during serial inoculations. Eur. J. Plant Pathol. 108, 585–591 (doi:10.1023/A:1019952907105)
41. Fereres A., Moreno A. 2009. Behavioural aspects influencing plant virus transmission by homopteran insects. Virus Res. 141, 158–168 (doi:10.1016/j.virusres.2008.10.020)
42. Fereres A., Kampmeier G. E., Irwin M. E. 1999. Aphid attraction and preference for soybean and pepper plants infected with *Potyviridae*. Ann. Entomol. Soc. Am. 92, 542–548
43. Frank S. A. 1996. Models of parasite virulence. Q. Rev. Biol. 71, 37–78 (doi:10.1086/419267)
44. Fraser C., Hollingsworth T. D., Chapman R., De Wolf F., Hanage W. P. 2007. Variation in HIV-1 set-point viral load: epidemiological analysis and an evolutionary hypothesis. Proc. Natl Acad. Sci. USA104, 17 441–17 446
45. Froissart R., Roze D., Uzest M., Galibert L., Blanc S., Michalakis Y. 2005. Recombination every day: abundant recombination in a virus during a single multi-cellular host infection. PLoS Biol. 3, e89 (doi:10.1371/journal.pbio.0030089)
46. Funayama-Noguchi S. 2001. Ecophysiology of virus-infected plants: a case study of *Eupatorium makinoi*infected by geminivirus. Plant Biol. 3, 251–262 (doi:10.1055/s-2001-15199)

47. Gal-on A. 2007. *Zucchini yellow mosaic virus*: insect transmission and pathogenicity: the tails of two proteins. Mol. Plant Pathol. 8, 139–150 (doi:10.1111/j.1364-3703.2007.00381.x)
48. Garcia-Arenal F., Fraile A., Malpica J. M. 2001. Variability and genetic structure of plant virus populations. Annu. Rev. Phytopathol. 39, 157–186 (doi:10.1146/annurev.phyto.39.1.157)
49. Gera A., Loebenstein G., Raccah B. 1979. Protein coats of two strains of *Cucumber mosaic virus* affect transmission by *Aphis gossypii*. Phytopathology 69, 396–399 (doi:10.1094/Phyto-69-396)
50. Gray S. M., Banerjee N. 1999. Mechanisms of arthropod transmission of plant and animal viruses.Microbiol. Mol. Biol. Rev. 63, 128–148
51. Gray S. M., Power A. G., Smith D. M., Seaman A. J., Altman N. S. 1991. Aphid transmission of *Barley yellow dwarf virus*: acquisition access periods and virus concentration requirements. Phytopathology81, 539–545 (doi:10.1094/Phyto-81-539)
52. Gray S. M., Smith D., Altman N. S. 1993. *Barley yellow dwarf virus* isolate-specific resistance in spring oats reduced virus accumulation and aphid transmission. Phytopathology 83, 716–720 (doi:10.1094/Phyto-83-716)
53. Gray S. M., Smith D., Sorrells M. 1994. Reduction of disease incidence in small field plots by isolate-specific resistance to *Barley yellow dwarf virus*. Phytopathology 84, 713–718 (doi:10.1094/Phyto-84-713)
54. Hare D. J., Dodds J. A. 1987. Survival of the *Colorado potato* beetle on virus-infected tomato in relation to plant nitrogen and alkaloid content. Entomol. Exp. Appl. 44, 31–35 (doi:10.1007/BF00361306)
55. Harris K. F. 1977. An ingestion–egestion hypothesis of non circulative virus transmission. In Aphids as virus vectors (eds Harris K. F., Maramorosch K., editors.). New York, NY, Academic Press
56. Hodge S., Powell G. 2008. Do plant viruses facilitate their aphid vectors by inducing symptoms that alter behavior

and performance? Environ. Entomol. 37, 1573–1581 (doi:10.1603/0046-225X-37.6.1573)

57. Hoffman T. K., Kolb F. L. 1998. Effects of *Barley yellow dwarf virus* on yield and yield components of drilled winter wheat. Plant Dis. 82, 620–624 (doi:10.1094/PDIS.1998.82.6.620)
58. Hogenhout S. A., Ammar E.-D., Whitfield A. E., Redinbaugh M. G. 2008. Insect–vector interactions with persistently transmitted viruses. Annu. Rev. Phytopathol. 46, 327–359 (doi:10.1146/annurev.phyto.022508.092135)
59. Hull R. 2001. Matthews› plant virology San Diego, CA: Academic Press
60. Hunt R. E., Nault L. R. 1990. Influence of life history of grasses and *Maize chlorotic dwarf virus* on the biotic potential of the leafhopper *Graminella nigrifrons* (Homoptera: Cicadellidae). Environ. Entomol.19, 76–84
61. Inoue T., Sakurai T. 2006. Infection of *Tomato spotted wilt virus* (TSWV) shortens the life span of thelytokous *Thrips tabaci* (Thysanoptera: Thripidae). Appl. Entomol. Zool. 41, 239–246 (doi:10.1303/aez.2006.239)
62. Jarosz A. M. 2002. Virulence management in plant–pathogen interactions. In Adaptive dynamics of infectious diseases: in pursuit of virulence management (eds Dieckmann U., Metz J. A., Sabelis M. W., Sigmund K., editors.). Cambridge, UK: Cambridge University Press
63. Jarosz A. M., Davelos A. L. 1995. Effects of disease in wild plant populations and the evolution of pathogen aggressiveness. New Phytol. 129, 371–387 (doi:10.1111/j.1469-8137.1995.tb04308.x)
64. Jensen K. H., Little T. J., Skorping A., Ebert D. 2006. Empirical support for optimal virulence in a castrating parasite. PLoS Biol. 4, e197 (doi:10.1371/journal.pbio.0040197)
65. Kalleshwaraswamy C. M., Kumar N. K. K. 2008. Transmission efficiency of *Papaya ringspot virus* by three aphid species. Phytopathology 98, 541–546
66. Lapidot M., Friedmann M., Lachman O., Yehezkel A., Nahon S., Cohen S., Pilowsky M. 1997.Comparison of resistance level to *Tomato yellow leaf curl virus* among commercial cultivars

and breeding lines. Plant Dis. 81, 1425–1428 (doi:10.1094/PDIS.1997.81.12.1425)

67. Lapidot M., Friedmann M., Pilowsky M., Ben-Joseph R., Cohen S. 2001. Effect of host plant resistance to*Tomato yellow leaf curl virus* (TYLCV) on virus acquisition and transmission by its whitefly vector.Phytopathology 91, 1209–1213 (doi:10.1094/PHYTO.2001.91.12.1209)

68. Levin B. R. 1996. The evolution and maintenance of virulence in microparasites. Emerge. Infect. Dis. 2, 93–102 (doi:10.3201/eid0202.960203)

69. Levin B. R., Bull J. J. 1994. Short-sighted evolution and the virulence of pathogenic microorganisms.Trends Microbiol. 2, 76–81 (doi:10.1016/0966-842X(94)90538-X)

70. Llamas-Llamas M. E., Zavaleta-Mejia E., Gonzalez-Hernandez V. A., Cervantes-Diaz L., Santizo-Rincon J. A., Ochoa-Martinez D. L. 1998. Effect of temperature on symptom expression and accumulation of*Tomato spotted wilt virus* in different host species. Plant Pathol. 47, 341–347 (doi:10.1046/j.1365-3059.1998.00249.x)

71. Mackinnon M. J., Read A. F. 1999. Selection for high and low virulence in the malaria parasite*Plasmodium chabaudi*. Proc. R. Soc. B 266, 741–748 (doi:10.1098/rspb.1999.0699)

72. Malmstrom C. M., Hughes C. C., Newton L. A., Stoner C. J. 2005. Virus infection in remnant native bunchgrasses from invaded California grasslands. New Phytol. 168, 217–230 (doi:10.1111/j.1469-8137.2005.01479.x)

73. Malmstrom C., Stoner C., Brandenburg S., Newton L. 2006. Virus infection and grazing exert counteracting influences on survivorship of native bunchgrass seedlings competing with invasive exotics. J. Ecol. 94, 264–275 (doi:10.1111/j.1365-2745.2006.01101.x)

74. Maris P. C., Joosten N. N., Goldbach R. W., Peters D. 2007. *Tomato spotted wilt virus* infection improves host suitability for its vector *Frankliniella occidentalis*. Phytopathology 94, 706–711 (doi:10.1094/PHYTO.2004.94.7.706)

75. Maskell L. C., Raybould A. F., Cooper J. I., Edwards M.-L., Gray A. J. 1999. Effects of *Turnip mosaic virus* and *Turnip yellow*

mosaic virus on the survival, growth and reproduction of wild cabbage (*Brassica oleracea*). Ann. Appl. Biol. 135, 401–407 (doi:10.1111/j.1744-7348.1999.tb00867.x)

76. Matsuura S., Hoshino S. 2009. Effect of *Tomato yellow leaf curl* disease on reproduction of *Bemisia tabaci* Q biotype (Hemiptera: Aleyrodidae) on tomato plants. Appl. Entomol. Zool. 44, 143–148 (doi:10.1303/aez.2009.143)
77. Mayer R. T., Inbar M., Mckenzie C. L., Shatters R., Borowicz V., Albrecht U., Powell C. A., Doostdar H. 2002. Multitrophic interactions of the silverleaf whitefly, host plants, competing herbivores, and phytopathogens. Arch. Insect. Biochem. Physiol. 51, 151–169 (doi:10.1002/arch.10065)
78. Mcelhany P., Real L. A., Power A. G. 1995. Vector preference and disease dynamics: a study of *Barley yellow dwarf virus*. Ecology 76, 444–457 (doi:10.2307/1941203)
79. Medina-Ortega K. J., Bosque-Perez N. A., Ngumbi E., Jimenez-Martinez E. S., Eigenbrode S. D. 2009.*Rhopalosiphum padi* (Hemiptera: Aphididae) responses to volatile cues from *Barley yellow dwarf virus*-infected wheat. Environ. Entomol. 38, 836–845 (doi:10.1603/022.038.0337)
80. Mehta P., Wyman J. A., Nakhla M. K., Maxwell D. P. 1994. Transmission of *Tomato yellow leaf curl geminivirus* by *Bemisia tabaci* (Homoptera: *Aleyrodidae*). J. Econ. Entomol. 87, 1291–1297
81. Mellor P. S., Kitching R. P., Wilkinson P. J. 1987. Mechanical transmission of *Capripox virus* and *African swine fever virus* by *Stomoxys calcitrans*. Res. Vet. Sci. 43, 109–112
82. Mideo N., Day T. 2008. On the evolution of reproductive restraint in malaria. Proc. R. Soc. B 275, 1217–1224 (doi:10.1098/rspb.2007.1545)
83. Moury B., Cardin L., Onesto J. P., Candresse T., Poupet A. 2001. Survey of *Prunus necrotic ringspot virus* in rose and its variability in rose and Prunus spp. Phytopathology 91, 84–91 (doi:10.1094/PHYTO.2001.91.1.84)
84. Moury B., Fabre F., Senoussi R. 2007. Estimation of the number of virus particles transmitted by an insect vector. Proc. Natl Acad. Sci. USA 104, 17 891–17 896

85. Musser R. O., Hum-Musser S. M., Felton G. W., Gergerich R. C. 2003. Increased larval growth and preference for virus-infected leaves by the Mexican bean beetle, *Epilachna varivestis* mulsant, a plant virus vector. J. Insect Behav. 16, 247–256 (doi:10.1023/A.1023919902976)

86. Ng J. C., Falk B. W. 2006. Virus–vector interactions mediating nonpersistent and semipersistent transmission of plant viruses. Annu. Rev. Phytopathol. 44, 183–212 (doi:10.1146/annurev.phyto.44.070505.143325)

87. Ng J. C. K., Tian T., Falk B. W. 2004. Quantitative parameters determining whitefly (*Bemisia tabaci*) transmission of *Lettuce infectious yellows virus* and an engineered defective RNA. J. Gen. Virol. 85, 2697–2707 (doi:10.1099/vir.0.80189-0)

88. Ngumbi E., Eigenbrode S. D., Bosque-Perez N. A., Ding H., Rodriguez A. 2007. *Myzus persicae* is arrested more by blends than by individual compounds elevated in headspace of PLRV-infected potato. J. Chem. Ecol. 33, 1733–1747 (doi:10.1007/s10886-007-9340-z)

89. Pacheco D. A., Rezende J. A. M., Piedade S. M. D. S. 2003. Biomass, virus concentration, and symptomatology of cucurbits infected by mild and severe strains of *Papaya ringspot virus*. Scientia Agricola 60, 691–698

90. Palacios I., Drucker M., Blanc S., Leite S., Moreno A., Fereres A. 2002. *Cauliflower mosaic virus* is preferentially acquired from the phloem by its aphid vectors. J. Gen. Virol. 83, 3163–3171

91. Pirone T. P. 1981. Efficiency and selectivity of the helper-component-mediated aphid transmission of purified potyviruses. Phytopathology 71, 922–924 (doi:10.1094/Phyto-71-922)

92. Pirone T. P., Megahed E. S. 1966. Aphid transmissibility of some purified viruses and viral RNAs.Virology 30, 631–637 (doi:10.1016/0042-6822(66)90168-1

93. Poulicard N., Pinel-Galzi A., Hebrard E., Fargette D. 2010. Why *Rice yellow mottle virus*, a rapidly evolving RNA plant virus, is not efficient at breaking rymv1-2 resistance. Mol. Plant Pathol. 11, 145–154 (doi:10.1111/j.1364-3703.2009.00582.x)

94. Power A. G. 1992. Patterns of virulence and benevolence in insect-borne pathogens of plants. Crit. Rev. Plant Sci. 11, 351–372

95. Raberg L., Graham A. L., Read A. F. 2009. Decomposing health: tolerance and resistance to parasites in animals. Phil. Trans. R. Soc. B 364, 37–49 (doi:10.1098/rstb.2008.0184)

96. Reynaud B., Peterschmitt M. 1992. A study of the mode of transmission of *Maize streak virus* by*Cicadulina mbila* using an enzyme-linked immunosorbent assay. Ann. Appl. Biol. 121, 85–94 (doi:10.1111/j.1744-7348.1992.tb03989.x)

97. Roberts M. G. 2007. The pluses and minuses of 0. J. R. Soc. Interface 4, 949–961 (doi:10.1098/rsif.2007.1031)

98. Rodriguez-Cerezo E., Klein P. G., Shaw J. G. 1991. A determinant of disease symptom severity is located in the 3′-terminal noncoding region of the RNA of a plant virus. Proc. Natl Acad. Sci. USA 88, 9863–9867 (doi:10.1073/pnas.88.21.9863)

99. Romanow L. R., Moyer J. W., Kennedy G. G. 1986. Alteration of efficiencies of acquisition and inoculation of *Watermelon mosaic virus* 2 by plant resistance to the virus and to an aphid vector. Phytopathology 76, 1276–1281 (doi:10.1094/Phyto-76-1276)

100. Rotenberg D., Kumar K. N. K., Ullman D. E., Montero-Astùa M., Willis D. K., German T. L., Whitfield A. E. 2009. Variation in tomato spotted wilt virus titer in *Frankliniella occidentalis* and its association with frequency of transmission. Phytopathology 99, 404–410 (http://dx.doi.org/10.1094/PHYTO-99-4-0404)

101. Sacristan S., Garcia-Arenal F. 2008. The evolution of virulence and pathogenicity in plant pathogen populations. Mol. Plant Pathol. 9, 369–384 (doi:10.1111/j.1364-3703.2007.00460.x)

102. Shi B.-J., Palukaitis P., Symons R. H. 2002. Differential virulence by strains of *Cucumber mosaic virus* is mediated by the 2b gene. Mol. plant Microbe Interact. 15, 947–955 (doi:10.1094/MPMI.2002.15.9.947)

103. Sinisterra X. H., Mckenzie C. L., Hunter W. B., Powell C. A., Shatters R. G., Jr 2005. Differential transcriptional activity of plant-pathogenic begomoviruses in their whitefly vector (*Bemisia tabaci*, Gennadius: Hemiptera *Aleyrodidae*). J. Gen. Virol. 86, 1525–1532 (doi:10.1099/vir.0.80665-0)

104. Sisterson M. S. 2008. Effects of insect–vector preference for healthy or infected plants on pathogen spread: insights from a model. J. Econ. Entomol. 101, 1–8 (doi:10.1603/0022-0493(2008)101[1:EOIPFH]2.0.CO;2)

105. Thurston M. I., Pallett D. W., Cortina-Borja M., Edwards M. L., Raybould A. F., Cooper J. I. 2001. The incidence of viruses in wild *Brassica nigra* in Dorset (UK). Ann. Appl. Biol. 139, 277–284 (doi:10.1111/j.1744-7348.2001.tb00140.x)

106. Untiveros M., Fuentes S., Salazar L. F. 2007. Synergistic interaction of *Sweet potato chlorotic stunt virus*(*Crinivirus*) with carla-, cucumo-, ipomo-, and potyviruses infecting Sweet Potato. Plant Dis. 91, 669–676 (doi:10.1094/PDIS-91-6-0669)

107. Van Den Heuvel J. F. J. M., Boerma T. M., Peters D. 1991. Transmission of *Potato leafroll virus* from plants and artificial diets by *Myzus persicae*. Phytopathology 81, 150–154

108. Wintermantel W. M., Cortez A. A., Anchieta A. G., Gulati-Sakhuja A., Hladky L. L. 2008. Co-infection by two criniviruses alters accumulation of each virus in a host-specific manner and influences efficiency of virus transmission. Phytopathology 98, 1340–1345 (doi:10.1094/PHYTO-98-12-1340)

109. Yahara T., Oyama K. 1993. Effects of virus infection on demographic traits of an agamospermous population of *Eupatorium chinense* (Asteraceae). Oecologia 96, 310–315 (doi:10.1007/BF00317499)

110. Yuan C., Ullman D. E. 1996. Comparison of efficiency and propensity as measures of vector importance in *Zucchini yellow mosaic potyvirus* transmission by *Aphis gossypii* and *A. craccivora*.. Phytopathology 86, 698–703 (doi:10.1094/Phyto-86-698)

111. Zaitlin M., Hull R. 2003. Plant virus–host interactions. Annu. Rev. Plant Physiol. 38, 291–315 (doi:10.1146/annurev.pp.38.060187.001451)

Chapter 6

Mechanisms of Arthropod Transmission of Plant and Animal Viruses

Stewart M. Gray[1,2] and Nanditta Banerjee[2]

[1]plant protection research unit, agricultural research service, U.S. department of agriculture and

[2]department of plant pathology, cornell university, ithaca, new york 14853.

ABSTRACT

A majority of the plant-infecting viruses and many of the animal-infecting viruses are dependent upon arthropod vectors for transmission between hosts and/or as alternative hosts. The viruses have evolved specific associations with their vectors, and we are beginning to understand the underlying mechanisms that regulate the virus transmission process. A majority of plant viruses are carried on the cuticle lining of a vector's mouthparts or foregut. This initially appeared to be simple mechanical contamination, but it is now known to be a biologically complex interaction between specific virus proteins and as yet unidentified vector cuticle-associated compounds. Numerous other plant viruses and the majority of animal viruses are carried within the body of the vector. These viruses have evolved specific mechanisms to enable them to be transported through multiple tissues and to evade vector defenses. In response, vector species have evolved so that not all individuals within a species are susceptible to virus infection or can serve as a competent vector. Not only are the virus components of the transmission process being identified, but also the genetic and physiological components of the vectors which determine their ability to be used successfully by the virus are being elucidated. The mechanisms of arthropod-virus associations are many and complex, but common themes are beginning to emerge which may allow the development of novel strategies to ultimately control epidemics caused by arthropod-borne viruses.

Nearly 100 years ago yellow fever virus was confirmed to be transmitted by mosquitoes (128). Shortly thereafter, leafhoppers were established as the vector of rice dwarf virus (145), although leafhopper transmission had been reported as early as 1895 (see reference 44 for details). In the following decades, numerous arthropod vectors of plant and animal viruses were identified (33). Today over 500 animal viruses are classified as arboviruses, i.e., viruses able to replicate in a blood-feeding arthropod and to infect a vertebrate host whenever the arthropod feeds on that host (109). Additionally, numerous vertebrate-infecting viruses are transmitted by arthropod vectors but do not replicate in the vector (23). Finally, there are many hundreds of plant viruses (18), most of which are dependent upon a vector for transmission between and inoculation into plant hosts. Plant-infecting viruses have evolved many interesting and biologically complex associations with their vectors, which include arthropods, nematodes, and fungi. The arthropod-plant virus associations are the focus of this review, but analogies and comparisons with animal-infecting viruses are discussed where possible.

Fifty years ago, relatively few arboviruses were known (33). Most did not infect humans, and many had evolved a stable, unobtrusive relationship with both their arthropod and animal hosts. As humans intruded into previously undisturbed ecosystems during their efforts to domesticate the land, they also intruded into virus-vector relationships that were quick to take advantage of the new animal (human) host. Hence, the number of arboviruses has increased exponentially and "new" viruses continue to emerge or reemerge into the headlines (see references 66 and 104 for discussions of emerging viruses), the most notable being yellows fever, equine encephalomyelitis, dengue, and other related hemorrhagic fever viruses.

The expansion of humans into new ecosystems has been fueled primarily by a need to develop and expand agricultural land. More often than not, the main agricultural practice has been monoculture, i.e., the planting of large acreages with a single monogenic crop. Modern agricultural techniques and practices have, in part, contributed to an explosion of newly discovered and emerging plant viruses, the most notable being the Gemini viruses, clostero viruses, and tospoviruses; the last group is a plant-infecting group within the otherwise animal-infecting *Bunyaviridae*. Similar to the emerging animal virus diseases, many of the emerging plant virus disease problems may be the result of humans disturbing a rather stable, unobtrusive relationship between viruses, insects, and their natural plant host. The development of new agroecosystems provides opportunities for viruses and vectors to exploit the newly and widely available cultivated plant host.

Despite the notable arboviruses that are responsible for devastating and horrific human suffering and death, as well as the arthropod-vectored plant viruses that are responsible for billions of dollars in annual crop losses, the mechanisms of virus transmission by arthropods are only now beginning to be understood. There is an enormous literature describing various virus-arthropod associations. However, little is known about the molecular and cellular mechanisms that regulate the transmission processes and determine the efficiency of transmission. The advent of molecular biology and the ability to genetically manipulate viruses, plants, and now insects has fueled a resurgence in studies on the mechanisms of insect transmission of viruses. Animal virologists and medical entomologists have focused the bulk of their efforts on understanding the vector, including the genetic and physiological parameters that influence the replication, survival, and transmission of the virus. This is an appropriate focus since most the animal-infecting viruses transmitted by arthropods also infect and replicate in the arthropod vector. In contrast, most the arthropod-transmitted plant viruses do not replicate in their vectors. Therefore, research has focused more on the viral genes and gene products required for the interactions of virus and vector. Although the interactions between medical entomologists, animal virologists, and plant virologists studying virus transmission have been limited in the past, a number of common themes are emerging that may facilitate a more interactive approach to understanding all virus-vector interactions in the future. The purpose of this review is to describe the current state of plant virus-insect vector research and to relate findings in the plant virus world to similar findings or reports from the animal virus world. It is not meant to be a comprehensive treatment of arbovirus transmission or even plant virus transmission.

GENERAL MECHANISMS OF VIRUS TRANSMISSION

In the early years, viruses were said to be either mechanically transmitted or biologically transmitted by their arthropod vectors (33). Mechanical transmission referred to the nonspecific transmission of viruses by single or multiple vector taxa, usually on contaminated mouthparts. The viruses were unable to replicate in the vector. Although it became clear early on that a simple "flying-pin" or "flying-needle" explanation often did not fully characterize the mechanical transmission process, the process was not considered to be a complex biological association. The mechanisms of mechanical transmission of animal viruses have not received much attention, since all of these viruses can spread between their hosts without an arthropod intermediary in nature or at least in the laboratory. Biological transmission referred to the specific association of a virus with a particular arthropod species or genus and, more important, to the fact that the virus was able to propagate within the vector. These definitions of mechanical and biological transmission came primarily from the animal virology community and are still in use today (23, 164). Most of the animal viruses that are associated with an arthropod vector would fall into the biological-transmission category. In fact, the definition of an arbovirus would specifically preclude mechanical transmission.

Plant virologists have long recognized the "mechanical" and "biological" terms to be an inadequate representation of the mechanisms of insect transmission of plant-infecting viruses and have struggled to produce terminology that accurately reflects the many general mechanisms that apply to plant virus-insect vector associations. Much of the early work on plant virus-insect vector associations was related to timing events, e.g., acquisition and inoculation periods, retention periods, and latent periods (the time between ingestion of the virus and the ability of the insect to inoculate a host). Therefore, the terminology evolved to describe time events (for reviews, see references 64, 65, 94, 141, 163).

Viruses were said to be nonpersistent if they were not retained by the vector for more than a few hours. Semipersistent viruses were retained for days or possibly weeks. Viruses in both these categories were acquired and inoculated within seconds or minutes, and did not require a latent period, and did not replicate in the vector. Persistent viruses, once acquired, were associated with the vector for the remainder of its life. These viruses required longer acquisition and inoculation times (hours to days) and latent periods of 1 day to several weeks.

As additional data on the mechanisms of transmission were generated, other variations of the terminology evolved. The nonpersistent and semipersistent viruses were found to specifically associate with the epicuticle that lines the stylets (mouthparts) or foreguts of their vectors, respectively, and were often referred to as stylet-borne or foregut-borne viruses. The cuticle (including the lining of the mouthparts and foregut) is shed during each molt, and therefore any acquired virus is also lost. Collectively, all of these viruses have been referred to as noncirculative. The viruses are not internalized by the vector in the sense that they do not enter the hemocoel of the vector or cross any vector cell membrane.

In contrast, successful transmission of persistent viruses requires that the ingested virus be internalized. Virus is actively transported across multiple cell membranes, is found in the hemocoel (vector body cavity), and ultimately must associate with the vector salivary system to be inoculated into a host. These viruses are now referred to as circulative viruses and can be further divided into propagative viruses, which replicate in their arthropod vector in addition to their plant hosts, and nonpropagative viruses, which replicate only in their plant hosts. The insect vector is only a conduit for the nonpropagative viruses to move between plant hosts, although very specific virus-vector interactions are required. All of the circulative viruses are retained by the vector following a molt.

All the above terms were developed for use with aphid and leafhopper vectors and are applicable to many plant viruses. Terminology problems arose, however, as additional arthropod, nematode, and especially fungal vectors (21) were discovered and virus-vector associations were studied. Watson (162) and later Hull (72) proposed a terminology including internally borne and externally borne viruses. The former would include persistent viruses, and the latter would include nonpersistent and semipersistent viruses. We suggested (58) that the use of "circulative" and "noncirculative" be retained, where "circulative" refers to viruses that are transmitted only if the virus is transported across cell membranes and carried internally within the vector body cavity or fungal cells. Noncirculative viruses do not cross vector cell membranes and are carried externally either on the vector surface (as for some fungi) or on the cuticle lining of the vector's mouthparts or foregut (as for some arthropods or nematodes). The noncirculative and circulative classification is simple and could be used for animal- and plant-infecting viruses that require a vector for optimal existence in nature. There is some loss of definition and categorization, but subgroupings such as nonpersistent and semipersistent could be added if they pertain to a particular vector taxon. There would, of course, be the paradoxical virus-vector associations that do not fit easily into the proposed scheme. For example, beetle-transmitted viruses and the myirid-bug-transmitted velvet tobacco mottle virus may use both circulative and noncirculative transmission mechanisms (46, 48).

VECTOR FEEDING: MECHANICS AND BEHAVIOR

A majority of arthropod and nematode vectors of plant viruses have a common feature: the mechanics of feeding. Their mouthparts are best described as piercing-sucking (5, 73, 125) (Fig. (Fig.11 and and2).2). The hollow, needle-like mouthparts can penetrate the plant cell wall, either by mechanical force and/or with the help of salivary and gut enzymes. The cell membrane is easily breached by mechanical force, making the cell contents available as food. The most significant feature of this type of feeding is that it does not always irreparably damage the plant cell. This nonlethal cell feeding is critical for survival of the virus, since it must be able to replicate in the cell to which it is delivered. Plant virus genomes encode movement proteins that enable them to move to neighboring cells (24). The fungal vectors do not have piercing-sucking mouthparts. Instead, the virus-carrying motile zoospores attach to the plant root surface, enzymatically and mechanically penetrate the cell wall and membrane, and then establish an infection within the plant cell cytoplasm (22). At some point after gaining entrance to the host cytoplasm, virus is released by the fungus. The mechanisms of virus release by fungi are unknown, but again virus is inoculated into a viable cell.

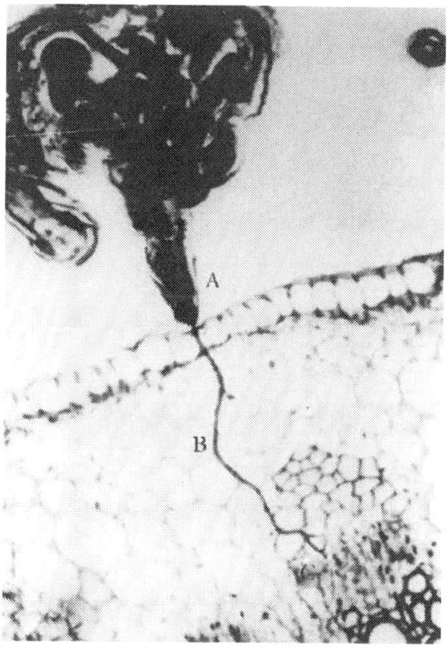

Figure 1: Light micrograph of a longitudinal section through an aphid head and leaf as the aphid is feeding on the plant. The aphid stylet protrudes from the proboscis (A) and penetrates intracellularly through the mesophyll cells (B) and into the vascular bundle (C).

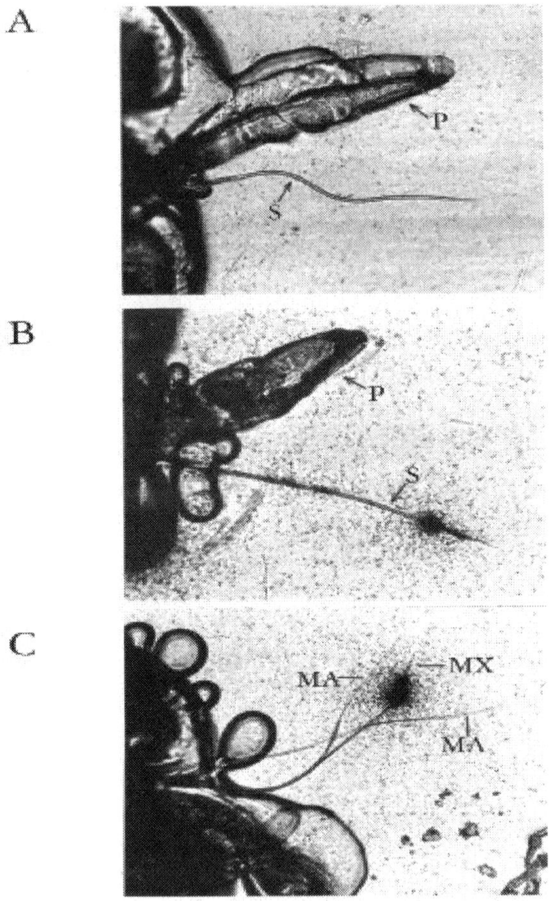

Figure 2: Autoradiographs of stylets of *Myzus persicae* given acquisition access to ^{125}I-labeled tobacco etch potyvirus virions. (A) Stylets of an aphid that has not fed on an infected plant. (B) Stylets of an aphid that acquired labeled virus through a plastic membrane. (C) Distribution of label in stylets that have separated, showing label associated only with the food canal formed by the maxillary stylets. MA, mandibular stylets; MX, maxillary stylets; P, proboscis; S, stylet. Magnification, ×420. Reproduced from reference 161a with permission of the publisher.

The general feeding behavior of many arthropod and nematode vectors also aids in virus transmission to plants (5, 125, 148). The acceptance or rejection of a plant host by a vector with piercing-sucking mouthparts is performed by a series of brief probes into multiple plant epidermal cells. These brief probes are sufficient to inoculate the noncirculative nonpersistent viruses. Another benefit of this type of transmission mechanism is that the plant need not be a host of the vector for the virus to establish an infection. That is, the virus and the vector do not require overlapping host ranges for the virus to be efficiently transmitted to a wide variety of plant hosts. In general, the noncirculative, nonpersistent plant viruses are not vector species specific but are vector taxon specific. For example, individual potyviruses are transmitted by numerous aphid species but are not transmitted by whiteflies or leafhoppers. These viruses have evolved a transmission strategy based on a numbers game: quantity rather than quality. A virus will associate with many vectors in the hope that a few vectors will rapidly move to and probe another plant that can serve as a host for the virus.

If brief feeding probes indicate the plant is an acceptable host or food source, the vector is likely to initiate prolonged feeding. This may occur in numerous epidermal or mesophyll cells, or, more often, the insect will seek out its preferred feeding site, the carbohydrate-rich phloem sap (Fig.1). Prolonged feeding allows for inoculation not only of the semi persistent, no circulative viruses but also of the circulative viruses. These viruses have evolved a very different transmission strategy from the noncirculative, nonpersistent viruses. In general, they are transmitted by a single or a few vector species. The mechanisms of transmission are such that the virus associates with the vector for longer periods. This ensures that the virus survives until the vector finds a suitable host. However, since the same plant must serve as a host for both the vector and the virus, the host range of the virus is determined by the vector.

Direct inoculation of plant viruses into the plant vascular tissue is somewhat analogous to inoculation of arboviruses into the bloodstream of an animal host. Most of the arbovirus vectors feed and transmit viruses by piercing or cutting minor blood vessels and sucking up blood while injecting salivary secretions into the feeding site to prevent the blood from coagulating (37). At the same time, viruliferous vectors are releasing saliva-associated or mouthpart-associated viruses. The question arises of why arboviruses are often efficiently mechanically transmitted by a simple mechanism of mouthpart contamination and without any appreciable vector specificity (23, 164) whereas even high-titer plant viruses are rarely or inefficiently transmitted on the contaminated mouthparts of insects (112, 120).

This differential ability of plant- and animal-infecting viruses to be mechanically transmitted by several insect taxa may be explained by a few fundamental properties. (i) Most plant viruses do not occur in the extremely high titers required for the nonspecific mechanical transmission of animal viruses. (ii) Inoculation into the plant vasculature or "bloodstream" takes time. Plant-feeding insects with piercing-sucking mouthparts require approximately 15 to 30 min to wind their stylets between cells to reach vascular bundles (Fig. 1). The enzymatic action of breaking down the intracellular material is likely to dislodge or inactivate any contaminating virus before it can be injected into the plant vascular system. In contrast, blood-feeding insects locate their feeding sites very quickly. (iii) Plant viruses must be inoculated directly into a viable cell. They are unable to independently cross the cell wall or cell membrane. In contrast, arboviruses are inoculated into the bloodstream, not cells. Virus can then attach to and infect vertebrate cells independent of the vector.

There are insect vectors (mainly beetles) of plant viruses that have chewing mouthparts and a more indiscriminate feeding behavior than the piercing-sucking insects and nematodes. Inoculation of plant viruses by beetles was once considered to be a mechanical process in which either virus contaminating the mouthparts was deposited into the wound or virus in the gut was regurgitated as the beetle fed (137). Recent work has shown this process to be extremely specific and biologically complex. The reader is referred to reference 46 for in-depth coverage of this process. Briefly, the beetle-transmitted viruses can be inoculated into a chewing wound because the virus can rapidly translocate in xylem elements away from the site of inoculation and infect cells at a distance from the feeding site. Several viruses that are not transmitted by beetles were found to be acquired by the beetles and to be present in the hemolymph as well as the gut regurgitant that is deposited into and around the wound. The nontransmissible virus was apparently inactivated at the wound site or was unable to gain entrance to a functional plant cell that was capable of sustaining a virus infection. The mechanism by which beetle-transmitted viruses infect cells at a distance from the wound is unknown.

The transmission of plant viruses is now known to be biologically complex even in situations where initially it appeared to be a simple, nonspecific mechanical inoculation. The details of many of these molecular and cellular mechanisms regulating the transmission of plant viruses are described in subsequent sections.

NONCIRCULATIVE TRANSMISSION

The noncirculative method of transmission is not widely associated with animal virus transmission, but it is the method of choice for a majority of plant viruses (Table (Table1).1). All of the major insect vector taxa, including aphids, whiteflies, and leafhoppers, as well as the nematode vectors, transmit plant viruses in a noncirculative manner. The necroviruses and some other members within the *Tombusviridae* are carried on the external surface of soil-borne fungal vectors (22). The fungus-transmitted viruses are not considered in this review, although the classification of circulative and noncirculative would hold true in terms of membrane transport and internalization.

Table 1: Mechanisms of transmission and principal vector species of plant virus families

Virus taxon	No. of members	Principal vector[a]	Helper required
Noncirculative, nonpersistent			
Caulimovirus	17	Aphids	Yes
Fabavirus	2	Aphids	No
Potyvirus	186	Aphids	Yes
Carlavirus	55	Aphids	No
Cucumovirus	3	Aphids	No
Alfamovirus	1	Aphids	No
Machlomovirus	1	Thrips, beetles	No
Macluravirus	2	Aphids	No
Potexvirus	55	Aphids (7/10), mites (2/10), mechanical	No
Noncirculative, semipersistent			
Badnavirus	16	Mealybugs (3/6), leafhoppers (1/6)	No
Closterovirus	25	Aphids (10/19), whiteflies (6/19), mealybugs (2/19)	—[b]
Nepovirus	39	Nematodes	—
Sequivirus	2	Aphids	No

Tobravirus	4	Nematodes	No
Trichovirus	6	Aphids (1/3), mealybugs (1/3), mites (1/3)	No
Waikavirus	3	Aphids (1/3), leafhoppers (2/3)	Yes
Noncirculative, (Other)			
Necrovirus	3	Fungi	No
Tombusvirus	12	Fungi (1/12), mechanical	No
Varicosavirus	4	Fungi	No
Circulative, nonpropagative			
Enamovirus	1	Aphids	No
Geminivirus			
Bigeminivirus	41	Whiteflies	—
Hybrigeminivirus	2	Treehoppers	No
Monogeminivirus	11	Leafhoppers	No
Luteovirus	27	Aphids	No
Nanavirus	5	Aphids	No
Umbravirus	10	Aphids	Yes
Bromovirus	6	Beetles	No
Carmovirus	22	Beetles (3/10)	No
Comovirus	14	Beetles	No
Sobemovirus	17	Beetles (6/8)	No
Tymovirus	21	Beetles	No
Bymovirus	6	Fungi	No
Furovirus	12	Fungi	No
Rymovirus	7	Mites	No
Circulative, propagative			
Bunyaviridae			
Tospovirus	5	Thrips	No
Marafivirus	3	Leafhoppers	No
Reoviridae			
Phytoveovirus	5	Leafhoppers	No
Fijivirus	6	Planthoppers	No
Oryzavirus	2	Planthoppers	No
Rhabdoviridae			
Phytorhabdovirus	32	Aphids (1/3), leafhoppers (1/3), planthoppers (1/3)	No
Cytorhabdovirus	17	Aphids (3/7), planthoppers (4/7)	No

Nucleorhabdovirus	38	Aphids (7/17), leafhoppers (4/17), planthoppers (6/17)	No
Tenuivirus	10	Planthoppers	No

[a]Numbers in parentheses indicate the number of viruses within the group that were reported to be transmitted by that vector divided by the total number of viruses within the group that were tested. Information was compiled from reference 18.

[b]—, there is information to indicate that a helper factor may be required for the transmission of some members of the group.

A Biological, Not a Mechanical Process

The noncirculative viruses transmitted by arthropod and nematode vectors can be further subdivided into semipersistent and nonpersistent viruses (17, 65, 93). These two groups share some characteristics, but in general, semipersistent viruses tend to be associated with the foregut of the vector and are retained for several days or weeks (months or years in some cases). Transmission efficiency increases as the acquisition feeding time increases, which suggests that the virus is stably bound and accumulates until binding sites are saturated. In contrast, the nonpersistent viruses are associated with the stylets of the vector (Fig. 2), are retained for only a few hours, and are easily lost during feeding probes. Furthermore, transmission efficiency rapidly decreases as the acquisition feeding time increases. This suggests that bound virus is easily dislodged during prolonged feeding and that subsequently ingested virus cannot be reacquired by the formerly occupied sites along the stylets.

The site of virus attachment for nonpersistent viruses was recently identified to be near the distal tip of the maxillary stylets (95, 161). Virus could also be found in the proximal regions of the stylet and foregut (3,161); however, there was no correlation between the amount of virus accumulated at these regions and transmission (124). In contrast, virus retention in the distal region of the stylets was highly correlated with virus transmission (161).

Three theories have been proposed for the mechanics of noncirculative transmission. (i) The stylet-borne theory, adapted from the mechanical-transmission theory of the animal virus literature, suggests that virus nonspecifically associates with or contaminates the distal tip of the stylet and is simply inoculated into the next plant as the vector begins to feed (79). In this mechanism, the vector is essentially a "needle." (ii) Harris (64) proposed an ingestion-egestion mechanism in which transmissible virus adheres to multiple sites along the anterior alimentary canal during ingestion of plant material and is subsequently released during periods of regurgitation and salivation. In this mechanism the vector acts as a "syringe" rather than a "needle." The ingestion-egestion hypothesis offered a potential mechanism of noncirculative transmission but did not distinguish between virus transported on the stylet tips or further inside the mouthparts or foregut. (iii) Recently developed technologies have led to a third hypothesis: ingestion-salivation (95). Virus can associate with multiple sites along the anterior alimentary canal, but the only virus to be transmitted is the virus attached to the proximal tip of the maxillary stylets, where the food and salivary canals are fused. Virus is released by the act of salivation rather than by regurgitation (Fig. 3). This could be viewed as a return to the "needle" analogy but not to the mechanical-transmission theory.

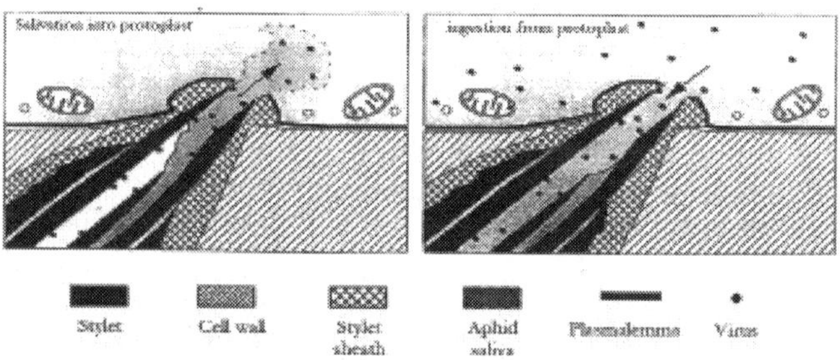

Figure 3: Model of the ingestion-salivation mechanism of noncirculative, nonpersistent transmission. Virus is ingested into the food canal (right), along with the cytoplasm. Virus adheres to the epicuticular lining of the food canal and the common duct at the very distal tip of the stylet, which is shared with the salivary canal. When the aphid first probes a cell after acquiring virus (left), saliva is injected into the cell. The watery salivary secretions will release virus from the cuticle lining the common duct, but virus farther inside the food canal would not be released by this mechanism. Reproduced from reference 95 with permission of the publisher.

Whether the insect or nematode acts as a needle or a syringe is perhaps not as important as the (now irrefutable) fact that the process is not a nonspecific mechanical transfer via contaminated mouthparts but, rather, a complex and very specific biological process (123). The most complete understanding of the mechanisms of noncirculative virus transmission comes from work on the aphid-transmitted potyviruses and caulimoviruses, both of which are nonpersistent (123). The reader is also directed to numerous other reviews on the subject of noncirculative transmission of plant viruses by arthropods and nematodes (17, 58, 65, 72,79, 93, 94, 141).

Several groups of viruses, including the potyviruses and caulimoviruses, require a nonstructural, virus-encoded protein referred to as a helper component, a helper factor, or a helper (Table 1). Purified virus fed to aphids through a Parafilm membrane sachet was not transmissible, but if aphids were given access to a solution of plant sap from an infected plant (virus removed) before or along with purified virus, transmission was possible (55). Sap from a healthy plant did not mediate the transmission of purified virus. Some viruses require another virus, referred to as a helper virus, to be transmitted (Table 1), but it is not known for all cases if the helper virus particle itself is required or if the helper virus simply provides a helper factor. In addition to functioning in vector transmission, helper proteins have other functions in the virus life cycle. The potyvirus helper functions in polyprotein processing, movement of the virus in its plant host, and viral genome amplification (92, 135). The caulimovirus helper can bind microtubules and was proposed to be involved in movement of the virus in its host (13). Although there are several hypotheses for the role of helper in virus-vector interactions (58, 123), one is emerging as the most plausible and will be the focus of discussion here. The "bridge" hypothesis, i.e., that the helper acts to mediate the attachment of virus to the vector, was first proposed by Govier and Kassanis (55), but only recently has direct evidence been established.

Ammar et al. (3) provided ultrastructural evidence that potyvirus fed to an aphid in the presence of purified helper was embedded in a matrix material associated with the epicuticle. Virus was not retained and the matrix material was absent in aphids fed on the potyvirus alone. Immunolabeling demonstrated that helper protein was associated with virus retained in the matrix. Direct evidence of virus-helper-aphid interactions came from the identification of specific domains in the potyvirus coat protein and helper component that are required for aphid transmission. The potyvirus coat protein contains a DAG amino acid motif located near the N terminus. Mutations within or adjacent to this domain prevented the binding of virus to helper in vitro (11) and were shown to render numerous potyviruses nontransmissible (11, 74, 123, 161). Recently, Wang et al. (161) used radiolabeled virus to observe the effects of mutations in the coat protein DAG motif on the retention of virus in the stylet food canal and found that mutations in this region prevented the accumulation of virus in the stylets and prevented transmission.

The potyvirus helper factor has two characteristic amino acid motifs, a KITC box and a PTK box (123). Natural or engineered mutations in or adjacent to these motifs rendered the virus nontransmissible by the natural vector (4, 71). A specific mutation of the KITC sequence to EITC abolished transmission but did not affect the in vitro binding of virus to the helper (122a). Furthermore, virus was not observed in the stylets when acquired with the EITC mutant helper but was observed when acquired along with wild-type (KITC) helper (161). These data indicate that the KITC box functions in aphid-helper interactions, specifically in retention of the virus in the stylet. Mutations in the PTK box abolished helper-virus interactions in vitro (116). Therefore, this domain may play a role in attachment of the virus to the helper. Alternatively, mutations in this domain may prevent dimerization of the helper to the active configuration (150). All of these results strongly support the hypothesis that the potyvirus helper acts as a bridge to bind virus to the aphid stylet.

Further evidence that indirectly supports the bridging function of helper proteins was provided by analysis of the cauliflower mosaic caulimovirus (CaMV) helper. The CaMV helper accumulated in paracrystals in the cytoplasm of infected plant cells from which active helper was solubilized (12). The predicted structure of the CaMV helper indicates an N-terminal -sheet domain and a C-terminal -helix. Random structure separates the two terminal domains. The C-terminal domain mediates binding of the helper to virions in vitro. Mutations in this region abolished helper-virus binding in vitro and aphid transmission. Mutations in the N terminus also abolished aphid transmission but did not abolish the ability of the helper to bind to virions in vitro (134). The current working model is that the C terminus of the helper protein binds to virus particles whereas the N terminus is free to bind to sites in the aphid alimentary canal and mediate or bridge the indirect association of the virus particles to the insect cuticle.

The requirement for helper has also been demonstrated or suggested for a number of other insect- and nematode-transmitted viruses carried in both a nonpersistent and semipersistent manner (Table 1). It is unknown if the helpers for these other viruses function in a manner similar to the potyvirus and caulimovirus helpers or if the "bridge" hypothesis will apply. A common feature of all helper-mediated viruses that have been observed in their vector is that the virus particles are embedded in a semiopaque matrix material associated with the epicuticle lining of the anterior alimentary canal (3, 17, 27). The origin and composition of the matrix material are unknown.

Not all viruses transmitted in a noncirculative manner require a helper protein or helper virus (Table (Table1).1). Purified virions of members of the alfamoviruses, carlaviruses, and cucumoviruses can be transmitted by aphids without helpers. Studies with cucumber mosaic cucumovirus have shown that transmission is regulated solely by the capsid protein (26, 118). It is not known if these viruses are retained in similar locations in the vector to those that contain the helper-dependent viruses.

Why, if viruses can evolve a seemingly simpler capsid-mediated transmission strategy, have a majority of the noncirculative viruses evolved a helper-dependent transmission strategy? Pirone and Blanc (123) suggest that helpers may offer a method to widen the evolutionary bottleneck imposed by vector-dependent transmission. They make the point that a majority of the helper-dependent plant viruses are RNA viruses or DNA pararetroviruses. The low fidelity of RNA polymerases and the reverse transcriptase replication strategy used by the pararetroviruses are primarily responsible for the development of quasispecies, i.e., populations of viruses with a continuum of genome variants and invariably a continuum of biological properties (1, 87). Interestingly, a majority of the arboviruses are RNA viruses or DNA retroviruses, and a similar concept of populations existing as a collection of variants has been applied to their evolution (109).

Pirone and Blanc (123) argue that helpers can mediate the transmission of not only the homologous virus particle but also those of a number of related species (86, 90, 121); therefore, helpers should mediate the transmission of a number of coat protein variants within a quasispecies. Similarly, a single coat protein species should be able to interact with several helper variants within a quasispecies. Therefore, mutations in either the coat protein or the helper genes that reduce the overall transmission fitness of a specific virus-helper pair may not be detrimental to the overall transmission of a quasispecies. An additional benefit is that the mutations in helper proteins may allow the variant access to a new species of vector, thereby increasing the chances of transmission out of a host and possibly into a different set of recipient hosts. The helper strategy may actually preserve the genomic diversity within a quasispecies rather than limiting the number of viable genomes. Helpers may also provide an efficient means of expanding the number of vector species that can efficiently transmit a noncirculative virus.

Clearly, we have much to learn about the mechanisms of noncirculative transmission. Semipersistent and nonpersistent viruses may share some attributes, but differences in the sites of virus retention in the vector and in the times of retention indicate major differences in release of virus, in addition to mechanisms of binding. There is little experimental data to explain how virus particles bound to the epicuticle substrate are released. The N terminus of the potyvirus coat protein which binds to the helper protein is often proteolytically cleaved in vitro without having any deleterious effect on viral infectivity (133). Similarly, the C terminus of the nematode-transmitted tobacco rattle tobravirus (98) can be cleaved from the particle without adversely affecting viral infectivity. Interestingly, the coat protein structure changes in response to pH and the C-terminal region does not appear to be part of the structural framework of the virus (98). It is possible that proteinases in the vector saliva or regurgitated gut secretions can act as the scissors that cut the virus particle loose.

Viruses retained at different sites in the vector are likely to be exposed to different enzymes and ionic conditions that may affect the surface structure of virions or the conformation of structural proteins. Similarly, the chemical makeup of salivary and/or digestive secretions is likely to differ among vector species or even among biotypes within a species. These differences could contribute to differences between non persistent and semipersistent viruses and to the differences in the specificity or transmission efficiency of vectors for the same virus.

Potential Connection to Animal Viruses

The mechanisms of noncirculative transmission described for plant viruses may also apply to animal viruses. As mentioned above, noncirculative transmission is not widely associated with animal viruses; however there are numerous reports of mechanically transmitted animal viruses (23, 151). Equine infectious anemia virus represents an extreme for animal viruses. This virus does not infect its tabanid fly vector, but it is apparently dependent upon the fly for transmission between equine hosts (23). Members of the *Poxviridae*, *Herpesviridae*, *Papovaviridae*, and *Retroviridae* are also mechanically transmitted by arthropods but are not totally dependent upon the vector to spread between hosts (23). There is general agreement that mechanical transmission is important in the epidemiology of numerous animal viruses (23, 151, 164), but there also seems to be a widespread belief that mechanical transmission is a nonspecific, short-term incidental association of a virus with a blood- or wound-feeding arthropod (62, 164). Is the mechanical transmission of animal viruses by arthropods just the result of contamination of mouthparts, or is the transmission process of some of these viruses more specifically mediated?

Myxoviruses are perhaps the best-studied "mechanically" transmitted animal viruses (reference 40 and references within). Laboratory studies indicated that there was no vector specificity, indeed not even taxonomic specificity for the myxoma virus. In addition to being transmitted by multiple arthropod species, the virus could be experimentally transmitted via pins or thorns. It is likely that the association of the myxoma virus with many vectors is a laboratory phenomenon and is not relevant to natural transmission and epidemic development. However, the virus-vector relationship may not involve strictly mechanical contamination for all the vectors of myxoma virus. The early successes of the myxomatosis epidemics in Australia, which were deliberately begun to control the rabbit host, were dependent upon several species of mosquito. Success was partly due to the behavior and ecology of the vector that placed it in close proximity to the rabbits. However, other data would argue for a more complex interaction between the virus and mosquito than the "flying-pin" model would suggest. For example, the virus was retained by several mosquito species for extended periods and multiple inoculations from a single insect were documented. Furthermore, there were differences in the efficiency of transmission by different species that were not correlated to the titer of virus imbibed. Virus was associated with the proboscis and head region but not with the body of the insect (40). All of this is similar to the noncirculative mode of transmission of plant viruses and suggests that the association of myxoma virus with its mosquito vectors may be more than just mouthpart contamination.

It is possible, perhaps even likely, that many animal-infecting viruses have evolved vector relationships that are biological but do not include virus replication in the vector. However, the commonly used methods of testing and classifying arboviruses would not identify these viruses. Generally, viruses that are isolated from arthropods are evaluated by being injected into insects to determine if they replicate in that host and thus can be classified as arboviruses. A similar strategy for plant viruses would have identified few "arthropod-transmitted viruses." Clearly, some animal viruses are mouthpart borne, and this type of transmission is important in the epidemiology of some viruses (23). Furthermore, animal viruses can be foregut borne, similar to the semipersistent, noncirculative plant viruses. For example, retroviruses can associate with and remain infectious in the foreguts of insects and subsequently can be transmitted to a new host after being regurgitated into the feeding site by the insect (82). This is not to say that insect transmission of retroviruses is important or common, only that noncirculative mechanisms of transmission similar to those described for insect-transmitted plant viruses, e.g., ingestion-egestion or ingestion-salivation, have been described for animal viruses. The noncirculative transmission of plant viruses is a very specific and complex biological process; perhaps the same is true for certain animal viruses. The noncirculative transmission of poxviruses may become even more important in light of recent findings that retroviruses (not normally efficiently transmitted by insects) can integrate into the poxvirus genome and can be efficiently transmitted by insects in a noncirculative manner (67).

CIRCULATIVE TRANSMISSION

Viruses transmitted in a circulative manner must be internalized by their vector to be successfully transmitted. That is, the virus must be transported across cell membranes. Members of the furoviruses and bymoviruses are transmitted internally by the motile zoospores of soil-borne fungi (36, 76, 132). These viruses are not discussed in this review, but by the definitions used here, they would be considered circulative viruses. All the remaining circulative plant viruses are transmitted by arthropods; there are no known circulative nematode-transmitted plant viruses (Table 1). As mentioned above, the circulative viruses are further divided into two subgroups, propagative viruses, i.e., those which replicate in their arthropod vectors (similar to the arboviruses) and nonpropagative viruses. The propagative viruses include members of five groups of viruses, three of which, the reoviruses, rhabdoviruses, and bunyaviruses, also have members that infect animals. There are no animal-infecting members of the tenuiviruses or marafiviruses. The nonpropagative viruses include the luteoviruses and the single-member enamovirus group. Geminiviruses are currently considered to be nonpropagative viruses, but the mechanism of transmission is undefined and they are discussed separately.

The general circulative pathway of virus movement through arthropod vectors (Fig. 4) is similar for both subgroups (and for arboviruses) and involves ingestion into the gut followed by association with and uptake by midgut or hindgut epithelial cells. Virus is then released into the hemocoel or secondarily infects other tissues. Eventually, all circulative viruses must associate with the salivary glands and be released into the salivary ducts. Once in the salivary duct, virus is free to be inoculated into plant (or animal) hosts as the insect salivates during feeding. Currently there is no evidence that saliva components contribute, negatively or positively, to the transmission of circulative plant viruses akin to the phenomenon of saliva-activated transmission (SAT) of arboviruses (110). SAT potentiates the transmission of some arboviruses through the release of pharmacologically active substances in saliva into the bloodstream of the vertebrate host. These substances have vasodilatory (117), antihemostatic (155), and host defense suppression (83) properties. SAT is also believed to be the underlying mechanism of "nonviremic transmission" of arboviruses between infected and uninfected vectors cofeeding in close proximity on a host that is not necessarily infected (84,110). We are unaware of any studies that have investigated the role of insect saliva in reducing a plant defense response and facilitating virus infection. Interestingly, Mowry (105) reported that aggregates of aphids placed on noninoculated leaves of plants previously inoculated with the circulative, nonpropagative potato leafroll luteovirus caused a significant increase in the amount of virus accumulating at the feeding site relative to the amount accumulating in aphid-free leaves on the same plant. As stated above, insect saliva is probably involved in the release of noncirculative viruses from vector mouthparts, but it would be interesting to determine if insect saliva can potentiate the transmission of circulative plant viruses by influencing the infection site in the plant.

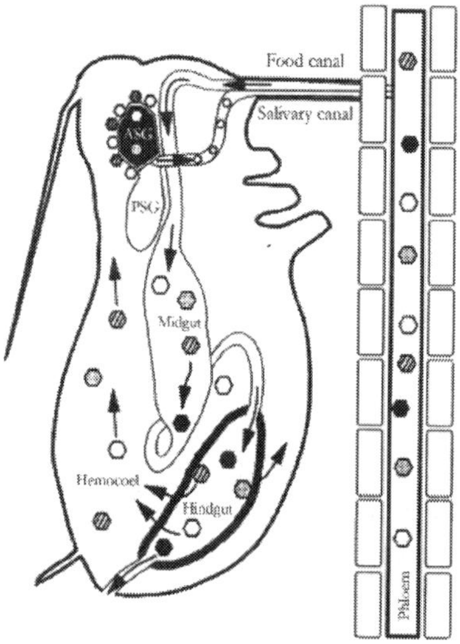

Figure 4: Circulative route of barley yellow dwarf luteoviruses (BYDVs) through aphids. All BYDV strains can be ingested from phloem into the aphid's alimentary canal and arrive in the hindgut intact. The hindgut epithelium is the first transmission barrier; most BYDVs can bind to hindgut epithelial cells and be transported into the hemocoel, but some are excluded (solid hexagons). BYDVs acquired in the hemocoel must migrate to the ASG. The basal lamina of the ASG may selectively filter BYDVs or may concentrate virions, thereby increasing the efficiency of transport into the ASG. BYDVs (gray hexagons) not concentrated at the ASG may be transported into the ASG if they encounter it, but the efficiency of transmission is low. BYDVs may be concentrated at the ASG but be prevented from entering the ASG by an inability to bind to the ASG plasmalemma and initiate endocytosis (striped hexagons). Efficiently transmitted BYDVs are concentrated at the ASG and efficiently transported in the ASG and the salivary canal (open hexagons). Reprinted from reference 127 with permission of the publisher.

Circulative, Nonpropagative Transmission

The luteoviruses and pea enation enamovirus (PEMV) have a common circulative pathway and biology within their aphid vectors. The members of the luteovirus group and PEMV are each efficiently transmitted by one or, at most, a few aphid species. The transmission pathway through the aphid and the biological factors contributing to the vector specificity were recently reviewed (34, 52) and are only briefly described here.

Ultrastructural studies have shown that virus is not degraded or inactivated in the gut and that entry of virus into the hemocoel occurs through either the midgut (45) or hindgut (50) epithelial cells by endocytosis (Fig .5). Virus is transported through the cytoplasm in vesicles that ultimately fuse with the basal plasmalemma, and particles are released into the space between the membrane and the basal lamina. Virus apparently moves rapidly across the basal lamina and into the hemocoel. In most virus isolate-aphid species combinations studied, virus was acquired in the hemocoel regardless of whether the aphid was a vector of that particular virus isolates (51). The gut does not appear to be a major barrier to luteovirus acquisition, although the process is specific for luteoviruses. Other morphologically similar viruses were observed in high concentrations in the gut lumen but were not acquired in the hemocoel (51).

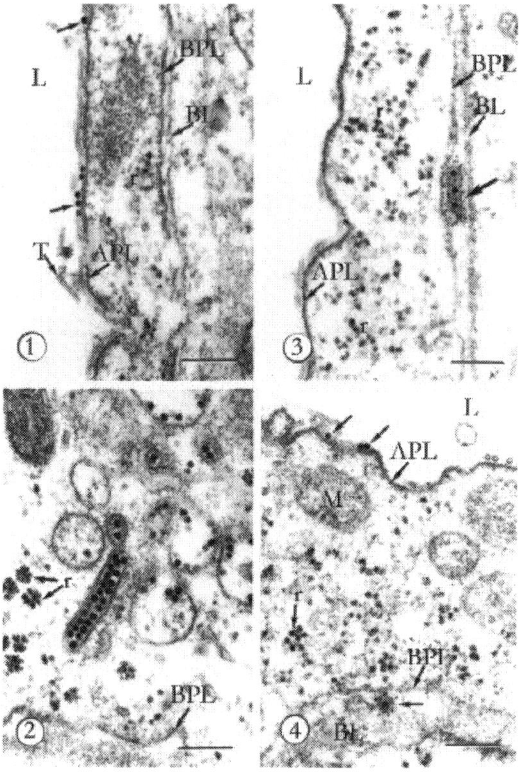

Figure 5: Electron micrographs of the hindgut of *Rhopalosiphum padi* microinjected with anti-barley yellow dwarf luteovirus (BYDV) antibodies for immunolabeling following acquisition feedings on Parafilm membranes containing purified BYDV or on oats infected with BYDV. (Panel 1) Ingested virions (arrows) in the hindgut lumen (L) adsorbed to the apical plasmalemma (APL). Note the longitudinal views of extracellular tubules (T), ribosomes (r), basal plasmalemma (BPL), and basal lamina (BL). (Panel 2) Unlabeled virions concentrated in receptosome-like vesicles and in a tubular vesicle adjacent to the basal plasmalemma (BPL) and basal lamina. Ribosomes (r) are also shown. (Panel 3) Ferritin-labeled virions (arrow) captured between the basal plasmalemma (BPL) and basal lamina (BL) upon release from the hindgut cell into the hemocoel. Apical plasmalemma (APL), hindgut lumen (L), and ribosomes (r) are also shown. (Panel 4) Unlabeled virions (arrows) in the hindgut lumen (L) adjacent to the apical plasmalemma (APL) and an anti-BYDV-labeled virion adjacent to the basal plasmalemma (BPL) following transport to the hemocoel. The basal lamina (BL), mitochondria (M), and ribosomes (r) are also shown. Bars, 200 nm. Reproduced from reference 51 with permission of the publisher.

Luteoviruses are able to survive in the aphid hemolymph despite potential insect immune responses that may be capable of neutralizing the invading virus. Potential mechanisms for this evasion are discussed below, but similar to the gut barrier, these mechanisms appear general to all luteoviruses and do not contribute to vector-specific transmission (156).

The salivary glands in aphids consist of two principal glands and two accessory salivary glands (ASG) (126). Luteoviruses and PEMV associate exclusively with the ASG and more specifically with the anterior portion of these four-celled glands (52). The ASG produce a watery secretion, containing few or no enzymes, that is thought to be involved in deposition of the stylet sheath during feeding (126). The highly invaginated apical plasmalemma of ASG cells suggests a rapid transport of water and ions, which would be consistent with the suggestions that the ASG function as an excretory organ and play a role in the removal of waxy material originating from degenerating fat cells in the hemolymph (126). The salivary glands of ticks have also been found to play a role in removal of foreign substances from hemolymph and may be part of the tick self-defense system (159). It is possible that luteoviruses have evolved to take advantage of specific excretory pathways to access the salivary ducts. Ultrastructural evidence indicates that the pathway of luteovirus through the ASG (Fig. (Fig.66 and and7)7) is similar to mechanisms used to cross the hindgut. An inability of luteovirus isolates to penetrate the ASG of nonvector aphids has long been known to contribute to vector specificity (130). Recently it was shown that the basal lamina and the basal plasmalemma function as independent barriers to transmission in different luteovirus isolate-aphid species combinations (Fig. (Fig.7)7) (51, 54a, 115). The two ASG-associated barriers and the hindgut barrier can function as the primary barrier of transmission for the same virus in different aphid species or in the same aphid for different virus isolates. This indicates that different membrane attachment sites (receptors) and different virus attachment protein domains are used at each transmission barrier by different virus isolate-aphid species combinations.

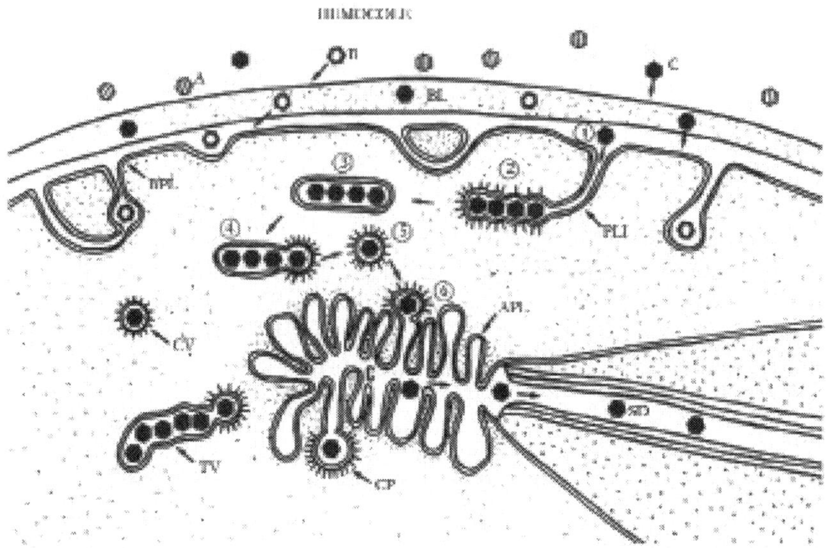

Figure 6: Model of the interactions of luteoviruses with the ASG of aphid vector species. Three types of interactions were observed when virions of the MAV isolate of barley yellow dwarf virus were acquired by aphids that fed on infected plants or were injected with purified virions into the hemocole. In the first type of interaction, MAV virions had no affinity for the salivary basal lamina (BL) of specific aphid species and did not attach to or penetrate the basal lamina (A, nonpenetrating, nontransmitted virions). In other species, MAV virions did exhibit affinity for the salivary basal lamina and were able to attach to and, in some cases, penetrate the basal lamina. However, these virions were unable to initiate endocytosis at the basal plasmalemma (BPL) and were not transmitted (B, penetrating, nontransmitted virions). In the third type of interaction, virions consistently penetrated the basal lamina (step 1), were aggregated in plasmalemma invaginations (PLI), and were endocytosed into the cell by coated-pit formation (step 2). Virions acquired in the cytoplasm accumulated at the apical end of the cell in tubular vesicles (step 3). Individual virions budded from the tubular vesicles by coated-pit formation (step 4) and were transported to the salivary canal (Cn) in coated vesicles (step 5) that fused to the apical plasmalemma (APL), releasing the virion into the canal lumen (step 6). Transcytosed virions were then able to move into the salivary duct (SD) (C, penetrating-transmitted virions; TV, tubular vesicle; CP, coated pit; CV, coated vesicle). Reproduced from reference 54a with permission of the publisher.

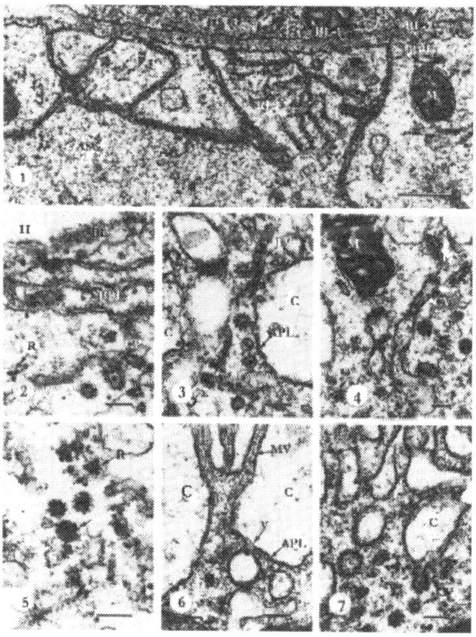

Figure 7: Ultrastructure of membranes associated with transcellular transport of microinjected virions of the MAV isolate of barley yellow dwarf virus through the ASG of *Sitobion avenae*. (Panel 1) Virions of MAV embedded in the ASG basal lamina (BL-2) and concentrated in basal plasmalemma (BPL) invaginations (arrows). Note the absence of virions in the basal lamina (BL-1) of the adjacent subesophageal nerve ganglion (SN). Particles in the cytoplasm are ribosomes associated with the rough endoplasmic reticulum (RER). M, mitochondria. Bar, 500 nm. (Panel 2) Virions penetrating the basal lamina (BL) from the hemocole (H) and in a coated pit (CP) during endocytosis through the basal plasmalemma (BPL). The small, irregularly shaped particles observed free in the cytoplasm are ribosomes (r), as determined by RNase digestion (3) and observation of ultrastructure under higher magnification. (Panel 3) Virions packaged in tubular vesicles (TV) adjacent to the apical plasmalemma (APL) lining a microvillus-lined canal (C). V, virion in canal. (Panel 4) Virions in tubular vesicles (TV) and associated coated vesicles (CV). M, mitochondria. (Panel 5) Comparison of a virion in a coated vesicle (arrow) to cytoplasmic ribosomes (R). (Panel 6) A virion (V) being released from the accessory salivary gland cell into the canal lumen (c) by exocytosis through the apical plasmalemma (APL). MV, microvilli. (Panel 7) Virions (arrows) in the canal lumen (C) released from coated pits (CP) following fusion of coated vesicles (CV) with the cell membrane. Bars, 100 nm. Reproduced from reference 54a with permission of the publisher.

The luteovirus- and PEMV-encoded proteins involved in aphid transmission have been studied, and the two virus groups share some features at the molecular level. The luteoviruses are currently divided into three taxonomic subgroups based on differences in genome organization, and all three are different from the bipartite PEMV. However, the luteoviruses all share a conserved arrangement of three open reading frames, two of which encode the structural proteins (102). The virus capsid contains a predominant coat protein (ca. 22 to 24 kDa) and a minor amount of a larger protein translated via a readthrough of the coat protein stop codon. The full-length luteovirus readthrough protein is ca. 72 to 74 kDa, but the carboxyl-terminal portion of the readthrough domain is proteolytically processed to yield a 55- to 58-kDa readthrough protein commonly associated with purified virus preparations (14, 42, 77, 160). It is not known if this type of processing actually occurs in vivo. Purified virus and virus produced from cloned cDNA copies of the virus that do not translate the carboxyl terminus of the readthrough domain are transmissible (19, 58a, 160). These findings indicated that the carboxyl-terminal portion of the readthrough domain was not required for aphid transmission and also that there is no requirement for a nonstructural helper in the transmission process. The PEMV readthrough protein is inherently smaller than its luteovirus counterpart and does not undergo further processing (35).

The readthrough protein was not required for particle assembly or plant infection (35, 42, 129), but particles containing only the 22- to 24-kDa coat protein were no longer transmissible by aphids to plants (14, 25, 35,156). This led to the widespread assumption that readthrough protein was responsible for the aphid transmission phenotype. However, virions without read through protein ingested by aphids were detected in the hemolymph, indicating that the coat protein contained all the determinants for uptake of the virus through the hindgut (25). There are a number of highly conserved domains in the coat proteins of all luteo viruses that are likely candidates for mediating virus attachment and transport through the aphid gut. This theory of a common virus sequence mediating gut uptake is consistent with the above-mentioned biological data that the hindgut does not contribute significantly to vector-specific transmission of luteoviruses. A detailed mutational analysis of the coat protein is needed to validate this hypothesis.

Luteovirus coat protein genes without the corresponding readthrough sequences have been expressed in insect cells by using a baculovirus vector, and virus-like particles (VLP) were observed (85). The read through-minus VLP were purified and either fed to aphids through a Parafilm membrane sachet or injected directly into the hemocoel. Ultrastructural examination of the aphids revealed the ingested particles were acquired through the gut into the hemocoel, and, surprisingly, VLP were observed in the accessory salivary gland cells and in the salivary ducts (54). These results are consistent with earlier studies showing that readthrough was not required for acquisition through the gut but contrasted with the hypothesis that readthrough determined vector specificity by regulating the transport of virus through the accessory salivary gland. What, then, is the function, if any, of the readthrough domain in the aphid transmission process?

It has long been assumed that the only barriers to luteovirus transmission were the tissue-associated membranes, e.g., the hindgut and accessory salivary gland. However, one potentially important aspect of the vector has been neglected in the search for aphid-virus interactions: the insect immune system. The effect of insect immune systems on parasite infection and transmission has received widespread attention (61, 97), but the effect on virus infection has not been as widely studied (106). The immune system of aphids has received little attention. Aphid hemolymph was reported to be void of hemocytes (126), but it is unknown if this is a general phenomenon for all aphids. Other types of defenses, such as humeral encapsulation (158) or the production of defense-related proteins such as interferon (29, 106), may exist. These types of defense systems are active in many insects (60), including Homopterans. How, then, are luteo viruses or PEMV able to survive for extended periods in the aphid hemolymph, an environment shown to be hostile to insect pathogens and parasites? The answer may be related to the read through protein.

Aphids harbor endosymbiotic bacteria of the genus *Buchnera* in specialized cells located in the abdomen, called mycetocytes (126). Neither the aphids nor the bacteria are able to survive and reproduce without the other. Not all the benefits that the bacteria provide for the aphid are known, but one function Is to provide essential amino acids that the aphid is unable to synthesize (7). In addition, the bacteria produce copious amounts of a chaperonin protein named symbionin, a homologue of the *Escherichia coli* GroEL protein (7,41). The role of this protein in aphid metabolism is unknown, but the chaperonin class of proteins generally functions in protein folding, translocation across membranes, and recovery from stress. Symbionin is produced and stored exclusively in the mycetocytes and is unlikely to be exported into the aphid hemolymph (43). The reported detection of symbionin in hemolymph (157) is most probably due to the degradation of the endosymbionts and mycetocytes as the aphid reaches maturity (7, 126).

Interestingly, symbionin has been shown to bind to purified luteoviruses in vitro or to a recombinant luteovirus readthrough polypeptide (41, 68, 156, 157). When aphids were cured of endosymbionts by treatment with antibiotic, their ability to transmit virus was significantly reduced and the amount of coat protein detected in the aphid was diminished. Strangely, the amount of readthrough was not affected (68,157). The results of these experiments must be interpreted carefully. The destruction of the endosymbionts is likely to have dramatic effects on the metabolism and physiology of the aphids, and these changes may be directly or indirectly responsible for the effects on luteovirus protein detection and virus transmission.

Recently, six luteoviruses and the related PEMV were all shown to bind specifically but differentially to *E. coli* GroEL and symbionin homologues from vector and nonvector aphids (156). The binding capacity was not correlated with transmission ability or efficiency, suggesting that if symbionin plays a role in transmission, it does not play a role in vector specificity. Furthermore, an analysis of the ability of a series of readthrough deletion mutants to bind symbionin in vitro indicated that the amino-terminal portion of the readthrough domain contained the determinants for symbionin binding. Finally, virions that did not contain readthrough protein and did not bind symbionin in vitro were less persistent in the aphid hemolymph than was wild-type virus. These studies provide convincing data that symbionin can interact specifically with luteoviruses and PEMV in the aphid hemolymph and can slow the degradation of virus. The mechanisms of degradation of virus in the hemolymph are unknown, and it is unknown if the attachment of symbionin to the virus protects the virus from targeting by the aphid immune system or, alternatively, if it facilitates virus movement into the accessory salivary gland.

The circulative, nonpropagative plant viruses have evolved several mechanisms to utilize insect cell membrane functions and to interact with the products of the aphid endosymbionts. Why develop such a complex and nonproductive association with the vector? The virus must maintain a number of defenses and tricks to move through various membranes and survive in several hostile environments. The virus does prolong its association with a vector, but it does not replicate and is constantly fighting a losing battle to remain viable in a hostile vehicle of transport. The luteoviruses and geminiviruses are phloem restricted and must be inoculated directly into phloem tissues to cause an infection. Aphids, whiteflies, leafhoppers, and planthoppers, the vectors of these viruses, are all phloem feeders. It takes time for the insects to reach the phloem, and they will feed on the phloem only if the plant is a host of the insect. Therefore, to ensure their long-term survival and maximize their chances of moving between host plants, these viruses have evolved a transmission strategy that requires that they have a long term relationship with the vector. Furthermore, this type of transmission means that the vector will determine the host range of the virus, since the virus will be inoculated into phloem tissues only if the plant is a host of the vector. The ability of the virus to survive for extended periods without replicating in the vector and being pathogenic to the vector is good for the vector, although long-term survival of a nonreplicating virus in the potentially hostile environment of a vector does not appear to be advantageous to the virus.

Luteoviruses, PEMV, and Gemini viruses appear to have used reassortment as a driving force in their evolution (15, 49, 96). The various luteovirus subgroups have ties to different virus supergroups relative to their replication, but they all have acquired and retained a conserved arrangement of structural and movement proteins.

Perhaps these viruses have not yet been able to acquire the genes that would allow them to replicate in their insect vector. Alternatively, they may be evolutionarily undecided whether to ultimately pursue a noncirculative mode of transmission or a circulative propagative mode. For example, PEMV is a bipartite virus; RNA 1 is luteovirus-like and, as discussed above, contains the genes encoding the transmission-associated structural proteins. This virus has acquired a second RNA which, in addition to other functions, has allowed the virus to escape its phloem limitation. It can be acquired from and inoculated into epidermal cells, a feature that allows it to be inoculated, perhaps even acquired, by aphids during brief feeding probes. This could lead to a broader host range of the virus, since it is not completely dependent upon the vector to determine its host range. Perhaps the virus will ultimately acquire a helper or a new capsid that will allow it to associate with the mouthparts of its aphid vectors and become noncirculative. One member of the geminiviruses may be moving in the opposite direction, toward becoming propagative in its vector (see below).

Geminivirus Transmission

Geminiviruses are single-stranded circular DNA viruses that have been divided into three taxonomic groups or genera (Table 1). The viruses within the monogeminivirus and hybrigeminivirus genera are each transmitted by a different species of leafhopper or treehopper. Viruses within the bigeminivirus genera are all transmitted by whiteflies, although there is likely to be more than one mechanism of transmission. The coat protein has been shown to be the sole determinant of transmission of some whitefly-borne viruses (113), a property that was recently mapped to the N terminus of the coat protein of abutilon mosaic bigeminivirus (166). The coat protein was also shown to be the sole determinant of whether a geminivirus is transmitted by a whitefly or a leafhopper (16). However, the coat protein does not solely determine the transmission phenotype of all geminiviruses. Recently the genomic analysis of another whitefly-transmitted bigeminivirus, tomato golden mosaic virus, indicated that although the coat protein was required for acquisition of the virus, both genomic components (DNA A and DNA B) were required for transmission. DNA B was essential for the accumulation of virus in the whitefly, while DNA A was required for the successful inoculation of plants by viruliferous insects (88).

The transmission of all geminiviruses has been classified as circulative and nonpropagative. Virus has been observed in the gut epithelial cells and associated with salivary glands of whitefly vectors, and it is assumed to follow a similar circulative strategy as the aphid-transmitted luteoviruses, although no detailed ultrastructural studies have been published (30). Whiteflies also possess endosymbionts (31), but it is not known if they produce a symbionin homologue, nor has the ability of geminiviruses to bind any of the characterized symbionin homologues been reported.

Several lines of evidence, in addition to the nonstructural gene requirement for transmission (88), suggest that some whitefly-transmitted geminiviruses have evolved interesting twists that may indicate a more complex transmission pathway than that of luteoviruses. Studies to determine virus titers over time in the insects have not conclusively shown an increase that would suggest virus replication, but the viral DNA does persist in the insect longer than its infectivity would suggest (20, 30, 131). No replicative forms of the viral DNA have been detected within the insect, which argues against the replication of virus in the insect. However, squash leaf curl virus was observed in several whitefly tissues, and the presence of virus was associated with cytopathological abnormalities in some tissues (119). Furthermore, the presence of the virus in the insect can have detrimental effects on the biology and reproduction of the vector (131). Both of these observations would suggest virus replication. No cytopathological or deleterious reproductive effects have been documented for aphids fed on luteovirus-infected plants.

Another interesting twist is the recent finding that a monopartite isolate of the tomato yellow leaf curl virus is transmitted transovarily in its whitefly vector (47). Although this is in contrast to previously published reports (30), the data are convincing that this tomato yellow leaf curl virus isolate can be transovarily passaged. One criterion for the classification as a nonpropagative, circulative plant virus is an inability to be transovarily transmitted (65), since this type of vertical transmission usually indicates that the virus is replicating in the vector. Geminiviruses may have evolved a mechanism to cross the transovarial transmission barriers without replicating in that tissue, or perhaps there is some low level of infection of reproductive tissues. A potential paradox (if the geminiviruses are found to replicate in their vectors) is that the complete genome organizations of the various groups of geminiviruses are known and specific and required functions in the plant infection process have been assigned to all genes and gene products. Therefore, the same genes would have to function in virus replication within both plant and insect hosts, although presumably any host components required by the virus would be different.

Circulative, Propagative Transmission

The plant-infecting viruses within the circulative, propagative classification (Table (Table1)1) are those most closely related to the arboviruses; indeed three of the five taxonomic groups considered here have animal-infecting members: rhabdoviruses, reoviruses, and bunyaviruses. The plant viruses within these groups could be considered plant-infecting arboviruses or phytoarboviruses (165). It is odd, however, that the arboviruses and phytoarboviruses are classified as vertebrate-infecting and plant-infecting viruses, respectively, rather than both being classified as invertebrate viruses. The arthropod host is more important in the evolution and survival of the virus because it will exert a greater selection pressure (109). The virus must evolve and maintain the ability to infect and survive in the arthropod, an accomplishment that requires the virus to surmount a number of barriers not present in the vertebrate host (see "Vector competence"). Furthermore, most of these viruses do not have a pronounced deleterious effect on their arthropod host and they depend on the arthropod host for long-term survival. In contrast, the animal or plant host is often a temporary host that serves only as a high-titer source to allow the efficient infection of more arthropod hosts (109, 164). There are, of course, exceptions to this general trend. Several arboviruses and phytoarboviruses adversely affect the longevity and fecundity of their vectors, while others are avirulent in their plant or vertebrate host (references2, 109, and 164 and references within).

Until recently, the phytoarboviruses had not received a great deal of attention. With few notable exceptions, such as the tomato spotted wilt tospovirus, many of these viruses are not economically important. Their genomes tend to be relatively large and complex, and most have remained recalcitrant to analyses by many of the modern molecular biology techniques. In addition, it has been difficult to generate sufficient numbers of stable mutants with phenotypes related to vector transmission. Although these problems have also plagued arbovirus research, it has benefited tremendously from the establishment of cultured vector cell lines (101) and the ability to conduct detailed genetic studies on vector populations (144, 164). Both of these research strategies have been difficult to develop and apply to the insect vectors of the phytoarboviruses.

Vector Competence

The individual arboviruses and phytoarboviruses tend to be transmitted by only one or a limited number of closely related vector species. Furthermore, intraspecific variation in susceptibility and the ability to transmit virus has been reported for populations of vectors of numerous viruses (69, 70, 109, 146,149). Consequently, much of the research on transmission has investigated the vector specificity of these viruses. The general pathway through the arthropod is similar for all these viruses. Virus is imbibed along with the plant sap or the bloodmeal. It then attaches to and infects midgut cells, usually reaching high titers in these tissues. It is released into the hemocoel and secondarily infects other tissues, including reproductive tissues, from which it can spread vertically to offspring. Horizontal transmission to other plant or animal hosts occurs following infection of salivary tissues and subsequent release of infectious virus in the salivary secretions that are injected into the host during feeding.

Vector competence (ability to transmit) is determined not only by the ability of the virus to infect the tissues of the vector but also by the ability of the virus to successfully enter and exit the critical tissues. Extensive studies have been done to identify the cellular barriers to transmission, and Ammar (2) has provided an excellent and comprehensive review of this topic for both phytoarboviruses and arboviruses. The barriers include the midgut infection barrier, which was first demonstrated for eastern equine encephalomyelitis alphavirus (99) and has subsequently been demonstrated for other animal- and plant-infecting viruses. An active midgut infection barrier will effectively render the arthropod immune to the virus. This barrier was once considered the reason why many potential vectors were not capable of virus transmission. However, there were several viruses that were able to infect a potential vector but were not transmitted. Hardy et al. (63) first reported the existence of two other barriers that could explain this phenomenon, a midgut escape barrier and a salivary gland infection barrier. A midgut escape barrier has been demonstrated for tomato spotted wilt tospovirus (*Bunyaviradae*) in the adult stage of the thrips vector. The virus must be acquired by the larval thrips to be transmitted. Virus can infect and replicate in midgut cells of both larval and adult thrips but can disseminate only from larval midgut cells into other thrips tissues (153). The wound tumor reovirus (57) and sowthistle yellow vein rhabdovirus (9), both phytoarboviruses, were able to invade and replicate in several tissues of their leafhopper or aphid vectors, respectively. However, in nontransmitting individuals, the viruses were not associated with the salivary glands. This suggests the existence of a salivary gland infection barrier but does not rule out the possibility that the virus is not able to survive in the hemolymph or hemolymph-associated cells that would come in contact with the salivary glands. There is also a salivary gland escape barrier, which has been demonstrated for some arboviruses in their mosquito vectors (59), but this has not been demonstrated for any phytoarbovirus. The phenomenon of saliva-activated transmission (110) appears to be yet another potential barrier to the successful transmission of some arboviruses, but it has not been investigated for phytoarboviruses. The successful transmission of any of these viruses requires the virus to run the gauntlet of potential barriers, each of which have been shown to be active in some virus-vector combination. Similar to the situation described above for the circulative, nonpropagative luteoviruses, the specific barrier may differ for any combination of virus and vector and no generalities seem to be applicable.

The molecular and physiological basis for virus-vector interactions that regulate transmission are not well understood, but it is clear that genetic elements within both the virus and the vector ultimately decide if a particular species or individual within a species of arthropod is able to be a vector for a particular virus strain. Environmental or abiotic factors also play a role in determining virus-vector interactions, but in general these factors seem to influence the efficiency of the interaction rather than to determine the ability of the interaction to take place (164).

The genetics of vector competence are receiving widespread attention, and results have begun to change the central dogma that all individuals within a vector species are potential vectors. A more enlightened concept states that populations within a species will differ in their ability to be efficient vectors for certain viruses (144). Intraspecific variation in vector capacity is not unique to arboviruses; it has long been known for vectors that transmit plant viruses by all of the mechanisms described thus far (138). Understanding why a vector is a vector and developing the tools to rapidly and accurately identify potential vectors is important for understanding the epidemiology of a virus and for developing control measures. Viruses are extremely difficult, if not impossible, to control once they have infected a susceptible animal or plant host. Current strategies for virus disease control are usually aimed at protecting the host, e.g., vaccines in animal hosts or pathogen-derived resistance strategies in plant hosts

(89, 114), but a more direct strategy would be to prevent the infection of the arthropod host and/or transmission of the virus.

Arbovirologists and medical entomologists have begun to develop systems to investigate the genetics of vector populations and have begun to develop the tools to allow the molecular mapping of elements that differ between individuals that are able to efficiently transmit viruses and individuals that are refractive to virus infection or transmission (144). In contrast to the simple monogenic control of vector susceptibility to malaria parasites or filarial infection, the competence of viral vectors appears to be a complex multigenic phenomenon in several instances (144, 147). However, a single locus that controls the susceptibility of *Culicoides variipennis* to bluetongue virus was identified (143). The inability of a strain of *Aedes aegypti* to transmit several flaviviruses was also found to be regulated by a single gene or set of closely linked genes (100). Similarly, the ability of rice hoja blanca tenuivirus to replicate in its planthopper host, *Sagosodes oryzicola*, is controlled by a single recessive gene (168).

Genetic maps are being constructed for several insect species that are the principal vectors of several important human and animal viruses (144). In addition, techniques are advancing so that the stable transformation of insects with foreign genes is now possible (75, 80). Analogous systems are beginning to be developed for the insect vectors of the phytoarboviruses. The routine generation of sexual forms and the sexual crossing of many important aphid vector species have been accomplished in several laboratories, and genetic polymorphisms are being identified (10, 136, 152). One of the problems in the analysis and mapping of genetic traits in insects such as mosquitoes has been in the relatively small amount of DNA that can be extracted from an insect for analysis. Aphids may offer a solution to this problem, since they reproduce parthenogenetically unless environmental factors induce a switch to sexual reproduction. The clonal propagation of aphids provides a limitless supply of identical individuals for genetic and biological study. Furthermore, the long-term stability of virus transmission phenotypes of clonal populations has been established (127). Although the genetic mechanisms regulating vector competence for arboviruses and phytoarboviruses remains largely unknown, modern molecular technologies are likely to allow for the identification of these genetic elements in the future. Similar technologies have been well developed and are very successful in the identification of genes and assignment of gene function in plants and animals.

Virus Competence

The genetics of virus transmission by vectors is not controlled solely by the vector; the virus also contributes to the overall process (58, 122). The current knowledge of virus genetics in relation to noncirculative transmission and circulative, nonpropagative transmission was described earlier in this review. Limited progress has been made in understanding the phytoarbovirus genes and gene products that influence vector transmission. A lack of stable cell lines from insect vector species and a difficulty in developing stable mutants with a transmission-deficient phenotype have contributed to the slow progress.

The establishment of continuous mosquito cell lines (56) has greatly facilitated our knowledge of arbovirus-vector interactions. The cell lines have allowed the study of virus entry into and release from insect cells and of virus replication and gene expression in insect cells relative to their animal host counterpart (101). It has been difficult to establish stable cell lines for many of the important phytoarbovirus vectors (32). Chiu and Black (28) established cell lines from the leafhopper vector of wound tumor reovirus, and, more recently, additional cell lines have been established for additional leafhopper vectors of other reoviruses (154) as well as for thrips vectors of tomato spotted wilt tospovirus (107). These successes, coupled with recent progress on the molecular biology of several reoviruses and the tospoviruses, is likely to allow significant progress to be made in the future in understanding how these viruses can infect their insect hosts.

Despite an absence of vector cell lines, progress on the identification of virus genes whose function is related to transmission has been made by studying virus associations with whole insects. Total-protein extracts from whole thrips or from thrips gut tissue were separated by sodium dodecyl sulfate-polyacrylamide gel electrophoresis and subsequently probed with tomato spotted wilt bunyavirus or its glycoproteins in a gel overlay assay. Two independent laboratories identified two different thrips proteins, one of which was associated with midgut tissues (6). The tissue association of the other was not determined (81). The animal-infecting LaCrosse bunyavirus glycoproteins have long been implicated in vector transmission (8), and recently it was shown that the GP1 interacts with both mosquito and vertebrate cells in culture but not with mosquito gut cells in vivo. GP2 binds only to mosquito cells. Both glycoproteins are most probably involved in cell attachment and virus entry (91).

Studies on whole, virus-infected insects have also identified differences in viral RNA and protein accumulation between the plant and insect hosts. Falk et al. (39) identified a nonstructural protein of maize stripe tenuivirus that accumulated in maize but not in the leafhopper vector. Similar results were recently reported for the related rice grassy stunt tenuivirus in rice and its leafhopper host (103). The function of the nonstructural protein is unknown. Perhaps it serves as a plant virus movement protein or aids in the initial uptake of virus by the vector but does not subsequently need to be produced by the vector. In contrast to the aforementioned studies, the RNAs encoding the two maize stripe tenuivirus glycoproteins are abundant in both insect and plant host cells (38). It is not known if the proteins accumulate to similar levels or are required for infection of both hosts, but they are integral membrane proteins and, by analogy to other viruses (91), are assumed to be involved in insect cell membrane attachment. All serologically detectable rice dwarf reovirus proteins are also present in both insect and plant hosts (140). Similar findings of no qualitative differences in viral RNAs or proteins have been reported for the alphaviruses (101, 139). However, posttranslational processing of viral proteins differed in mosquito and vertebrate hosts. Differences in glycosylation pathways in mosquito cells and vertebrate cells resulted in differences in attached oligosaccharides and subsequent differences in proteolytic cleavage. These differences do not appear to alter transport of the protein but apparently affect budding of the virions through cell membranes (101, 139). In addition, differences in methylation and RNA-capping pathways in invertebrate and vertebrate cells apparently affect alphavirus replication and accumulation rates (139). These fundamental differences are likely to contribute to the distinct differences in pathologic findings induced by alphaviruses in mosquito and vertebrate cell cultures (78).

Another major problem in developing an understanding of phytoarbovirus-vector interactions has been in the development or identification of stable mutants that have altered vector transmission phenotypes. The viruses have all remained recalcitrant to manipulation by many of the modern molecular biology techniques. Infectious DNA clones have not been produced, and therefore neither a directed mutational strategy nor a reverse genetic approach to identifying gene function is possible. A limited number of transmission mutants have been obtained by repeated mechanical inoculation of plant hosts without going through the insect host. A strain of the rice dwarf reovirus maintained for 12 years in vegetatively propagated rice plants lost the P2 outer capsid protein. The genomic sequence encoding P2 was present in the rice dwarf reovirus-infected plants, but a point mutation that introduced a termination codon in the open reading frame prevented translation of the protein. The P2 protein was not required for infection of the plant host, but the lack of P2 protein did prevent infection of the insect host, perhaps due to an inability of the virus to attach to the vector cells (111, 167). Consequently the virus was not transmitted by the insects to plants.

Vegetative propagation of wound tumor reovirus-infected plants also resulted in leafhopper transmission-defective virus isolates. This was later found to result from the generation of defective RNAs of 4 of the 12 genomic segments. These defective viruses were not able to infect leafhopper vector cells but were able to maintain a near-wild-type infection of the plant host (108). Presumably all of the virus functions necessary to infect the plant host were contained on the eight remaining genomic segments whereas one or more of the four defective segments provided as yet undefined functions specific for infection of the insect host. The data generated thus far points to the conclusion that outer capsid proteins of the phytoarboviruses are, as would be predicted, involved in the infection of insect cells, i.e., attachment proteins. These would not be necessary for plant hosts due to the cell wall, which, along with the cell membrane, must be breached by the insect vector stylet.

There are very few references to the continued serial passage of phytoarboviruses in their insect vector. Sonchus yellow vein rhabdovirus was mechanically passaged by injecting virus into the hemocoel of aphid vectors. Continuous serial passage did give rise to virus isolates that were difficult to transmit to plants and also were more pathogenic to the vector (142). The reasons for the low probability of transmission were not determined and might have been associated with a deficiency in systemic plant infection or an inability to move through all the transmission barriers in the aphid.

The technique of mechanically passaging the virus in either the insect or plant host is apparently useful in the generation of mutants. With the advances in technologies that now allow further characterization of such mutants, there should be advances in our understanding of virus-vector interactions despite the difficulties with vector cell cultures and a lack of infectious clones of the viruses.

FUTURE DIRECTIONS AND CHALLENGES

Except for the phytoarbo viruses and a few other notable examples, genetic analysis of viral gene expression and function is currently possible and is progressing rapidly. We will soon know which viral genes and gene products are required for vector transmission, but for the most part we will not understand their exact role. The challenges ahead lie in our ability to understand the interactions of the viruses inside the arthropod (or other) vector and to determine what genetic factors the vector contributes to the overall transmission process. The obstacle for most researchers studying virus transmission involves the present inability to get inside the vector and observe what is going on. New technologies must be and are being developed (e.g., transformation of insects and genetic manipulation of aphids). The sensitivity and detection limits of existing technologies are being improved (e.g., detection and visualization of potyvirus particles on aphid stylets, or the association of symbionin with luteovirus readthrough proteins). However, roadblocks are ever present. For example, it is likely that virus particles undergo conformational changes in their vectors as they are exposed to various environments within the gut, hemocole, or salivary system. These changes are likely to be critical for certain aspects of virus-vector interactions and the virus transmission process. The presence of relatively few virus particles in relatively few vector cells or on a small area of vector cuticle presents a problem for analysis of biological interactions. The production of continuous vector cell lines may provide the tools to answer some of these questions for researchers studying phytoarbo viruses, but it will not provide definitive experimental systems for those studying viruses which do not replicate in their vectors.

Insect vectors cannot always be controlled by chemical means, and with the increasing sensitivity to the environment and the loss of many chemical control measures, vector control is not at present a long-term option. Protective measures of vector control are not really even an option for many of the nonpersistent plant viruses or perhaps even the mechanically transmitted animal viruses, since the infection process is too quick. Understanding the mechanisms of virus transmission is the key to developing effective strategies to block virus-vector interactions. If the virus can no longer be transmitted or even if the efficiency of transmission can be reduced to manageable levels, the disease will be less of a problem. The answer surely lies in our ability to render the host immune to infection or in our ability to control the transmission process. Genetic engineering and plant breeding have produced many virus-resistant plants, but immunity is the exception rather than the rule, and therefore genetically engineered resistance may not be the silver bullet that will solve all the problems. Our ability to control virus transmission is dependent upon our ability to first understand the transmission process and to effectively predict steps in the process that are vulnerable to intervention. Arthropod-borne viruses are likely to continue to emerge or reemerge and become more, rather than less, problematic. Success will depend on the continued integration of the expertise of animal and plant virologists along with entomologists, molecular biologists and geneticists.

REFERENCES

1. Al K N, Covey S N. Variation in biological properties of cauliflower mosaic virus clones. J Gen Virol.1994;75:3137–3145.
2. Ammar E D. Propagative transmission of plant and animal viruses by insects: factors affecting vector specificity and competence. Adv Dis Vector Res. 1994;10:289–331.
3. Ammar E D, Jarlfors U, Pirone T P. Association of potyvirus helper component protein with virions and the cuticle lining the maxillary food canal and foregut of an aphid vector. Phytopathology. 1994;84:1054–1060.
4. Atreya C D, Pirone T P. Mutational analysis of the helper component proteinase gene of a potyvirus: effects of amino acid substitutions, deletions, and gene replacement on virulence and

aphid transmissibility.Proc Natl Acad Sci USA. 1993;90:11919–11923.

5. Backus E A. Anatomical and sensory mechanisms of planthopper and leafhopper feeding behavior. In: Nault L R, Rodriguez J G, editors. The leafhoppers and planthoppers. New York, N.Y: John Wiley & Sons, Inc.; 1985. pp. 163–194.
6. Bandla M D, Campbell L, Ullman D E, Sherwood J L. Interaction of tomato spotted wilt tospovirus glycoproteins with a thrips midgut protein, a potential cellular receptor for TSWV. Phytopathology.1998;88:98–104.
7. Baumann P, Baumann L, Lai C, Rouhbakhsh D, Moran N A, Clark M A. Genetics, physiology and evolutionary relationships of the genus *Buchnera*: intracellular symbionts of aphids. Annu Rev Microbiol.1995;49:55–94.
8. Beaty B J, Holterman M, Tabachnick W, Shope R E, Rozhon E J, Bishop D H L. Molecular basis of bunyavirus transmission by mosquitoes: role of the middle-sized RNA segment. Science. 1981;211:1433–1435.
9. Behncken G M. Evidence of multiplication of sowthistle yellow vein virus in an inefficient aphid vector,*Macrosiphum euphorbiae*. Virology. 1973;53:405–412.
10. Birch A N E, Fenton B, Malloch G, Jones A T, Phillips M S, Harrower B E, Woodford J A T, Catley M A. Ribosomal spacer length variability in the large raspberry aphid, *Amphorophora idaei* (Aphidinae: Macrosiphini) Insect Mol Biol. 1994;3:239–245.
11. Blanc S, Lopez Moya J J, Wang R, Garcia Lampasona S, Thornbury D W, Pirone T P. A specific interaction between coat protein and helper component correlates with aphid transmission of a potyvirus.Virology. 1997;231:141–147.
12. Blanc S, Schmidt I, Kuhl G, Esperandieu P, Lebeurier G, Hull R, Cerutti M, Louis C. Paracrystalline structure of cauliflower mosaic virus aphid transmission factor produced both in plants and in a heterologous system and relationship with a solubilized active form. Virology. 1993;197:283–292.
13. Blanc S, Schmidt I, Vantard M, Scholthof H B, Kuhl G, Esperanddieu P, Cerutti M, Louis C. The aphid transmission factor of cauliflower

mosaic virus forms a stable complex with microtubules in both insect and plant cells. Proc Natl Acad Sci USA. 1996;93:15158–15163.

14. Brault V, et al. Aphid transmission of beet western yellows luteovirus requires the minor capsid read-through protein P74. EMBO J. 1995;14:650–659.
15. Briddon R W, Bedford I D, Tsai J H, Markham P G. Analysis of the nucleotide sequence of the treehopper-transmitted geminivirus, tomato pseudo-curly top virus, suggests a recombinant origin. Virology.1996;219:387–394.
16. Briddon R W, Pinner M S, Stanley J, Markham P G. Geminivirus coat protein replacement alters insect specificity. Virology. 1990;177:85–94.
17. Brown D J F, Robertson W M, Trudgill D L. Transmission of viruses by plant nematodes. Annu Rev Phytopathol. 1995;33:223–249.
18. Brunt A A, Crabtree K, Dallwitz M J, Gibbs A J, Watson L. Viruses of plants. Cambridge, United Kingdom: CAB International; 1996.
19. Bruyere A, Brault V, Ziegler Graff V, Simonis M T, Van Den Heuvel J F J M, Richards K, Guilley H, Jonard G, Herrbach E. Effects of mutations in the beet western yellows virus readthrough protein on its expression and packaging and on virus accumulation, symptoms, and aphid transmission. Virology.1997;230:323–334.
20. Caciagli P, Bosco D. Quantitation over time of tomato yellow leaf curl geminivirus DNA in its whitefly vector. Phytopathology. 1997;87:610–613.
21. Campbell R N. Persistence: A vector relationship not applicable to fungal vectors. Phytopathology.1993;83:363.
22. Campbell R N. Fungal transmission of plant viruses. Annu Rev Phytopathol. 1996;34:87–108.
23. Carn V M. The role of dipterous insects in the mechanical transmission of animal viruses. Br Vet J.1996;152:377–393.
24. Carrington J C, Kasschau K D, Mahajan S K, Schaad M C. Cell-to-cell and long-distance transport of viruses in plants. Plant Cell. 1996;8:1669–1681.
25. Chay C A, Gunasinge U B, Dinesh K S P, Miller W A, Gray S M. Aphid transmission and systemic plant infection determinants

of barley yellow dwarf luteovirus-PAV are contained in the coat protein readthrough domain and 17-kDa protein, respectively. Virology. 1996;219:57–65.

26. Chen B, Francki R I B. Cucumovirus transmission by the aphid *Myzus-persicae* is determined solely by the viral coat protein. J Gen Virol. 1990;71:939–944.

27. Childress S A, Harris K F. Localization of virus-like particles in the foreguts of viruliferous *Graminella nigrifrons* leafhoppers carrying the semi-persistent maize chlorotic dwarf virus. J Gen Virol. 1989;70:247–251.

28. Chiu R J, Black L M. Monolayer cultures of insect cell lines and their inoculation with a plant virus.Nature. 1967;215:1076–1078.

29. Cohen S. *In vivo* effects in whiteflies of a possible antiviral factor. Virology. 1967;37:448–454

30. Cohen S, Antignus Y. Tomato yellow leaf curl virus, a whitefly-borne geminivirus of tomatoes. Adv Dis Vector Res. 1994;10:259–288.

31. Costa H S, Westcot D M, Ullman D E, Rosell R, Brown J K, Johnson M W. Morphological variation in Bemisia endosymbionts. Protoplasma. 1995;189:194–202.

32. Creamer R. Invertebrate tissue culture as a tool to study insect transmission of plant viruses. In Vitro Cell Dev Biol. 1993;29A:284–288.

33. Day M F, Bennetts M J. A review of problems of specificity in arthropod vectors of plant and animal viruses. Canberra, Australia: Division of Entomology, CSIRO; 1954.

34. Demler S A, de Zoeten G A, Adam G, Harris K F. Pea enation mosaic enamovirus: properties and aphid transmission. In: Harrison B D, Murant A F, editors. The plant viruses. 5. Polyhedral virions and bipartite RNA genomes. New York, N.Y: Plenum Press; 1996. pp. 303–344.

35. Demler S A, Rucker Feeney D G, Skaf J S, De Zoeten G A. Expression and suppression of circulative aphid transmission in pea enation mosaic virus. J Gen Virol. 1997;78:511–523.

36. Dubois F, Sangwan R S, Sangwan N B S. Immunogold labeling

and electron microscopic screening of beet necrotic yellow vein virus in the fungus Polymyxa betae infecting Beta vulgaris root cortical parenchyma cells. Int J Plant Sci. 1994;155:545–552.

37. Edman J D, Spielman A. Blood feeding by vectors: physiology, ecology, behavior, and vertebrate defense. In: Monath T P, editor. The arboviruses: epidemiology and ecology. Boca Raton, Fla: CRC Press, Inc.; 1988. pp. 153–190.

38. Estabrook E M, Suyenaga K, Tsai J H, Falk B W. Maize stripe tenuivirus RNA2 transcripts in plant and insect hosts and analysis of pvc2, a protein similar to the Phlebovirus virion membrane glycoproteins. Virus Genes. 1996;12:239–247.

39. Falk B W, Tsai J H, Lommel A. Differences in levels of detection for the maize stripe virus capsid and major non-capsid proteins in plant and insect hosts. J Gen Virol. 1987;68:1801–1812.

40. Fenner F, Ratcliffe F N. Myxomatosis. Cambridge, United Kingdom: Cambridge University Press; 1965.

41. Filichkin S A, Brumfield S, Filichkin T P, Young M J. In vitro interactions of the aphid endosymbiotic symL chaperonin with barley yellow dwarf virus. J Virol. 1997;71:569–577.

42. Filichkin S A, Lister R M, McGrath P F, Young M J. *In vivo* expression and mutational analysis of the barley yellow dwarf virus readthrough gene. Virology. 1994;205:290–299.

43. Fukatsu T, Ishikawa H. Synthesis and localization of symbionin an aphid endosymbiont protein. Insect Biochem Mol Biol. 1992;22:167–174.

44. Fukushi T. Relationship between propagative rice viruses and their vectors. In: Maramorosch K, editor.Viruses, vectors and vegetation. New York, N.Y: John Wiley & Sons, Inc.; 1969. pp. 279–301.

45. Garret A, Kerlan C, Thomas D. The intestine is a site of passage for potato leafroll virus from the gut lumen into the haemocoel in the aphid vector *Myzus-persicae*. Arch Virol. 1993;131:377–392.

46. Gergerich R C, Scott H A. Determinants in the specificity of virus transmission by leaf-feeding beetles.Adv Dis Vector Res. 1991;8:1–14.

47. Ghanim M, Morin S, Zeidan M, Czosnek H. Evidence for transovarial transmission of tomato yellow leaf curl virus by its

vector, the whitefly *Bemesia tabaci*. Virology. 1998;240:295–303.

48. Gibb K S, Randles J W. Transmission of velvet tobacco mottle virus and related viruses by the Mirid*Cyrtopeltis nicotianae*. Adv Dis Vector Res. 1991;7:1–18.
49. Gibbs M J, Cooper J I. A recombinational event in the history of luteoviruses probably induced by base-pairing between the genomes of two distinct viruses. Virology. 1995;206:1129–1132.
50. Gildow F E. Virus-membrane interactions involved in circulative transmission of luteoviruses by aphids.Adv Dis Vector Res. 1987;4:93 120.
51. Gildow F E. Evidence for receptor-mediated endocytosis regulating luteovirus acquisition by aphids.Phytopathology. 1993;83:270–277.
52. Gildow, F. E. Luteovirus transmission and mechanisms regulating vector-specificity. *In* Luteoviridea, in press. CAB International, Wallingford, United Kingdom.
53. Gildow F E, Damsteegt V D, Smith O P, Gray S M. Cellular mechanisms regulating circulative transmission and aphid vector specificity of soybean dwarf luteoviruses. Phytopathology. 1994;84:1155–1156.
54. Gildow F E, Reavy B, Mayo M A, Woodford T, Duncan G H. Potato leafroll virus-like particles lacking read through protein are transmitted by *Myzus persicae*. Phytopathology. 1997;87:S33.
55. 54a. Gildow F E, Gray S M. The aphid salivary gland basal lamina as a selective barrier associated with vector-specific transmission of barley yellow dwarf luteovirus. Phytopathology. 1993;83:1293–1302.
56. Govier D A, Kassanis B. A virus induced component of plant sap needed when aphids acquire potato virus Y from purified preparations. Virology. 1974;78:420–426.
57. Grace T D C. Establishment of a line of mosquito cells grown in vitro. Nature. 1966;211:366–367.
58. Granados R R, Hirumi H, Maramorosch K. Electron microscopic evidence for wound tumor virus accumulation in various organs of an inefficient leafhopper vector, *Agalliopsis novella*. J Invertebr Pathol.1967;9:147–159.

59. Gray S M. Plant virus proteins involved in natural vector transmission. Trends Microbiol. 1996;4:253–294.

60. 58a. Gray, S. M., et al. Unpublished data.

61. Grimstad P R, Paulson S L, Craig G B. Vector competence of *Aedes hendersoni* for La Crosse virus and evidence of a salivary-gland escape barrier. J Med Entomol. 1985;22:447–453.

62. Gupta A P. Immunology of insects and other arthropods. Boca Raton, Fla: CRC Press, Inc.; 1991.

63. Ham P J. Immunity in haematophagous insect vectors of parasitic infection. Adv Dis Vector Res.1992;9:41–66.

64. Hardy J L. Susceptibility and resistance of vector mosquitoes. In: Monath T P, editor. The arboviruses: epidemiology and ecology. I. Boca Raton, Fla: CRC Press, Inc.; 1988. pp. 127–152.

65. Hardy J L, Houk E J, Kramer L D, Reeves W C. Intrinsic factors affecting vector competence of mosquitoes for arboviruses. Annu Rev Entomol. 1983;28:229–262.

66. Harris K F. An ingestion-egestion hypothesis of noncirculative virus transmission. In: Harris K F, Maramorosch K, editors. Aphids as virus vectors. New York, N.Y: Academic Press, Inc.; 1977. pp. 165–220.

67. Harris K F. Aphid transmission of plant viruses. In: Mandahar C L, editor. Plant viruses. II. Pathology. Boca Raton, Fla: CRC Press, Inc.; 1990. pp. 177–204.

68. Henig R M. A dancing matrix: voyages along the viral frontier. New York, N.Y: Alfred Knopf; 1993.

69. Hertig C, Coupar B E H, Gould A R, Boyle D B. Field and vaccine strains of fowlpox virus carry integrated sequences from the avian retrovirus, reticuloendotheliosis virus. Virology. 1997;235:367–376

70. Hogenhout S A, Verbeek M, Hans F, Houterman P M, Fortass M, Van Der Wilk F, Huttinga H, Van Den Heuvel J F J M. Molecular bases of the interactions between luteoviruses and aphids. Agronomie.1996;16:167–173.

71. Holbrook F R, Tabachnick W J. *Culicoides variipennis* (Diptera: Ceratopogonidae) complex in California. J Med Entomol. 1995;32:413–419.

72. Holbrook F R, Tabachnick W J, Brady R. Genetic variation in populations of *Culicoides variipennis*complex in the six New England states, USA. Med Vet Entomol. 1996;10:173–180.

73. Huet H, Gal O A, Meir E, Lecoq H, Raccah B. Mutations in the helper component protease gene of zucchini yellow mosaic virus affect its ability to mediate aphid transmissibility. J Gen Virol. 1994;75:1407–1414.

74. Hull R. Molecular biology of plant virus-vector interactions. Adv Dis Vector Res. 1994;10:361–386.

75. Hunter W B, Ullman D E. Anatomy and ultrastructure of the piercing-sucking mouthparts and paraglossal sensilla of Frankliniella-Occidentalis Pergande Thysanoptera Thripidae. Int J Insect Morphol Embryol. 1992;21:17–35.

76. Husted K. Reason for non-aphid transmissibility in a strain of Kalanchoe mosaic potyvirus. Virus Genes.1995;11:59–61.

77. Jasinskiene N, Coates C J, Benedict M Q, Cornel A J, Rafferty C S, James A A, Collins F H. Stable transformation of the yellow fever mosquito, *Aedes aegypti,* with the Hermes element from the housefly.Proc Natl Acad Sci USA. 1998;95:3743–3747.

78. Jianping C, Swaby A G, Adams M J, Yili R. Barley mild mosaic virus inside its fungal vector polymyxa-graminis. Ann Appl Biol. 1991;118:615–622.

79. Jolly C A, Mayo M A. Changes in the amino acid sequence of the coat protein readthrough domain of potato leafroll luteovirus affect the formation of an epitope and aphid transmission. Virology. 1994;201:182–185.

80. Karpf A R, Brown D T. Comparison of Sindbis virus-induced pathology in mosquito and vertebrate cell cultures. Virology. 1998;240:193–201.

81. Kennedy J S, Day M F, Eastop V F. A conspectus of aphids as vectors of plant viruses. London, United Kingdom: Commonwealth Institute of Entomology; 1962.

82. Kidwell M G, Wattam A R. An important step forward in the genetic manipulation of mosquito vectors of human disease. Proc Natl Acad Sci USA. 1998;95:3349–3350.

83. Kikkert M, Meurs C, van de Wetering F, Dorfmuller S, Peters D, Kormelink R, Goldbach R. Binding of tomato spotted wilt virus to a 94-kDa thrips protein. Phytopathology. 1998;88:63–69.

84. Kloft W J. Radioisotopes in vector research. Adv Dis Vector Res. 1992;9:41–66.

85. Kubes M, Fuchsberger N, Labuda M, Zuffova E, Nuttall P A. Salivary gland extracts of partially fed*Dermacentor reticulatus* ticks decrease natural killer cell activity in vitro. Immunology. 1994;82:113–116.

86. Labuda M, Austyn J M, Zuffova E, Kozuch O, Fuchsberger N, Lysy J, Nuttall P A. Importance of localized skin infection in tick-borne encephalitis virus transmission. Virology. 1996;219:357–366.

87. Lamb J W, Duncan G H, Reavy B, Gildow F E, Mayo M A, Thay R T. Assembly of virus-like particles in insect cells infected with a baculovirus containing a modified coat protein gene of potato leafroll luteovirus. J Gen Virol. 1996;77:1349–1358.

88. Lecoq H, Pitrat M. Specificity of the helper component-mediated aphid transmission of three potyviruses infection muskmelon. Phytopathology. 1985;75:890–893.

89. Legavre T, Maia I G, Casse Delbart F, Bernardi F, Robaglia C. Switches in the mode of transmission select for or against a poorly aphid-transmissible strain of potato virus Y with reduced helper component and virus accumulation. J Gen Virol. 1996;77:1343–1347.

90. Liu S, Bedford I D, Briddon R W, Markham P G. Efficient whitefly transmission of African cassava mosaic geminivirus requires sequences from both genomic components. J Gen Virol. 1997;78:1791–1794

91. Lomonossoff G P. Pathogen-derived resistance to plant viruses. Annu Rev Phytopathol. 1995;33:323–343.

92. Lopez Moya J J, Canto T, Diaz Ruiz J R, Lopez Abella D. Transmission by aphids of a naturally non-transmissible plum pox virus isolate with the aid of potato virus Y helper component. J Gen Virol.1995;76:2293–2297.

93. Ludwig G V, Israel B A, Christensen B M, Yull T M, Schultz K T. Role of La Crosse virus glycoproteins in attachment of virus to host cells. Virology. 1991;181:564–571.

94. Maia I G, Haenni A, Bernardi F. Potyviral HC-Pro: a multifunctional protein. J Gen Virol.1996;77:1335–1341.

95. Mandahar C L. Virus transmission. In: Mandahar C L, editor. Plant viruses. II. Pathology. Boca Raton, Fla: CRC Press; 1990. pp. 205–254.

96. Maramorosch K. Arthropod transmission of plant viruses. Annu Rev Entomol. 1963;8:369–414.

97. Martin B, Collar J L, Tjallingii W F, Fereres A. Intracellular ingestion and salivation by aphids may cause the acquisition and inoculation of non-persistently transmitted plant viruses. J Gen Virol.1997;78:2701–2705.

98. Martin R R, Keese P K, Young M J, Waterhouse P M, Gerlach W L. Evolution and molecular biology of luteoviruses. Annu Rev Phytopathol. 1990;28:341–364.

99. Maudlin I. Transmission of African trypanosomiasis: interactions among Tsetse immune system, symbionts, and parasites. Adv Dis Vector Res. 1991;7:117–148.

100. Mayo M A, Brierley K M, Goodman B A. Developments in the understanding of the particle structure of tobraviruses. Biochimie (Paris) 1993;75:639–644.

101. Merrill M H, TenBroeck C. The transmission of equine encephalomyelitis virus by *Aedes aegypti*. J Exp Med. 1935;62:687–695.

102. Miller B R, Mitchell C J. Selection of a flavivirus-refractory strain of the yellow fever mosquito *Aedes aegypti*. Am J Trop Med Hyg. 1991;45:399–407

103. Miller M L, Brown D T. Alphavirus infection in cultured tissue cells. Adv Dis Vector Res. 1991;8:107–142.

104. Miller W A, Dinesh K S P, Paul C P. Luteovirus gene expression. Crit Rev Plant Sci. 1995;14:179–211.

105. Miranda G J, Koganezawa H. Identification, purification, and serological detection of the major noncapsid protein of rice grassy stunt virus. Phytopathology. 1995;85:1530–1533.

106. Morse S S. Examining the origins of emerging viruses. In: Morse S S, editor. Emerging viruses. New York, N.Y: Oxford University Press; 1993. pp. 10–28.

107. Mowry T M. Within-plant accumulation of potato leafroll virus by aggregated green peach aphid feeding. Phytopathology. 1995;85:859–863.

108. Murphy F A, Whitfield S G, Sudia W D, Chamberlain R W. Interaction of vector with vertebrate pathogenic viruses. In: Maramorosch K, Shope R E, editors. Invertebrate immunity. New York, N.Y: Academic Press, Inc.; 1975. pp. 25–53.

109. Nagata T, Storms M M H, Goldbach R, Peters D. Multiplication of tomato spotted wilt virus in primary cell cultures derived from two thrips species. Virus Res. 1997;49:59–66.

110. Nuss D L, Summers D. Variant dsRNAs associated with transmission-defective isolates of wound tumor virus represent terminally conserved remnants of genome sequences. Virology. 1984;133:276–288.

111. Nuttall P A, Jones L D, Davies C R. The role of arthropod vectors in arbovirus evolution. Adv Dis Vector Res. 1991;8:15–45.

112. Nuttall P A, Jones L D, Labuda M, Kaufman W R. Adaptations of arboviruses to ticks. J Med Entomol.1994;31:1–9.

113. Omura T, Maruyama W, Ichimi K, Fukui Y, Yan J, Zhu Y, Kamiunten H. Involvement in virus infection to insect vector cells of the P2 outer capsid proteins of rice gall dwarf and rice dwarf phytoreoviruses. Phytopathology. 1997;87:S72.

114. Orlob G B. Reappraisal of transmission of tobacco mosaic virus by insects. Phytopathology.1963;53:822–830.

115. Ozzam O, Frazer J, De La Rosa D, Beaver J S, Ahlquist P, Maxwell D P. Whitefly transmission and efficient ssDNA accumulation of bean golden mosaic geminivirus require functional coat protein. Virology.1994;204:289–296.

116. Pappu H R, Niblett C L, Lee R F. Application of recombinant DNA technology to plant protection: molecular approaches to engineering virus resistance in crop plants. World J Microbiol Biotechnol.1995;11:426–437

117. Peiffer M L, Gildow F E, Gray S M. Two distinct mechanisms regulate luteovirus transmission efficiency and specificity at the aphid salivary gland. J Gen Virol. 1997;78:495–503.

118. Peng Y H, Kadoury D, Gal On A, Huet H, Wang Y, Raccah B. Mutations in the HC-Pro gene of zucchini yellow mosaic

potyvirus: effects on aphid transmission and binding to purified virions. J Gen Virol.1998;79:897–904.

119. Perez de Leon A A, Ribeiro J M C, Tabachnick W J, Valenzuela J G. Identification of a salivary vasodilator in the primary North American vector of bluetongue viruses, *Culicoides variipennis*. Am J Trop Med Hyg. 1997;57:375–381.

120. Perry K L, Zhang L, Shintaku M H, Palukaitis P. Mapping determinants in cucumber mosaic virus for transmission by *Aphis gossypii*. Virology. 1994;205:591–595.

121. Pesic-van Esbroeck Z, Harris K F, Duffus J E. Immunocytochemical localization of squash leaf curl virus in squash and the sweet potato whitefly. Phytopathology. 1995;85:1180.

122. Pirone T P. Does tobacco mosaic virus infect plant through wounds produced by aphid stylets?Virology. 1972;49:801–803.

123. Pirone T P. Efficiency and selectivity of the helper component mediated aphid transmission of purified potyviruses. Phytopathology. 1981;71:922–924.

124. Pirone T P. Viral genes and gene products that determine insect transmissibility. Semin Virol.1991;2:81–87.

125. 122a. Pirone, T. P. Personal communication.

126. Pirone T P, Blanc S. Helper-dependent vector transmission of plant viruses. Annu Rev Phytopathol.1996;34:227–247.

127. Pirone T P, Thornbury D W. Quantity of virus required for aphid transmission of a potyvirus.Phytopathology. 1988;78:104–107.

128. Pollard D G. Aphid penetration of plant tissues. In: Harris K F, Maramorosch K, editors. Aphids as virus vectors. New York, N.Y: Academic Press, Inc.; 1977. pp. 165–220.

129. Ponsen M B. The site of potato leafroll virus multiplication in its vector, *Myzus persicae*: an anatomical study. Meded Landbouwhogesch Wageningen. 1972;72-16:1–147.

130. Power A G, Gray S M. Aphid transmission of barley yellow dwarf viruses: interactions between viruses, vectors, and host plants. In: D'Arcy C J, Burnett P A, editors. Barley yellow dwarf: 40 years of progress. St. Paul, Minn: APS Press; 1995. pp. 259–291.

131. Reed W. Recent researches concerning the etiology, propagation and prevention of yellow fever by the United States Army Commission. J Hyg. 1902;2:101–119.

132. Reutenauer A, Ziegler G V, Lot H, Scheidecker D, Guilley H, Richards K, Jonard G. Identification of beet western yellows luteovirus genes implicated in viral replication and particle morphogenesis. Virology.1993;195:692–699.

133. Rochow W F, Foxe M J, Muller I. A mechanism of vector specificity for circulative aphid-transmitted plant viruses. Ann New York Acad Sci. 1975;266:293–301.

134. Rubinstein G, Czosnek H. Long-term association of tomato yellow leaf curl virus with its whitefly vector *Bemisia tabaci*: effect on the insect transmission capacity, longevity and fecundity. J Gen Virol.1997;78:2683–2689.

135. Rysanek P, Stocky G, Haeberle A M, Putz C. Immunogold labelling of beet necrotic yellow vein virus particles inside its fungal vector *Polymyxa betae*. Agronomie (Paris) 1992;12:651–659.

136. Salomon R. Proteolytic cleavage of the N-terminal region of potyvirus coat protein and its relation to host recovery and vector transmission. Arch Virol Suppl. 1992;5:75–76.

137. Schmidt I, Blanc S, Esperandieu P, Kul G, Devauchelle G, Louis C, Cerutti M. Interaction between the aphid transmission factor and virus particles is a part of the molecular mechanism of cauliflower mosaic virus aphid transmission. Proc Natl Acad Sci USA. 1994;91:8885–8889.

138. Shi X M, Miller H, Verchot J, Carrington J C, Vance V B. Mutations in the region encoding the central domain of helper component-proteinase (HC-Pro) eliminate potato virus X-potyviral synergism. Virology.1997;231:35–42.

139. Shufran K A, Peters D C, Webster J A. Generation of clonal diversity by sexual reproduction in the greenbug, *Schizaphis graminum*. Insect Mol Biol. 1997;6:203–209.

140. Smith C E. Transmission of cowpea mosaic by the bean leaf beetle. Science. 1924;60:268.

141. Smith K M. Plant virus-vector relationships. Adv Virus Res. 1965;11:61–96.

142. Stollar V. Insect-transmitted vertebrate viruses: alphatogaviruses. In Vitro Cell Dev Biol.1993;29A:289–295.

143. Suzuki N, Sugawara M, Kusano T, Mori H, Matsuura Y. Immunodetection of rice dwarf phytoreoviral proteins in both insect and plant hosts. Virology. 1994;202:41–48.

144. Swenson K G. Plant virus transmission by insects. Methods Virol. 1967;1:267–307.

145. Sylvester E S, Richardson J. Decreased survival of *Hypermyzus lactucae* inoculated with serially passed sowthistle yellow vein virus. Virology. 1971;46:310–317.

146. Tabachnick W J. Genetic control of oral susceptibility to infection of *Culicoides variipennis* for bluetongue virus. Am J Trop Med Hyg. 1991;45:666–671.

147. Tabachnick W J. Genetics of insect vector competence for arboviruses. Adv Dis Vector Res.1994;10:93–108.

148. Takami N. On dwarf disease of rice plant and "tsumaguro-yokabai." J Jpn Agric Soc. 1901;241:22–30.

149. Tardieux I, Poupel O, Lapchin L, Rodhain F. Variation among strains of *Aedes aegypti* in susceptibility to oral infection with dengue type 2. Am J Trop Med Hyg. 1990;43:308–313.

150. Tardieux I, Poupel O, Lapchin L, Rodhain F. Analysis of inheritance of oral susceptibility of *Aedes aegypti* to dengue-2 virus using isofemale lines. J Med Entomol. 1991;28:518–521.

151. Taylor C E. Nematodes. In: Harris K F, Maramorosch K, editors. Vectors of plant pathogens. New York, N.Y: Academic Press, Inc.; 1980. pp. 375–416.

152. Tesh R B, Gubler D J, Rosen L. Variation among geographic strains of *Aedes albopictus* in susceptibility to infection with chikungunya virus. Am J Trop Med Hyg. 1976;25:326–333.

153. Thornbury D W, Hellman G M, Rhodes R E, Pirone T P. Purification and characterization of potyvirus helper component. Virology. 1985;144:260–267.

154. Turell M J. Horizontal and vertical transmission of viruses by insect and tick vectors. In: Monath T P, editor. The arboviruses: epidemiology and ecology. I. Boca Raton, Fla: CRC Press, Inc.; 1988. pp. 127–152.

155. Ullah F, Peters D C. Sexual reproduction capabilities of greenbugs (Homoptera: Aphididae) J Kans Entomol Soc. 1996;69:153–159.

156. Ullman D E, Cho J J, Mau R F L, Westcot D M, Custer D M. A midgut barrier to tomato spotted wilt virus acquisition by adult western flower thrips. Phytopathology. 1992;82:1333–1342.

157. Uyeda I, Kimura I, Shikata E. Characterization of genome structure and establishment of vector cell lines for plant reoviruses. Adv Virus Res. 1995;45:249–279.

158. Valenzuela J G, Chuffe O M, Ribeiro J M C. Apyrase and anti-platelet activities from the salivary glands of the bed bug *Cimex lectularius*. Insect Biochem Mol Biol. 1996;26:557–562.

159. Van Den Heuvel J F J M, Bruyere A, Hogenhout S A, Ziegler Graff V, Brault V, Verbeek M, Van Der Wilk F, Richards K. The N-terminal region of the luteovirus readthrough domain determines virus binding to Buchnera GroEL and is essential for virus persistence in the aphid. J Virol. 1997;71:7258–7265.

160. Van Den Heuvel J F J M, Verbeek M, Van Der Wilk F. Endosymbiotic bacteria associated with circulative transmission of potato leafroll virus by *Myzus persicae*. J Gen Virol. 1994;75:2559–2565.

161. Vey A. Humeral encapsulation. In: Pathak J P N, editor. Insect immunity. Dordrecht, The Netherlands: Kluwer Academic Publishers; 1993. pp. 59–68.

162. Wang H, Nuttall P A. Excretion of host immunoglobulin in tick saliva and detection of IgG-binding proteins in tick haemolymph and salivary glands. Parasitology. 1994;109:525–530.

163. Wang J Y, Chay C, Gildow F E, Gray S M. Readthrough protein associated with virions of barley yellow dwarf luteovirus and its potential role in regulating the efficiency of aphid transmission. Virology.1995;206:954–962.

164. Wang R Y, Ammar E D, Thornbury D W, Lopez Moya J J, Pirone T P. Loss of potyvirus transmissibility and helper-component activity correlate with non-retention of virions in aphid stylets. J Gen Virol. 1996;77:861–867.

165. 161a. Wang R Y, Pirone T P. Mineral oil interferes with retention of tobacco etch potyvirus in the stylets of*Myzus persicae*. Phytopathology. 1996;86:820–823.

166. Watson M A. Seventh Commonwealth Entomological Conference. London, United Kingdom: Eastern Press, Ltd.; 1960. The ways in which plant viruses are transmitted by vectors.

167. Watson M A, Plumb R T. Transmission of plant-pathogenic viruses by aphids. Annu Rev Entomol.1972;17:425–452.

168. Weaver S C. Vector biology in arboviral pathogenesis. In: Nathanson N, editor. Viral pathogenesis.Philadelphia, Pa: Lippincott-Raven Publishers; 1997. pp. 329–352.

169. Whitcomb R F, Davis R E. Mycoplasma and phytoarboviruses as plant pathogens persistently transmitted by insects. Annu Rev Entomol. 1970;15:405–464.

170. Wu Z C, Hu J S, Polston J F, Ullman D E, Hiebert E. Complete nucleotide sequence of a nonvector-transmissible strain of abutilon mosaic geminivirus in Hawaii. Phytopathology. 1996;86:608–613.

171. Yan J, Tomaru M, Takahashi A, Kimura I, Hibino H, Omura T. P2 protein encoded by genome segment S2 of rice dwarf phytoreovirus is essential for virus infection. Virology. 1996;224:539–541.

172. Zeigler R S, Morales F J. Genetic determination of replication of rice hoja blanca virus within its planthopper vector, *Sogatodes oryzicola*. Phytopathology. 1990;80:559–566.

Chapter 7

Potential Influence of Climate Change on Vector-Borne and Zoonotic Diseases: A Review and Proposed Research Plan

James N. Mills, Kenneth L. Gage, and Ali S. Khan

National Center for Emerging and Zoonotic Infectious Diseases, Centers for Disease Control and Prevention, Atlanta, Georgia, USA.

ABSTRACT

Background

Because of complex interactions of climate variables at the levels of the pathogen, vector, and host, the potential influence of climate change on vector-borne and zoonotic diseases (VBZDs) is poorly understood and difficult to predict. Climate effects on the nonvector-borne zoonotic diseases are especially obscure and have received scant treatment.

Objective

We described known and potential effects of climate change on VBZDs and proposed specific studies to increase our understanding of these effects. The nonvector-borne zoonotic diseases have received scant treatment and are emphasized in this paper.

Data Sources and Synthesis

We used a review of the existing literature and extrapolations from observations of short-term climate variation to suggest potential impacts of climate change on VBZDs. Using public health priorities on climate change, published by the Centers for Disease Control and Prevention, we developed six specific goals for increasing understanding of the interaction between climate and VBZDs and for improving capacity for predicting climate change effects on incidence and distribution of VBZDs.

Conclusions

Climate change may affect the incidence of VBZDs through its effect on four principal characteristics of host and vector populations that relate to pathogen transmission to humans: geographic distribution, population density, prevalence of infection by zoonotic pathogens, and the pathogen load in individual hosts and vectors. These mechanisms may interact with each other and with other factors such as anthropogenic disturbance to produce varying effects on pathogen transmission within host and vector populations and to humans. Because climate change effects on most VBZDs act through wildlife hosts and vectors, understanding these effects will require multidisciplinary teams to conduct and interpret ecosystem-based studies of VBZD pathogens in host and vector populations and to identify the hosts, vectors, and pathogens with the greatest potential to affect human populations under climate change scenarios.

The concept that weather and climate are linked to the incidence of infectious diseases in humans has been recognized since the time of Hippocrates (National Research Council 2001). Understanding the link between climate and disease has increasing urgency. According to the Intergovernmental Panel on Climate Change (IPCC 2007), warming of the earth's climate is "unequivocal." Global changes already documented include increased global surface temperature, rising sea level, decreased arctic and alpine snow and ice, and evidence of plants and animals responding to these changes by moving to higher elevations or closer to the poles. Precipitation has increased in some parts of the world while decreasing in others. These changes are predicted to continue into the foreseeable future (IPCC 2007).

Climate change is predicted to have a variety of impacts on human health, many of which have been extensively reviewed (Confalonieri et al. 2007; Ebi et al. 2006, 2008; Frumkin et al. 2008; Patz and Olson 2006). Some of these effects are easily intuited: increasing temperatures will likely increase the incidence of heat-related mortality (and decrease the risk mortality from cold exposure); increased drought will result in increased food and water shortages, whereas more frequent and more severe heavy precipitation events will increase the incidence of flood-related injuries and deaths, water-and food-borne illness, and other infectious, respiratory, and skin diseases.

Another class of potential impacts on human health often cited as a consequence of climate change is less direct, less intuitive, and less predictable: Those caused by infectious diseases acquired by humans from invertebrate and vertebrate animals—the vector-borne and zoonotic diseases (VBZDs). Zoonotic diseases are those caused by pathogens that are transmitted between vertebrate animals and humans. Vector-borne diseases are those for which the pathogen is transmitted to or among humans by an arthropod vector. Zoonotic diseases may be vector borne (transmitted to humans from a vertebrate reservoir by an arthropod vector such as Lyme disease) or nonvector borne [transmitted to humans by direct or indirect contact with the vertebrate host without the participation of an arthropod vector such as hantavirus pulmonary syndrome (HPS)]. Vector-borne diseases, in turn, may be zoonotic, as in the Lyme disease example, or nonzoonotic (transmitted by an arthropod vector from human to human without the involvement of a nonhuman reservoir such as malaria). We have used the inclusive term "VBZD" to include all three possible categories [for additional definitions, examples, and background information, see Table 1 and Supplemental Material (doi:10.1289/ehp.0901389)]. Making predictions concerning the effects of VBZDs adds additional complexity to forecasts. Although understanding the transmission of any infectious pathogen requires knowledge of the interactions between the pathogen and humans, in the case of VBZDs we must also understand the interactions of the pathogen with the arthropod vector and with the vertebrate host. Thus, a complete understanding of VBZDs requires in-depth knowledge of the ecology and natural history of the host or vector (Gage et al. 2008; Mills and Childs 1998).

Table 1: Some of the important VBZDs mentioned in this review, with their etiological agents, vectors, and vertebrate hosts

Disease	Pathogen	Vector	Vertebrate host
Vector-borne zoonotic diseases			
Lyme disease	*Borrelia burgdorferi* (bacterium)	*Ixodes* spp. (tick)	White-footed deer mouse (*Peromyscus leucopus*) and eastern chipmunk (*Tamias striatus*)[a]
Tick-borne encephalitis (TBE)	TBE virus	*Ixodes* spp. (tick)	Rodents
Rift Valley fever	Rift Valley fever virus	*Aedes* and *Culex* spp. (mosquito)	Livestock[b]
Plague	*Yersinia pestis* (bacterium)	*Xenopsylla cheopis* (flea)	Rodents
Tularemia	*Francisella tularensis*	Ticks (several species)[c]	Rodents, lagomorphs[c]
West Nile fever	West Nile virus	*Culex* spp. (mosquito)	Birds, especially crows and jays
Leishmaniasis	*Leishmania* spp. (protozoan)	*Phlebotomus* and *Lutzomyia* spp. (sand fly)	Many mammal species
Chagas disease	*Trypanosoma cruzi* (parasite)	Triatomine bugs	Many wild and domestic mammals

Vector-borne nonzoonotic diseases			
Malaria	*Plasmodium* spp. (protozoan)	*Anopheles* spp. (mosquito)	Humans
Dengue fever	Dengue virus	*Aedes aegypti*	Humans
Non vector-borne zoonotic diseases			
Hantavirus pulmonary syndrome (HPS)	Sin Nombre virus	None	North American deer mouse (*Peromyscus maniculatus*)
	New York virus	None	White-footed deer mouse (*Peromyscus leucopus*)
	Black Creek Canal virus	None	Hispid cotton rat (*Sigmodon hispidus*)
	Numerous viruses in South and Central America	None	Rodents of subfamily Sigmodontinae
Hemorrhagic fever with renal syndrome	Seoul virus (and other Eurasian hantaviruses)	None	Norway rat (*Rattus norvegicus*; for Seoul virus) and several other rodents of subfamily Murinae
South American hemorrhagic fevers	Arenaviruses	None	Rodents of subfamily Sigmodontinae
Monkeypox	Monkeypox virus	None	Terrestrial rodent species
Filovirus hemorrhagic fevers	Marburg virus and Ebola virus	None	Egyptian fruit bat (*Rousettus aegyptiacus*) and likely other bat species
Nipah virus encephalitis	Nipah virus	None	Fruit bats (*Pteropus* spp.)

[a]Principal hosts in eastern North America; other rodent species are hosts in western North America, Europe, and Asia.

[b]Virus survives in eggs of infected mosquitoes; vertebrate reservoir not required for viral maintenance.

[c]Vectors, hosts, and routes of transmission are highly variable.

In this article, we have proposed four primary mechanisms by which climate change is likely to affect pathogen, host, and vector populations; summarized current evidence that these mechanisms affect host and vector populations; and assessed how these effects are likely to influence human health. We also have attempted to identify important gaps in our knowledge and have suggested studies that are needed to fill those gaps and provide reliable information about the ultimate effects of climate change on VBZDs.

Expected Changes

If climate change is to affect the frequency of VBZDs through acting on nonhuman hosts, vectors, and pathogens, it is likely to act by one (or a combination) of four primary mechanisms: *a*) range shifts in host or vector distribution that bring these hosts and vectors into contact with new human populations; *b*) changes in the population density of the host or vector that would result in increased or decreased frequency of contact with humans or with other hosts and vectors; *c*) changes in the prevalence of infection by the pathogen in the host or vector population that would increase or decrease the frequency of human (or other host or vector) contact with an infected host or vector; and *d*) changes in pathogen load brought about by changes in rates of pathogen reproduction, replication, or development in hosts or vectors that would affect the likelihood that a human (or other host or vector) contact would result in pathogen transmission.

The Evidence: What do Existing Studies Portend? Range Shifts

Geographic changes in the distributions of wildlife species in response to climate change are difficult to document because of the absence of current and historic data on distributions of many species and populations (Jannett et al. 2007; Thomas et al. 2006). Nevertheless, range shifts have been observed for a variety of taxa, including important mammalian hosts and arthropod vectors. These range shifts have generally been poleward and upward (toward higher elevations) (Hickling et al. 2006; Rosenzweig et al. 2007), and they have resulted in overall expansions, contractions, or no change in the total area occupied by a population or species. Altitudinal and latitudinal range shifts have occurred for *Ixodes ricinus*, the vector of the agents of Lyme disease and tick-borne encephalitis (TBE) in Europe (reviewed by Gage et al. 2008), and these shifts are associated with ("association" as used throughout this review is not proof of causation) new foci of disease and an increase in incidence of TBE (Kerr 2001;Lindgren and Gustafson 2001). Northerly range shifts also have been observed for *Ixodes scapularis*, a vector of Lyme disease, human granulocytic anaplasmosis, and babesiosis in North America. Models indicate that this species will extend its range farther into Canada while contracting its southern range (Brownstein et al. 2005; Ogden et al. 2006, 2010).

The hispid cotton rat (*Sigmodon hispidus*), which occurs in the southern United States, is the host of Black Creek Canal hantavirus (Table 1), a known cause of HPS (Rollin et al. 1995) as well as Muleshoe hantavirus (Rawlings et al. 1996), and Tamiami arenavirus (Calisher et al. 1970). The distribution of the hispid cotton rat is climate limited, and precise temperature minima for the species' distributional limits have been described (Mohlhenrich 1961). Nevertheless, that distribution has undergone a northward expansion (Cameron and Spencer 1981; Schmidly 2002) in the last few decades, and a new altitudinal record was described for hispid cotton rats in New Mexico (Dunnum 2002). The white-footed deer mouse (*Peromyscus leucopus*), a host for the agents of Lyme disease, human granulocytic anaplasmosis, babesiosis, and HPS, has extended its range northward in Wisconsin (Long 1996) and Minnesota (Jannett et al. 2007). Hispid cotton rats and white-footed deer mice are common species in the United States and have been studied by generations of mammalogists. Little or no baseline data are available for the huge number of rodents in the tropics, the area where hosts (especially rodents and bats), vectors, and pathogens have their greatest diversity, yet they are the least studied [for a discussion of tropical disease diversity, rodents, and bats, see Supplemental Material (doi:10.1289/ehp.0901389)]. Known and unknown tropical host and pathogen systems are likely to shift their ranges closer to subtropical and temperate population centers as climate changes at higher latitudes.

Altitudinal temperature gradients are about 1,000 times steeper than latitudinal gradients (Colwell et al. 2008), which makes altitudinal transects more practical models for studying the effects of temperature change on plant and animal distributions. A recent range survey of small mammals in Yosemite National Park, California (USA), serves as a model (Moritz et al. 2008). Compared with similar surveys conducted approximately 100 years earlier (when minimum temperatures were 3°C lower), half of the 28 species monitored showed large (average = 500 m) upward changes in elevational limits (Figure 1). Low-altitude species shifted both their lower and upper range limits upslope (e.g., the piñon deer mouse, *Peromyscus truei*) or expanded their upper range upslope while maintaining a stable lower range limit (e.g., the California pocket mouse, *Chaetodipus californicus*). High-altitude species such as the alpine chipmunk (*Tamias alpinus*) showed overall range contractions because of upslope shifts in their lower limits. A continuation of this pattern suggests the ultimate extinction of some high-altitude species.

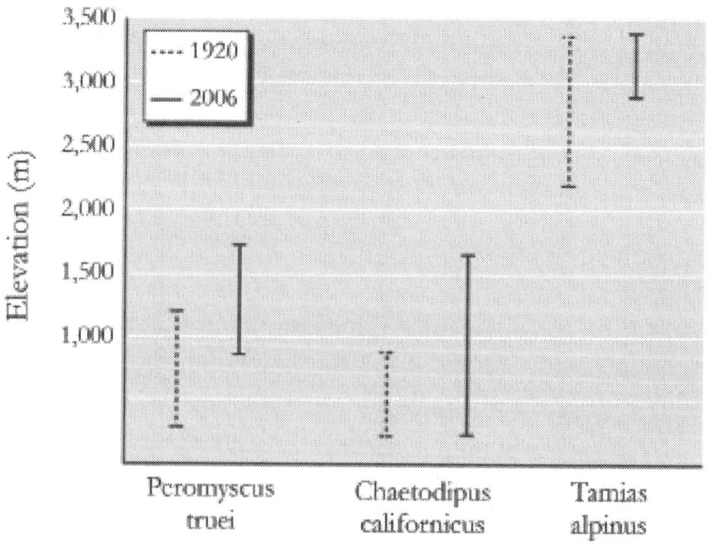

Figure 1: Elevational distribution of the piñon deer mouse (*Peromyscus truei*), the California pocket mouse (*Chaetodipus californicus*), and the alpine chipmunk (*Tamias alpinus*) in Yosemite National Park, California, 1920 and 2006 (Moritz et al. 2008).

The latitudinal temperature gradient in the tropics is relatively shallow. Not only does this make latitudinal studies more difficult, but it portends relatively higher extinction rates for midtropical species of restricted geographic range and limited dispersal capabilities. Elevational shifts provide the only published data for range shifts in the tropics, where upslope range shifts have been demonstrated for plants and vertebrate animals (Colwell et al. 2008; Pounds et al. 2005). Unlike most temperate areas, in the lowland tropics there is no community of species adapted to even hotter areas available to replace those species that shift their ranges upslope or poleward. Thus, the species diversity of lowland tropical areas is expected to decrease as global temperatures rise (Colwell et al. 2008). However, extinctions are likely to be selective. Specialist species with relatively narrow niche breadth (especially in terms of physiological tolerances, habitat, and diet requirements) are most likely to suffer, whereas more adaptable generalist species may thrive, with potentially important consequences for pathogen transmission (Mills 2006).

Range shifts may not be restricted to latitudinal and elevational dimensions. Several host and vector species are restricted to specific habitat types. The frequency of occurrence of hosts, vectors, or pathogens in these habitat types helps to define relative risk of disease to humans associated with these habitats (Mills and Childs 1998). Effects of climate change on the species composition of plant and animal communities are poorly understood. Range shifts in response to climate change are unlikely to affect entire communities or assemblages in unison (Root and Schneider 2002). Species will migrate at different rates and according to their own motility, tolerances, and physiological constraints. Thus, species assemblages are likely to change: Some species in new areas will experience increased population densities and competitive release, allowing colonization of habitats from which they were formerly excluded, whereas others may experience increased pressures and decreased population densities as new competitors or predators move into their ranges or they are unable to migrate as climate change leaves them stranded on shrinking islands of suitable habitat. This concept was illustrated by several high-altitude rodent and insectivore species in Yosemite National Park that are now restricted to only a portion of their former range (Moritz et al. 2008) (Figure 1).

Changes in Population Density

Climate change has been associated with conditions that alter the carrying capacity of ecosystems for some plant or animal populations (Gage et al. 2008; Sutherst 2004). Such changes can result in dramatic increases, or sometimes decreases, in host or vector population densities. Examples from vector-borne diseases are numerous. Populations of *Aedes* mosquitoes (vector for the agent of Rift Valley fever in East Africa) (Table 1) increase dramatically after periods of high rainfall associated with El Niño Southern Oscillation (ENSO) events (Anyamba et al. 2001; Linthicum et al. 1999). Increases in mosquitoes and mosquito-borne malaria were associated with ENSO events in South America (Barrera et al. 1999; Bouma and Dye 1997; Bouma et al. 1997) and southern Africa (Mabaso et al. 2007). Increasing temperatures also can decrease the development time of mosquitoes allowing greater population densities to be reached (Gage et al. 2008). Increased incidence of malaria was linked to precipitation and higher temperatures in Kenya (Githeko and Ndegwa 2001) and Madagascar (Bouma 2003). Conversely, reduced rainfall in Senegal and Niger was associated with decreases in malaria (Julvez et al. 1997; Mouchet et al. 1996), presumably resulting from decreased mosquito reproduction.

The effects of environmental extremes on vertebrate host populations can be pronounced. High summer temperatures have resulted in increased mortality of hosts, such as bats in tropical or subtropical areas (Welbergen et al. 2008) or increased overwinter survivorship of species in temperate areas (Straile and Stenseth 2007). After an ENSO event in 1997, investigators recorded increased rainfall, improved quality of vegetation, and increased population density of North American deer mice (*Peromyscus maniculatus*) in the southwestern United States. These events preceded increased numbers of HPS cases in the area over 3 years (Yates et al. 2002). Increased rainfall was also associated with outbreaks of HPS in Paraguay (Williams et al. 1997) and Panama (Ruedas et al. 2004). Similarly, human plague (a flea-borne zoonotic disease caused by the bacterium *Yersinia pestis*; Table 1) in the western United States was influenced by the effects of above-normal temperatures and status of the Pacific Decadal Oscillation (PDO). The PDO resulted in precipitation increases (Ari et al. 2008) that were believed to enhance small-mammal food resources and flea survival (Enscore et al. 2002; Parmenter et al. 1999). Although less attention has been paid to decreases in host populations, lower rainfall is accompanied by decreasing populations of North American deer mice in the southwestern United States (Yates et al. 2002), whereas increasing rainfall during cold periods was associated with abrupt population declines in some ecosystems (Calisher et al. 2005).

Changes in Prevalence of Infection in Host or Vector Populations

The increases in host or vector populations discussed above can lead to increased frequency of contact between hosts or between hosts and vectors (density-dependent transmission) (Begon et al. 2002) and increased prevalence of infection in host or vector populations. The increased North American deer mouse population density in the southwestern United States that followed the 1997 ENSO was followed, a year later, by increased prevalence of hantavirus infection in North American deer mouse populations [Centers for Disease Control and Prevention (CDC) 1999; Yates et al. 2002]. This delayed density-dependent increase in infection in host populations may be a general phenomenon affecting horizontally transmitted pathogens in wildlife hosts in strongly seasonal climates (Madhav et al. 2007; Mills et al. 1999). Similarly, as rodent populations increase above certain thresholds, the likelihood of plague epizootics also may increase (Davis et al. 2004). Precipitation and temperature influence the appearance of plague epizootics among Asian gerbils (Stenseth et al. 2006) and epizootics among prairie dogs in Colorado were linked to ENSO events (Stapp et al. 2004).

Prevalence of infection for other VBZDs might be increased by other mechanisms besides density-dependent transmission. Environmental changes that lead to increased stress in hosts can decrease host immune response, resulting in increased probability of infection as well as higher pathogen loads and increased pathogen shedding by a variety of host species (Nelson et al. 1995), including hosts for hantaviruses (Demas and Nelson 1998; Klein et al. 2004; Lehmer et al. 2007) and arenaviruses (Barnard et al. 1996).

Changes in Pathogen Load

Temperatures can have profound effects on the development of pathogens and pathogen loads in arthropod vectors (Gage et al. 2008; Sutherst 2004). Malaria parasites develop in mosquito vectors only within certain temperature ranges (Patz and Olson 2006). Similarly, *Y. pestis*, the etiological agent of plague, develops and expresses biofilm efficiently only at temperatures < 28°C. Biofilm facilitates *Y. pestis* transmission by causing infected fleas to increase feeding attempts and regurgitate *Y. pestis* back into host animals during feeding (Gage and Kosoy 2005; Jarrett et al. 2004). Survival of *Y. pestis* also is influenced by temperature with many fleas clearing infection as temperatures increase above 28°C (Gage and Kosoy 2005; Hinnebusch et al. 1998).

Recurrence of viral replication (recrudescence) under stress, including heat stress, has been documented for human viral diseases (Halford et al. 1996; Mehta et al. 2004) and is likely to occur within zoonotic host populations also. Replication and shedding of Sin Nombre virus (Table 1) are detected intermittently in infected North American deer mice (Botten et al. 2003; Kuenzi et al. 2005). Although mechanisms for the reactivation of viral replication are poorly understood, stress-related immunosuppression has been suggested (Botten et al. 2002; Kuenzi et al. 2005). The relationship between stress and pathogen transmission, replication, persistence, and shedding in hosts and vectors is poorly studied. A clearer understanding of this relationship would lead to more accurate predictions of the effects of climate change on VBZD risk to humans.

Interactions among Climate Variables

The amplitude and even the direction of effects of climate on host and vector populations are locally variable and depend upon interactions with other variables (Mills 2005). Contrary to what was observed in New Mexico, the 1997 ENSO did not lead to a net increase in North American deer mouse populations at a high-altitude site in Colorado. Increases in abundance of North American deer mice in Colorado from 1995 to 2000 were associated with increased rainfall during warm periods, but populations crashed after increased rainfall during cold periods (Calisher et al. 2005). Similarly, the combined effects of temperature and humidity affect the behavior, survival, and reproduction of many vector species. Survival of ticks and fleas are negatively affected by the combination of hot and dry conditions (Gage and Kosoy 2005; Randolph 2004). The same conditions limit the ability of ticks to quest for hosts in exposed environments.

These examples indicate that host responses to climate change are multifactorial and their quantitative prediction must consider multiple variables simultaneously, including temperature, precipitation, altitude, and location. The separation and independent measurement of these interacting effects have been identified as a research priority (Harvell et al. 2002). Nevertheless, because these factors contribute to overall effects interactively and often operate synergistically, predictions using single variables must be subject to cautious interpretation.

Interactions of Climate Change with Anthropogenic Factors

Just as the interaction effects between various aspects of climate change (e.g., temperature and precipitation) must be considered to accurately predict the influence of climate on VBZDs, so too must the interactions between climate change and other anthropogenic and natural factors. Human activities facilitate host or vector range shifts by transporting hosts or vectors to new geographic areas (Benedict et al. 2007), including new continents, as was the case with vectors of plague (Parmenter et al. 1999) and West Nile virus (Komar 2003) and hosts of monkeypox in the United States (Likos et al. 2005). Human migrations in response to climate change may make them more vulnerable to some VBZDs. For example, increases in leishmaniasis were associated with drought-related clustering of humans near water supplies where sand fly vectors were concentrated (Thompson et al. 2002). Human cultural and behavioral differences will alter the end effect of all of the mechanisms discussed above. Although *Aedes aegypti*, the primary vector of Dengue virus, is likely to achieve northward range expansions in the United States as winter temperatures become warmer, this may not result in dengue epidemics in the United States. In southern Texas, where *Ae. aegypti* is already established, dengue has remained rare despite epidemics on the Mexican side of the border. This is thought to be due to human-related factors, such as the greater use of air conditioning in the United States, which decreases exposure to mosquitoes (Reiter et al. 2003). Finally, the degree of human intervention to prevent or mitigate adverse effects of climate change on health will affect the eventual outcomes of all of the mechanisms discussed above. This is a large field of study (Confalonieri et al. 2007) but is outside the scope of our discussion.

Anthropogenic disturbance of ecosystems will modify the response of many species to climate change. As mentioned, the distributional range of many wildlife species and vectors is predicted to shift poleward and toward higher altitudes as the climate warms, perhaps bringing hosts, vectors, and diseases currently restricted to the tropics within the range of temperate population centers. Similar species migrations occurred at the transition from the last ice age to the current interglacial period (Wright et al. 1993). Nevertheless, not all species and populations will have the option of moving. Nonvolant species on mountain tops or other habitat islands will have nowhere to go. Similarly, isolated foci of some vector-borne diseases that rely on the continued presence of certain hosts and vectors could disappear if movement of either is restricted. Although climate change might result in suitable climatic conditions elsewhere, these areas will remain disease-free unless all components of the system (host, vector, pathogen) reach and occur simultaneously in these sites for sufficient time to establish transmission cycles. Anthropogenic habitat fragmentation as a result of deforestation, agriculture, road building, construction of towns and cities, and other land use changes will impede migration, jeopardizing the existence of some populations and species (Root and Schneider 2002). A mathematical model was used to predict that > 400 (relatively mobile) bird species will suffer > 50% range contractions and > 50 species will become extinct because of combined effects of climate change and anthropogenic habitat loss (Jetz et al. 2007). According to the IPCC's *Fourth Assessment Report*, 20–30% of plant and animal species are likely to be at increasingly high risk of extinction as global mean temperatures exceed 2–3°C above preindustrial levels (Fischlin et al. 2007).

It seems intuitive that extinctions resulting in fewer species of host animals should decrease the number of potential zoonotic pathogens and thus the incidence of VBZDs. Several scientists have suggested that high biodiversity is causally related to high levels of infectious disease, both locally and regionally (Sattenspiel 2000; Wolfe et al. 2005). Indeed, some highly specific pathogens are likely to disappear with their hosts. Nevertheless, extinction and biodiversity loss may have some counterintuitive affects on the incidence of some VBZDs. Extinctions will occur selectively with habitat and dietary specialists being affected first (MacDonald and Brown 1992; Warren et al. 2001). Meanwhile more opportunistic, generalist species may not only survive but thrive in the absence of competition from specialists. In their study of climate change and altitudinal migration in Yosemite National Park, Moritz et al. (2008) found that opportunistic small mammal species (those that were short-lived and had more litters per year) were more likely to expand their range upward than were their long-lived, less fecund counterparts. The host species for most of the known rodent-borne hemorrhagic fever viruses that affect humans are opportunistic species (Mills 2006). Although it is possible that this pattern is due, at least in part, to sampling error (diseases associated with anthropophilic species would be the first to come to our attention), the pattern could be the logical consequence of several characteristics of opportunistic species (high vagility, rapid growth, early reproduction, high fecundity, and capacity to sustain high population densities that are conducive to the transmission of pathogens) that would facilitate the evolution and maintenance of pathogens. Further, decreases in the species diversity of potential host assemblages have been associated with increased prevalence of infection by zoonotic pathogens in host populations both for vector-borne diseases (Ostfeld and Keesing 2000) and for nonvector-borne zoonoses (Mills 2005). Thus, selective extinctions associated with climate change can result in a net increase in the risk of some zoonotic infections in both wildlife and humans.

Other Interactions and Confounders

In addition to barriers caused by anthropogenic changes, natural barriers to dispersal such as mountain ranges or bodies of water can preclude species from reaching suitable habitats. Stronger competitors or predators or the absence of prey or other food sources could prevent species from occupying otherwise suitable habitats.

Behavioral adaptation such as changing activity patterns or nesting sites can alter the responses of individuals and populations to climate change. One factor facilitating the northward range expansion of hispid cotton rats has likely been a switch to occupancy of deeper burrows that extend below the frost line (Dunnum 2002).

Species with the genetic capacity to undergo evolutionary adaptation to a changing environment can withstand or even benefit from climate change. The photoperiodic response of the pitcher plant mosquito (*Wyeomyia smithii*) has shifted toward shorter, more southern day lengths in response to an extended growing season, demonstrating an adaptive evolutionary response to global warming in eastern North America (Bradshaw and Holzapfel 2001). The capacity for such adaptation will vary among species, and those that lack adaptive capacity may be forced to migrate in order to survive.

Some investigators believe recent increases in malaria incidence in the highlands of East Africa were associated with a warming trend that began in the 1970s (Pascual et al. 2006; Patz 2002); others have linked the increases to other factors, including drug resistance (Hay et al. 2002a, 2002b; Shanks et al. 2002). However, the reality may involve the interaction of multiple factors.

Climate changes do not satisfactorily explain the temporal and spatial patterns of increases in incidence of tick-borne disease in Europe. Other factors likely include demographic changes, increases in deer abundance, and changes in land use after the end of communist rule in Eastern Europe (reviewed by Gage et al. 2008).

Finally, in this review, we have often used observations of short-term responses of hosts, vectors, and pathogens to climate variability to conjecture about possible responses to long-term climate change. Responses of host, vector, and pathogen populations to temporary—natural or experimental—changes in environmental conditions (wet or dry periods, warm or cold periods) are clues to how populations will respond to long-term climate change, but these inferences must be made cautiously. North American deer mice, an opportunistic species, quickly respond to increasing moisture in the southwestern United States. Their rapid population growth allows them to escape predators and competitors in the short term. However, if such changes are longer term, competitors will respond to the same changing climatic conditions and predators will adapt to the increased density of prey. The new long-term equilibrium is likely to be much different from what was observed during the initial short-term response. Longer term behavioral, social, and genetic adaptation to the new biotic and abiotic environment will ultimately modify outcomes in ways that may not have been predicted from short-term observations. This important issue, and other caveats for predicting climate change effects on disease, are treated in detail in an earlier review (National Research Council 2001).

In summary, host and vector "responses" that are correlated with (or "associated with," to use our terminology throughout this review) changing climate variables do not prove cause and effect. Potential confounding variables including behavioral changes, interspecific interactions, intrinsic population phenomena, anthropogenic factors, and evolutionary changes should be considered when appropriate.

What Kinds of Studies Will Be Useful?

The CDC policy on climate change and public health (CDC 2010) sets forth 11 priority public health actions that address research, prediction, training, communication, preparedness, and prevention to prepare the nation and the world for confronting potential health problems associated with climate change. Using these general priorities, we propose six specific goals that we believe would lead to a better understanding of the interaction between climate and VBZDs and an improved capability for predicting how climate change will affect the incidence and distribution of VBZDs.

Pathogen Identification and Characterization

Our knowledge of tropical biota and the pathogens associated with them is inadequate [see Supplemental Material (doi:10.1289/ ehp.0901389)]. Calls for the study of worldwide (and especially tropical) biodiversity have come from a variety of sources [e.g., the United Nations, the U.S. National Science Foundation (NSF), and the Ecological Society of America]. Understanding biodiversity of plants and animals has scientific, economic, and esthetic appeal and has attracted much support (e.g., NSF's Planetary Biodiversity Inventories program; NSF 2003). Understanding the diversity of tropical pathogens has obvious practical importance yet has received little attention. Although a complete survey of potential pathogens in nature is an overwhelming task, a useful beginning would be to select the most likely potential hosts and vectors (e.g., bats and rodents, ticks and mosquitoes) and catalog those groups of pathogens with known propensities for causing disease in humans (e.g., hemorrhagic fever viruses, arboviruses, rickettsiae, and some bacteria).

Establish baseline data on the geographic and habitat distribution of recognized zoonotic and vector-borne pathogens and their hosts and vectors

Accurate information on the current distribution of these agents and their hosts and vectors defines current potential disease-endemic areas and helps to quantify relative risk among habitat types. These data also are prerequisite to documenting spatial changes in the distribution of pathogens associated with climate change. Because pathogen distributions do not always coincide with host and vector distributions (Mills and Childs 1998), studies cannot be limited to documenting host and vector presence or absence but must include sampling hosts and vectors for pathogen presence. Finally, because distinct pathogens may be associated with genetically distinct populations of hosts or vectors (e.g., at the subspecies level) (Mills and Childs 1998), accompanying taxonomic studies will be required. Collection of accurate baseline data is the first step in the establishment of long-term monitoring programs.

Establish Longitudinal Monitoring Programs

A major impediment to accurate prediction has been the lack of long-term monitoring programs (Harvell et al. 2002; Jannett et al. 2007; Pascual and Bouma 2009; Sagarin 2002). These studies would track changes in zoonotic disease risk to humans by following changes in population dynamics and infection prevalence of a few zoonotic pathogens in their host and vector populations. These studies, whose length should be measured in decades, would monitor changes in environmental variables using field-based and remote-sensing platforms and identify factors associated with changes in host, vector, and pathogen dynamics at selected sites. Long-term sampling should also monitor changes in the distribution of hosts and vector populations and their distribution across latitudinal, elevational, and environmental gradients. Although only a few agents, hosts, and vectors can be addressed this way, these studies might be applied to other pathogens, even those yet to be discovered, that have the same or similar host or vector associations.

A few long-term databases describing temporal dynamics of animal populations or disease incidence already exist (e.g., data from long-term ecological research sites and records of reportable diseases), and a few more are proposed (e.g., NSF's National Ecological Observatory Network), but such ecological data were rarely collected for the purposes of infectious disease studies. Conversely, surveillance records for human diseases rarely contain significant amounts of useful ecological data. Nevertheless, some of these data sets might be paired with long-term weather data to provide insight into climate effects (Pascual et al. 2002; Stenseth et al. 2006).

Track data on the geographic distribution, severity, and frequency of outbreaks of wildlife diseases and VBZDs in humans

This is another type of longitudinal monitoring program, but the list of pathogens and hosts would be broader and the data collected more restricted (e.g., geographic coordinates, dates, number of cases). These data can be used to track geographic and temporal trends in VBZD incidence, identify vulnerable populations, and test predictions based on forecasting models. Several existing databases provide useful formats (e.g., U.S. Geological Service's Global Wildlife Disease News Map; National Biological Information Infrastructure 2010), the CDC's ArboNet, and the Global Early Warning System for Major Animal Diseases including Zoonoses [World Health Organization (WHO) 2010]. Integration of such formats with the monitoring, data gathering, and data dissemination capacity of CDC and WHO networks would provide a powerful tool, making geographic and incidence data quickly available to the broad community of public health professionals, researchers, and modelers.

Conduct experimental laboratory and field studies of effects of climate change on hosts and vectors and their abilities to maintain and transmit pathogens

Laboratory studies and manipulative field studies (Post et al. 2008) can be used to test mechanisms of climate change effects on hosts, vectors, and pathogens or to provide hypotheses for field testing. Because specific environmental factors cannot be isolated and controlled in the field, laboratory studies will be the best way to test the effects of specific changes in temperature, humidity, or physiological stress on host, vector, or pathogen populations. For example, stress-related immunosuppression has been suggested as an explanation for increased rates of transmission and for viral recrudescence including increases in pathogen load in hantavirus hosts observed in field studies (Botten et al. 2003; Kuenzi et al. 2005). Laboratory experiments provided preliminary evidence in support of this hypothesis in the case of Seoul hantavirus infection in Norway rats (*Rattus norvegicus*) (Klein et al. 2004). Additional controlled laboratory experiments will be necessary to confirm this hypothesis for other VBZD pathogens and to help quantify the environmental and social factors (temperature, crowding, aggression, breeding, etc.) associated with transmission and recrudescence.

Neither field nor laboratory studies alone can provide complete answers to these questions. Physiological patterns observed in the laboratory must be tested under natural field conditions and the physiological mechanisms for patterns observed in the field must be tested in the laboratory.

Use data from laboratory and field studies, epidemiological studies, and remote sensing to develop predictive models of changes in zoonotic disease risk and the projected distribution and abundance of major hosts and vectors

The utility of such predictive models has been proven. Long-term direct monitoring of host population density and prevalence of hantavirus infection in North American deer mice provided early warning of elevated risk for HPS in the southwestern United States (CDC 1998, 1999; Yates et al. 2002). Models have used rainfall and temperature data to identify high-risk areas for plague and HPS in the same geographic area (Eisen et al. 2007; Enscore et al. 2002; Parmenter et al. 1999). Remote sensors have demonstrated climate-associated changes in vegetation or other environmental parameters that foretold increased risk for Rift Valley fever (Anyamba et al. 2001) or HPS (Glass et al. 2002). Ecological niche modeling has been used to provide evidence for climate change-mediated range shifts for plague and tularemia and to provide predictions of continued future poleward expansion (Nakazawa et al. 2007). Ecological niche models also used climatic data and other environmental datasets to predict the geographic distribution of the hosts and vectors for Chagas disease and the filovirus hemorrhagic fevers (Peterson et al. 2002, 2004). Another model predicted the northward spread of the Lyme disease and anaplasmosis vector *I. scapularis* under proposed climate change scenarios (Brownstein et al. 2005). Recent surveillance has confirmed that expansion (Ogden et al. 2010). Continued data collection from long-term field studies combined with laboratory data providing measured physiological tolerances for specific hosts and vectors and effects of stressors on pathogen transmission can be used to develop increasingly accurate models of range expansions and effects of increased population density on heat stress and pathogen transmission.

Although predictive models may accurately identify the changes in suitable physical habitat for host and vector species, it is important to remember that the realized niche (actual range of conditions occupied by a species) is always smaller than the fundamental niche (potential range in the absence of predators, competitors, and other limiters); the many nonclimatic confounders discussed above (barriers to dispersal, predation, competition) will need to be included in accurate models (Lafferty 2009).

An Ecosystem Approach

Over the last few decades it has become clear that effective disease prevention must consider the whole environment in which disease occurs. The maintenance of healthy people requires the maintenance of healthy ecosystems. Understanding ecosystem changes in relation to climate change will require not only a clear understanding of future changes in the physical environment but also a precise understanding of the physiological, ecological, and evolutionary responses to these changes by pathogens, vectors, and vertebrate hosts. Because of the complexity of pathogen–vector–host interactions, the multiple interactions involved, and the environment in which these interactions are occurring, studies must be multidisciplinary, long term, spatially diverse, and sufficiently replicated to provide conclusions that are reliable and generalizable. No single institution has the expertise and resources to establish multiple, intensive, long-term field monitoring programs and appropriate laboratory experiments, collect and interpret satellite images, and apply these data to the development of mathematical simulation models and forecasting tools. Collaborative partnerships among government and nongovernmental organizations and universities will have the best chance of achieving these goals. In order for broad collaborations to be most effective, mechanisms must be developed for effective communication, data sharing, and research integration among institutions and disciplines.

Application to Public Health

An important product of these studies would be an enhanced ability to initiate mitigation strategies, promulgate early warning information, and target response capabilities. Predictions based on long-term monitoring programs and forecasting models should be quickly disseminated to local, state, and international public health partners. In consultation with those partners, intervention strategies should be developed to mitigate the impact of disease on human populations. In response to predictions of increased risk of HPS in the southwestern United States in 1998 and 1999, the CDC, in partnership with several southwestern States, developed and promulgated prevention messages via television, radio, pamphlets and posters. Despite large increases in local rodent host populations, numbers of human cases were lower than in the previous HPS outbreak in 1993/1994 (CDC 1998, 1999).

Prediction and promulgation efforts can be enhanced through integration with several existing U.S. government initiatives directed at climate change, including *a*) Climate Mapper, which makes the results of climate change models accessible to a broad user community; *b*) the Malaria Early Warning System, which recently examined rainfall patterns in sub-Saharan Africa using meteorological station data, rainfall estimated from satellite images, and malaria incidence; and *c*) the Global Earth Observation System of Systems, which is an ambitious undertaking to coordinate disparate earth-observation systems across the world including improved sharing of remote-sensing data.

CONCLUSIONS

Reliable data on the effects of climate change on VBZDs are scant. We have summarized the data from preliminary studies and used these data to extrapolate to logical conclusions concerning potential consequences of climate change on VBZDs. Nevertheless, these conclusions will remain speculative until tested by rigorous field and laboratory studies. We emphasize the importance of such studies and propose a series of goals that we believe would lead to improvements in our understanding of, and our ability to mitigate, the effects of climate change on VBZDs.

The goals of the actions outlined above are to form the multidisciplinary relationships that are need to conduct and interpret ecosystem-based studies of VBZD pathogens in host and vector populations; identify the hosts, vectors, and pathogens (likely to be largely tropical) with the greatest potential to affect human populations under climate change scenarios; and conduct studies that will increase our understanding of the four potential mechanisms by which climate change may affect VBZD incidence. The value of these studies is not limited to the context of climate change. We believe that most, if not all, of these goals are important in their own right and should be undertaken regardless of the additional urgency added by the unknown effects of climate change. The goals we propose are broad and general. For each of these goals, a research plan with specific objectives, methods, and deliverables should be developed. Such research plans will be most effectively conceived in a multidisciplinary environment where experts in ecology, wildlife and vector biology, and public health sit together at the planning table. The requirements for multiinstitutional and multidisciplinary studies are important. Understanding and mitigating the effects of VBZDs cannot be accomplished by the public health community without the collaboration of ecologists and wildlife biologists. The primary focus of our proposals is discovering and predicting the consequences of climate change on VBZDs and driving public health action for the development of more effective disease-prevention strategies. We are not the first to suggest research goals to address the understanding and mitigation of climate change effects on VBZDs and other infectious diseases. However, for many aspects there is a clear convergence of conclusions and research recommendations (see, for example, National Research Council 2001; Semenza and Menne 2009). The sooner these studies are undertaken, the sooner intervention strategies can be developed and instituted.

FOOTNOTES

Supplemental Material is available online (doi:10.1289/ehp.0901389 via http://dx.doi.org/).

We thank C. Manning for assistance with graphics and B. Ellis and P. Rollin for discussions and comments that improved the manuscript.

The findings and conclusions in this report are those of the authors and do not necessarily represent the views of the Centers for Disease Control and Prevention or the Department of Health and Human Services.

REFERENCES

1. Anyamba A, Linthicum KJ, Tucker CJ. Climate-disease connections: Rift Valley fever in Kenya. Cad Saude Publica. 2001;17(suppl):133–140.
2. Ari TB, Gershunov A, Gage KL, Snäll T, Ettestad P, Kausrud KL, et al. Human plague in the USA: the importance of regional and local climate. Biol Lett. 2008;4:737–740.
3. Barnard CJ, Behnke JM, Sewell J. Social status and resistance to disease in house mice (*Mus musculus*): status-related modulation of hormonal responses in relation to immunity costs in different social and physical environments. Ethology. 1996;102:63–84.
4. Barrera R, Grillet ME, Rangel Y, Berti J, Ache A. Temporal and spatial patterns of malaria reinfection in northeastern Venezuela. Am J Trop Med Hyg. 1999;61:784–790.
5. Begon M, Bennett M, Bowers RG, French NP, Hazel SM, Turner J. A clarification of transmission terms in host-microparasite models: numbers, densities and areas. Epidemiol Infect. 2002;129:147–153.
6. Benedict MQ, Levine RS, Hawley WA, Lounibos LP. Spread of the tiger: global risk of invasion by the mosquito *Aedes albopictus*. Vector Borne Zoonotic Dis. 2007;7:76–85.
7. Botten J, Mirowsky K, Kusewitt D, Ye C, Gottlieb K, Prescott J, et al. Persistent Sin Nombre virus infection in the deer mouse (*Peromyscus maniculatus*) model: sites of replication and strand-specific expression. J Virol. 2003;77:1540–1550.
8. Botten J, Mirowsky K, Ye C, Gottlieb K, Saavedra M, Ponce L, et al. Shedding and intracage transmission of Sin Nombre hantavirus in the deer mouse (*Peromyscus maniculatus*) model. J Virol.2002;76:7587–7594.

9. Bouma MJ. Methodological problems and amendments to demonstrate effects of temperature on the epidemiology of malaria. A new perspective on the highland epidemics in Madagascar, 1972–1989.Trans R Soc Trop Med Hyg. 2003;97:133–139.
10. Bouma MJ, Dye C. Cycles of malaria associated with El Nino in Venezuela. JAMA. 1997;278:1772–1774.
11. Bouma MJ, Poveda G, Rojas W, Chavasse D, Quinones M, Cox J, et al. Predicting high-risk years for malaria in Colombia using parameters of El Nino Southern Oscillation. Trop Med Int Health.1997;2:1122–1127.
12. Bradshaw WE, Holzapfel CM. Genetic shift in photoperiodic response correlated with global warming.Proc Natl Acad Sci USA. 2001;98:14509–14511.
13. Brownstein JS, Holford TR, Fish D. Effect of climate change on Lyme disease risk in North America.Ecohealth. 2005;2:38–46.
14. Calisher CH, Mills JN, Sweeney WP, Root JJ, Reeder SA, Jentes ES, et al. Population dynamics of a diverse rodent assemblage in mixed grass–shrub habitat, southeastern Colorado, 1995–2000. J Wildl Dis. 2005;41:12–28.
15. Calisher CH, Tzianabos T, Lord RD, Coleman PH. Tamiami virus, a new member of the Tacaribe group.Am J Trop Med Hyg. 1970;19:520–526.
16. Cameron GN, Spencer SR. Sigmodon hispidus. Mammal Species. 1981;158:1–9.
17. CDC (Centers for Disease Control and Prevention) Hantavirus pulmonary syndrome—Colorado and New Mexico, 1998. MMWR. 1998;47:449–452.
18. CDC (Centers for Disease Control and Prevention) Update: hantavirus pulmonary syndrome—United States, 1999. MMWR. 1999;48:521–525.
19. CDC (Centers for Disease Control and Prevention) Climate Change and Public Health. 2010. [[accessed 16 June 2010]]. Available: http://www.cdc.gov/nceh/climatechange/
20. Colwell RK, Brehm G, Cardelus CL, Gilman AC, Longino JT. Global warming, elevational range shifts, and lowland biotic attrition in the wet tropics. Science. 2008;322:258–261.
21. Confalonieri U, Menne B, Akhtar R, Ebi KL, Hauengue M, Kovats

RS, et al. Human health. In: Parry ML, Canziana OF, Palutikof JP, van der Linden PJ, Hanson CE, editors. Climate Change 2007: Impacts, Adaptation and Vulnerability. Contribution of Working Group II to the Fourth Assessment Report of the Intergovernmental Panel on Climate Change. Cambridge: Cambridge University Press; 2007. pp. 391–431.

22. Davis S, Begon M, De Bruym L, Ageyev VS, Klassovskiy NL, Pole SB, et al. Predictive thresholds for plague in Kazakhstan. Science. 2004;304:736–738.
23. Demas GE, Nelson RJ. Photoperiod, ambient temperature, and food availability interact to affect reproductive and immune function in adult male deer mice (*Peromyscus maniculatus*) J Biol Rhythms.1998;13:253–262.
24. Dunnum JL. Elevational range extension for the hispid cotton rat, *Sigmodon hispidus* (Rodentia: Muridae)Southwest Nat. 2002;47:637–639.
25. Ebi KL, Balbus J, Kinney PL, Lipp E, Mills D, O'Neill MS, et al. Effects of global change on human health. In: Gamble JL, editor. Analyses of the Effects of Global Change on Human Health and Welfare and Human Systems. Washington, DC: U.S. Environmental Protection Agency; 2008. pp. 39–87.
26. Ebi KL, Mills DM, Smith JB, Grambsch A. Climate change and human health impacts in the United States: an update on the results of the U.S. national assessment. Environ Health Perspect.2006;114:1318–1324.
27. Eisen RJ, Glass GE, Eisen L, Cheek J, Enscore RE, Ettestad P, et al. A spatial model of shared risk for plague and hantavirus pulmonary syndrome in the southwestern United States. Am J Trop Med Hyg.2007;77:999–1004.
28. Enscore RE, Biggerstaff BJ, Brown TL, Fulgham RF, Reynolds PJ, Engelthaler DM, et al. Modeling relationships between climate and the frequency of human plague cases in the southwestern United States, 1960–1997. Am J Trop Med Hyg. 2002;66:186–196.
29. Fischlin A, Midgley GF, Price JT, Leemans R, Gopal B, Turley C, et al. Ecosystems, their properties, goods, and services. In: Parry ML, Canziani OF, Palutikof JP, van der Linden PJ, Hanson CE, editors.

Climate Change 2007: Impacts, Adaptation and Vulnerability. Contribution of Working Group II to the Fourth Assessment Report of the Intergovernmental Panel on Climate Change. Cambridge: Cambridge University Press; 2007. pp. 211–272.

30. Frumkin H, Hess J, Luber G, Malilay J, McGeehin M. Climate change: the public health response. Am J Public Health. 2008;98:435–445.
31. Gage KL, Burkot TR, Eisen RJ, Hayes EB. Climate and vectorborne diseases. Am J Prev Med.2008;35:436–450.
32. Gage KL, Kosoy MY. Natural history of plague: perspectives from more than a century of research. Annu Rev Entomol. 2005;50:505–528.
33. Githeko AK, Ndegwa W. Predicting malaria epidemics in the Kenyan highlands using climate data: a tool for decision makers. Global Change Hum Health. 2001;2:54–63.
34. Glass GE, Yates TL, Fine JB, Shields TM, Kendall JB, Hope AG, et al. Satellite imagery characterizes local animal reservoir populations of Sin Nombre virus in the southwestern United States. Proc Natl Acad Sci USA. 2002;99:16817–16822.
35. Halford WP, Gebhardt BM, Carr DJ. Mechanisms of herpes simplex virus type 1 reactivation. J Virol.1996;70:5051–5060.
36. Harvell CD, Mitchel CE, Ward JR, Altizer S, Dobson AP, Ostfeld RS, et al. Climate warming and disease risks for terrestrial and marine biota. Science. 2002;296:2158–2162.
37. Hay SI, Cox J, Rogers DJ, Randolph SE, Stern DI, Shanks GD, et al. Climate change and the resurgence of malaria in the East African highlands. Nature. 2002a;415:905–909.
38. Hay SI, Rogers DJ, Randolph SE, Stern DI, Cox J, Shanks GD, et al. Hot topic or hot air? Climate change and malaria resurgence in East African highlands. Trends Parasitol. 2002b;18:530–534.
39. Hickling R, Roy DB, Hill JK, Fox R, Thomas CD. The distributions of a wide range of taxonomic groups are expanding polewards. Glob Chang Biol. 2006;12:450–455.
40. Hinnebusch BJ, Fischer ER, Schwan TG. Evaluation of the role of the *Yersinia pestis* plasminogen activator and other plasmid-encoded factors in temperature-dependent blockage of the flea. J Infect Dis. 1998;178:1406–1415. [PubMed]

41. IPCC (Intergovernmental Panel on Climate Change) Climate Change 2007: Synthesis Report. Geneva: IPCC; 2007.
42. Jannett FJ, Broschart MR, Grim LH, Schaberl JP. Northerly range extensions of mammalian species in Minnesota. Am Midl Nat. 2007;158:168–176.
43. Jarrett CO, Deak E, Isherwood KE, Oyston PC, Fischer ER, Whitney AR, et al. Transmission of *Yersinia pestis* from an infectious biofilm in the flea vector. J Infect Dis. 2004;190:783–792.
44. Jetz W, Wilcove DS, Dobson AP. Projected impacts of climate and land-use change on the global diversity of birds. PLoS Biol. 2007;5:e157. doi: 10.1371/journal.pbio.0050157.
45. Julvez J, Mouchet J, Michault A, Fouta A, Hamidine M. The progress of malaria in Sahelian eastern Niger. An ecological disaster zone. Bull Soc Pathol Exot. 1997;90:101–104.
46. Kerr C. Swedish TBE increase. Trends Microbiol. 2001;9:413. doi: 10.1016/S0966-842X(01)02183-7.[Online 5 September 2001]
47. Klein SL, Cernetich A, Hilmer S, Hoffman EP, Scott AL, Glass GE. Differential expression of immunoregulatory genes in male and female Norway rats following infection with Seoul virus. J Med Virol. 2004;74:180–190.
48. Komar N. West Nile virus: epidemiology and ecology in North America. Adv Virus Res. 2003;61:185–234.
49. Kuenzi AJ, Douglass RJ, Bond CW, Calisher CH, Mills JN. Long-term dynamics of Sin Nombre viral RNA and antibody in deer mice in Montana. J Wildl Dis. 2005;41:473–481.
50. Lafferty KD. The ecology of climate change and infectious diseases. Ecology. 2009;90:888–900.
51. Lehmer EM, Clay CA, Wilson E, St Jeor S, Dearing MD. Differential resource allocation in deer mice exposed to Sin Nombre virus. Physiol Biochem Zool. 2007;80:514–521.
52. Likos AM, Sammons SA, Olson VA, Frace AM, Li Y, Olsen-Rasmussen M, et al. A tale of two clades: monkeypox viruses. J Gen Virol. 2005;86:2661–2672.
53. Lindgren E, Gustafson R. Tick-borne encephalitis in Sweden and climate change. Lancet. 2001;358:16–18.
54. Linthicum KJ, Anyamba A, Tucker CJ, Kelley PW, Myers MF,

Peters CJ. Climate and satellite indicators to forecast Rift Valley fever epidemics in Kenya. Science. 1999;285:397–400.

55. Long CA. Ecological replacement of the deer mouse, *Peromyscus maniculatus*, by the white-footed mouse, *P. leucopus*, in the Great Lakes region. Can Field Nat. 1996;110:271–277.

56. Mabaso ML, Kleinschmidt I, Sharp B, Smith T. El Nino Southern Oscillation (ENSO) and annual malaria incidence in Southern Africa. Trans R Soc Trop Med Hyg. 2007;101:326–330.

57. MacDonald KA, Brown JH. Using montane mammals to model extinctions due to global change. Conserv Biol. 1992;6:409–425.

58. Madhav NK, Wagoner KD, Douglass RJ, Mills JN. Delayed density-dependent prevalence of Sin Nombre virus antibody in Montana deer mice (*Peromyscus maniculatus*) and implications for human disease risk. Vector Borne Zoonotic Dis. 2007;7:353–364.

59. Mehta SK, Cohrs RJ, Forghani B, Zerbe G, Gilden DH, Pierson DL. Stress-induced subclinical reactivation of varicella zoster virus in astronauts. J Med Virol. 2004;72:174–179.

60. Mills JN. Regulation of rodent-borne viruses in the natural host: implications for human disease. Arch Virol Suppl. 2005;19:45–57.

61. Mills JN. Biodiversity loss and emerging infectious disease: an example from the rodent-borne hemorrhagic fevers. Biodiversity. 2006;7:9–17.

62. Mills JN, Childs JE. Ecologic studies of rodent reservoirs: their relevance for human health. Emerg Infect Dis. 1998;4:529–537.

63. Mills JN, Ksiazek TG, Peters CJ, Childs JE. Long-term studies of hantavirus reservoir populations in the southwestern United States: a synthesis. Emerg Infect Dis. 1999;5:135–142.

64. Mohlhenrich JS. Distribution and ecology of the hispid and least cotton rats in New Mexico. J Mamm.1961;42:13–24.

65. Moritz C, Patton JL, Conroy CJ, Parra JL, White GC, Beissinger SR. Impact of a century of climate change on small-mammal communities in Yosemite National Park, USA. Science. 2008;322:261–264.

66. Mouchet J, Faye O, Juivez J, Manguin S. Drought and malaria retreat in the Sahel, West Africa. Lancet.1996;348:1735–1736.
67. Nakazawa Y, Williams R, Peterson AT, Mead P, Staples E, Gage KL. Climate change effects on plague and tularemia in the United States. Vector Borne Zoonotic Dis. 2007;7:529–540.
68. National Biological Information Infrastructure. Global Wildlife Disease News Map. 2010. [[accessed 16 June 2010]]. Version 2.0. Available: http://wildlifedisease.nbii.gov/wdinNewsDigestMap.jsp.
69. National Research Council. Under the Weather: Climate, Ecosystems, and Infectious Disease.Washington, DC: National Academy Press; 2001.
70. Nelson RJ, Demas GE, Klein SL, Kriegsfeld LJ. The influence of season, photoperiod, and pineal melatonin on immune function. J Pineal Res. 1995;19:149–165.
71. NSF (National Science Foundation) Planetory Biodiversity Inventories. 2003. [[accessed 16 June 2010]]. Available: http://www.nsf.gov/news/news_summ.jsp?cntn_id=103065.
72. Ogden NH, Bouchard C, Kurtenbach K, Margos G, Lindsay LR, Trudel L, et al. Active and passive surveillance and phylogenetic analysis of *Borrelia burgdorferi* elucidate the process of Lyme disease risk emergence in Canada. Environ Health Perspect. 2010;118:909–914.
73. Ogden NH, Maarouf A, Barker IK, Bigras-Poulin M, Lindsay LR, Morshed MG, et al. Climate change and the potential for range expansion of the Lyme disease vector *Ixodes scapularis* in Canada. Int J Parasitol. 2006;36:63–70.
74. Ostfeld RS, Keesing F. Biodiversity and disease risk: the case of Lyme disease. Conserv Biol.2000;14:722–728.
75. Parmenter RR, Yadav EP, Parmenter CA, Ettestad P, Gage KL. Incidence of plague associated with increased winter-spring precipitation in New Mexico. Am J Trop Med Hyg. 1999;61:814–821.
76. Pascual M, Ahumada JA, Chaves LF, Rodó X, Bouma M. Malaria resurgence in the East African highlands: temperature trends revisited. Proc Natl Acad Sci USA. 2006;103:5829–5834.

77. Pascual M, Bouma MJ. Do rising temperatures matter? Ecology. 2009;90:906–912.
78. Pascual M, Bouma MJ, Dobson AP. Cholera and climate: revisiting the quantitative evidence. Microbes Infect. 2002;4:237–245.
79. Patz JA. A human disease indicator for the effects of recent global climate change. Proc Natl Acad Sci USA. 2002;99:12506–12508.
80. Patz JA, Olson SH. Climate change and health: global to local influences on disease risk. Ann Trop Med Parasitol. 2006;100:535–549.
81. Peterson AT, Bauer JT, Mills JN. Ecologic and geographic distribution of filovirus disease. Emerg Infect Dis. 2004;10:40–47.
82. Peterson AT, Sánchez-Cordero V, Beard CB, Ramsey JM. Ecologic niche modeling and potential reservoirs for Chagas disease, Mexico. Emerg Infect Dis. 2002;8:662–667.
83. Post ES, Pedersen C, Wilmers CC, Forchhammer MC. Phenological sequences reveal aggregate life history response to climate warming. Ecology. 2008;89:363–370.
84. Pounds JA, Fogden MPL, Masters KL. Responses of natural communities to climate change in a highland tropical forest. In: Lovegoy TE, Hanna L, editors. Climage Change and Biodiversty. New Haven, CT: Yale University Press; 2005. pp. 70–74.
85. Randolph SE. Tick ecology: processes and patterns behind the epidemiological risk posed by ixodid ticks as vectors. Parasitology. 2004;129(suppl):S37–S65.
86. Rawlings JA, Torrez-Martinez N, Neill SU, Moore GM, Hicks BN, Pichuantes S, et al. Cocirculation of multiple hantaviruses in Texas, with characterization of the small (S) genome of a previously undescribed virus of cotton rats (*Sigmodon hispidus*) Am J Trop Med Hyg. 1996;55:672–679.
87. Reiter P, Lathrop S, Bunning M, Biggerstaff B, Singer D, Tiwari T, et al. Texas lifestyle limits transmission of dengue virus. Emerg Infect Dis. 2003;9:86–89.
88. Rollin PE, Ksiazek TG, Elliott LH, Ravkov EV, Martin ML, Morzunov S, et al. Isolation of Black Creek Canal virus, a new hantavirus from *Sigmodon hispidus* in Florida. J Med Virol. 1995;46:35–39.

89. Root TL, Schneider SH. Climate change: overview and implications for wildlife. In: Schneider SH, Root TL, editors. Wildlife Responses to Climate Change: North American Case Studies. Washington, DC: Island Press; 2002. pp. 1–56.

90. Rosenzweig C, Casassa G, Karoly DJ, Imeson A, Liu C, Menzel A, et al. Assessment of observed changes and responses in natural and managed systems. In: Parry ML, Canziani OF, Palutikof JP, van der Linden PJ, Hanson CE, editors. Climate Change 2007: Impacts, Adaptation and Vulnerability. Contribution of Working Group II to the Fourth Assessment Report of the Intergovernmental Panel on Climate. Cambridge: Cambridge University Press; 2007. pp. 79–131.

91. Ruedas LA, Salazar-Bravo J, Tinnin DS, Armien B, Caceres L, Garcia A, et al. Community ecology of small mammal populations in Panama following an outbreak of Hantavirus pulmonary syndrome. J Vector Ecol. 2004;29:177–191.

92. Sagarin R. Historical studies of species' response to climate change: promise and pitfalls. In: Schneider SH, Root TL, editors. Wildlife Responses to Climate Change: North American Case Studies.Washington, DC: Island Press; 2002. pp. 127–163.

93. Sattenspiel L. Tropical environments, human activities, and the transmission of infectious diseases. [[accessed 18 September 2010]];Yearb Phys Anthropol. 2000 43:3–31. Available:http://www.eeescience.utoledo.edu/faculty/gottgens/webpapers/DISEASEarticle.pdf.

94. Schmidly DJ. Texas Natural History: A Century of Change. Lubbock, TX: Texas Tech University Press; 2002.

95. Semenza JC, Menne B. Climate change and infectious diseases in Europe. Lancet Infect Dis. 2009;9:365–375.

96. Shanks GD, Hay SI, Stern DI, Biomndo K, Snow RW. Meteorologic influences on *Plasmodium falciparum* malaria in the highland tea estates of Kericho, western Kenya. Emerg Infect Dis.2002;8:1404–1408.

97. Stapp P, Antolin MF, Ball M. Patterns of extinction in prairie dog metapopulations: plague outbreaks follow El Nino events. Front Ecol Environ. 2004;2:235–240.

98. Stenseth NC, Samia NI, Viljugrein H, Kausrud KL, Begon M, Davis S, et al. Plague dynamics are driven by climate variation. Proc Natl Acad Sci USA. 2006;103:13110–13115.

99. Straile D, Stenseth NC. The North Atlantic Oscillation and ecology: links between historical time-series, and lessons regarding future climate warming. Clim Res. 2007;34:259–262.

100. Sutherst RW. Global change and human vulnerability to vector-borne diseases. Clin Microbiol Rev.2004;17:136–173.

101. Thomas CD, Franco AM, Hill JK. Range retractions and extinction in the face of climate warming. Trends Ecol Evol. 2006;21:415–416.

102. Thompson RA, Wellington de Oliveira Lima J, Maguire JH, Braud DH, Scholl DT. Climatic and demographic determinants of American visceral leishmaniasis in northeastern Brazil using remote sensing technology for environmental categorization of rain and region influences on leishmaniasis.Am J Trop Med Hyg. 2002;67:648–655.

103. Warren MS, Hill JK, Thomas JA, Asher J, Fox R, Huntley B, et al. Rapid responses of British butterflies to opposing forces of climate and habitat change. Nature. 2001;414:65–69.

104. Welbergen JA, Klose SM, Markus N, Eby P. Climate change and the effects of temperature extremes on Australian flying-foxes. Proc Biol Sci. 2008;275:419–425.

105. WHO (World Health Organization) Global Early Warning System for Major Animal Diseases, Including Zoonoses (GLEWS) 2010. [[accessed 16 June 2010]]. Available:http://www.who.int/zoonoses/outbreaks/glews/en/

106. Williams RJ, Bryan RT, Mills JN, Palma RE, Vera I, de Velasquez F, et al. An outbreak of hantavirus pulmonary syndrome in western Paraguay. Am J Trop Med Hyg. 1997;57:274–282.

107. Wolfe ND, Daszak P, Kilpatrick AM, Burke DS. Bushmeat hunting, deforestation, and prediction of zoonoses emergence. Emerg Infect Dis. 2005;11:1822–1827.

108. Wright HE, Kutzbach JE, Webb T, Ruddiman WE, Street-Perrott FA, Bartlein PJ. Global Climates since the Last Glacial Maximum. Minneapolis: University of Minnesota Press; 1993.

109. Yates TL, Mills JN, Parmenter CA, Ksiazek TG, Parmenter RR, Vande Castle JR, et al. The ecology and evolutionary history of an emergent disease: hantavirus pulmonary syndrome. Bioscience.2002;52:989–998.

Citations

CHAPTER 1

Robert W. Sutherst, Global Change and Human Vulnerability to Vector-Borne Diseases, doi: 10.1128/CMR.17.1.136-173.2004

CHAPTER 2

Laura L. Ingwell, Sanford D. Eigenbrode, and Nilsa A. Bosque-Pérez, Plant viruses alter insect behavior to enhance their spread, doi: 10.1038/srep00578.

CHAPTER 3

Neil Vora, Impact of Anthropogenic Environmental Alterations on Vector-Borne Diseases

CHAPTER 4

Suzie Key, Julian K-C Ma, and Pascal MW Drake, Genetically modified plants and human health, doi: 10.1258/jrsm.2008.070372.

CHAPTER 5

R. Froissart, J. Doumayrou, F. Vuillaume, S. Alizon, and Y. Michalakis, The virulence–transmission trade-off in vector-borne plant viruses: a review of (non-)existing studies, doi: 10.1098/rstb.2010.0068.

CHAPTER 6

Gray, Stewart M., and Nanditta Banerjee. "Mechanisms of Arthropod Transmission of Plant and Animal Viruses." Microbiology and Molecular Biology Reviews 63.1 (1999): 128–148.

CHAPTER 7

James N. Mills, Kenneth L. Gage, and Ali S. Khan, Potential Influence of Climate Change on Vector-Borne and Zoonotic Diseases: A Review and Proposed Research Plan, doi: 10.1289/ehp.0901389.

Index

E

F

G

H

I

L

M

N

O

P

R